Clinical Pharmacology: Anti-Cancer and Anti-HIV Drugs

Clinical Pharmacology: Anti-Cancer and Anti-HIV Drugs

Editor: Horatio Finley

AMERICAN
MEDICAL PUBLISHERS
www.americanmedicalpublishers.com

AMERICAN
MEDICAL PUBLISHERS
www.americanmedicalpublishers.com

Cataloging-in-Publication Data

Clinical pharmacology : anti-cancer and anti-HIV drugs / edited by Horatio Finley.
p. cm.
Includes bibliographical references and index.
ISBN 979-8-88740-005-1
1. Clinical pharmacology. 2. Antineoplastic agents. 3. HIV Infections--Chemotherapy.
4. Cancer--Chemotherapy. 5. AIDS (Disease)--Chemotherapy. 6. HIV (Viruses)--Treatment.
I. Finley, Horatio.
RM301.28 .C553 2023
615.1--dc23

American Medical Publishers,
41 Flatbush Avenue,
1st Floor, New York,
NY 11217, USA

ISBN 979-8-88740-005-1 (Hardback)

Contents

Preface

Clinical pharmacology comprises all the aspects of interactions between drugs and humans. Cancer and HIV are major public health issues and the development of anti-cancer and anti-HIV drugs is an important area of study within clinical pharmacology. An anticancer drug is a drug that is effective in the treatment of cancerous or malignant disease. Alkylating agents, antimetabolites, natural products, and hormones are the four major classes of anticancer drugs. Antiretroviral drugs are used for the treatment of HIV, which work by preventing the replication of virus in the body. They are used in a combination of two or more drugs, as HIV can become resistant to a single drug. There are several classes of anti-HIV drugs namely, non-nucleoside reverse transcriptase inhibitors (NNRTIs), nucleoside reverse transcriptase inhibitors (NRTIs), protease inhibitors (PIs), fusion inhibitors, CCR5 antagonists, integrase strand transfer inhibitors (INSTIs) and post-attachment inhibitors. This book contains some path-breaking studies in the field of clinical pharmacology with a focus on anti-cancer and anti-HIV drugs. The readers would gain knowledge that would broaden their perspective about these drugs. With state-of-the-art inputs by acclaimed experts of this field, this book targets medical students and professionals.

This book is a comprehensive compilation of works of different researchers from varied parts of the world. It includes valuable experiences of the researchers with the sole objective of providing the readers (learners) with a proper knowledge of the concerned field. This book will be beneficial in evoking inspiration and enhancing the knowledge of the interested readers.

In the end, I would like to extend my heartiest thanks to the authors who worked with great determination on their chapters. I also appreciate the publisher's support in the course of the book. I would also like to deeply acknowledge my family who stood by me as a source of inspiration during the project.

Editor

1

Synthesis and Biological Evaluation of Phaeosphaeride A Derivatives as Antitumor Agents

Victoria Abzianidze [1,*], Petr Beltyukov [2], Sofya Zakharenkova [1], Natalia Moiseeva [3], Jennifer Mejia [4], Alvin Holder [4], Yuri Trishin [5], Alexander Berestetskiy [6] and Victor Kuznetsov [1]

1 Laboratory of Chemical Modeling, Research Institute of Hygiene, Occupational Pathology and Human Ecology, Federal Medical Biological Agency, p/o Kuz'molovsky, 188663 Saint Petersburg, Russia; sofya.zakharenkova@gmail.com (S.Z.); kuznetsov_va1956@bk.ru (V.K.)

2 Laboratory of Molecular Toxicology and Experimental Therapy, Research Institute of Hygiene, Occupational Pathology and Human Ecology, Federal Medical Biological Agency, p/o Kuz'molovsky, 188663 Saint Petersburg, Russia; biochem2005@rambler.ru

3 N.N. Blokchin National Medical Research Center of Oncology, 115478 Moscow, Russia; n.i.moiseeva@gmail.com

4 Department of Chemistry and Biochemistry, Old Dominion University, 4541 Hampton Boulevard, Norfolk, VA 23529, USA; jmatt024@odu.edu (J.M.); aholder@odu.edu (A.H.)

5 Saint Petersburg State University of industrial technologies and design, Ivana Chernyh str., 4, 198095 Saint Petersburg, Russia; trish@yt4470.spb.edu

6 All-Russian Institute of Plant Protection, Russian Academy of Agricultural Sciences, Pushkin, 196608 Saint Petersburg, Russia; aberestetski@yahoo.com

* Correspondence: vvaavv@mail.ru

Abstract: New derivatives of phaeosphaeride A (PPA) were synthesized and characterized. Anti-tumor activity studies were carried out on the HCT-116, PC3, MCF-7, A549, K562, NCI-H929, Jurkat, THP-1, RPMI8228 tumor cell lines, and on the HEF cell line. All of the compounds synthesized were found to have better efficacy than PPA towards the tumor cell lines mentioned. Compound **6** was potent against six cancer cell lines, HCT-116, PC-3, K562, NCI-H929, Jurkat, and RPMI8226, showing a 47, 13.5, 16, 4, 1.5, and 7-fold increase in anticancer activity comparative to those of etoposide, respectively. Compound **1** possessed selectivity toward the NCI-H929 cell line (IC_{50} = 1.35 ± 0.69 μM), while product **7** was selective against three cancer cell lines, HCT-116, MCF-7, and NCI-H929, each having IC_{50} values of 1.65 μM, 1.80 μM and 2.00 μM, respectively.

Keywords: natural phaeosphaeride A; antitumor activity; human tumor cell lines; HEF cell line; acute toxicity

1. Introduction

Modern chemotherapeutic treatment of malignant tumors is widely considered to have begun approximately 75 years ago when researchers found that nitrogen mustard displayed anti-tumor activity [1]. In more recent decades, leading research approaches have focused on the development of new antitumor agents for targeted therapy, as well as combined treatment with immunotherapeutic and chemotherapeutic agents [2]. Diversity, and in many cases, the genetic uniqueness of tumors, does not allow for the development of universal and specific therapeutic treatment. As a result, the use of non-specific chemotherapeutic treatment is still the principal therapeutic option used in patients. Despite advances in cancer treatments, the disabling side effects and relative effectivity of these broad antitumor drugs plagues scientists to urgently develop improved chemotherapeutic agents.

Many chemotherapeutic agents used in clinical practice are developed from natural compounds or their derivatives and analogs, e.g., etoposide, eribulin, paclitaxel, vincristine, vinblastine, topotecan, cytarabine, doxorubicin, dactinomycin, and bleomycin [3–5]. These also include medicines developed and introduced into clinical practice from the 1950s–1960s (vincristine, vinblastine, cytarabine, etc.), as well as modern agents developed in the 2000's (topotecan, eribulin). Many chemotherapeutic agents based on natural analogs continue to undergo clinical studies to evaluate their effectiveness in the treatment of various types of tumors, as drugs developed from natural compounds often show lower toxicity and have higher target values towards malignant tumor cells [3]. While scientists continue to research these compounds, these naturally derived drugs are already relevant in the market today, with close to 40% of antitumor drugs approved by the FDA being of natural origin or semi-synthetic derivatives of natural compounds. When we reexamine this number and consider only the use of synthetic drugs, the analogues of natural compounds, the proportion of these antitumor agents are estimated at 70% [6]. Clearly, nature remains an inexhaustible source of new substances and has vast potential to aid in the fight against various tumors.

Here, phaeosphaeride A, produced by endophytic fungi from the genus *Phaeosphaeria*, was chosen for its ability to inhibit the Signal Transducer and Activator of Transcription 3 (STAT3) signaling pathway. The stereochemical configuration of this natural product had been established by total synthesis of ent-phaeosphaeride A and phaeosphaeride A [7,8] and by X-ray diffraction [9]. High incidence of STAT3 protein is characteristic of several oncological diseases like leukemia, multiple myeloma, cancers of the breast and lung, as well as multiple carcinomas such as renal, prostate, hepatocellular, ovarian, and pancreatic [10,11]. STAT3 also is shown to play an important role in regulating cell growth and viability [10,12–15]. Therefore, phaeosphaeride A, and its derivatives, are potentially promising anticancer agents for targeted therapy and combined treatments [10,11].

The results of the study in this article include information on the methods for the synthesis of the phaeosphaeride A derivatives and their biological evaluation, including the measurements of the cytotoxic effects and a preliminary assessment of acute toxicity in mice.

2. Results and Discussion

2.1. Chemistry

The synthesis of target compounds **1–8** is presented in Scheme 1. Mesylation of PPA with $MeSO_2Cl$ and Et_3N in CH_2Cl_2 gave the mesylate as a sole product, which was used in the next step without purification.

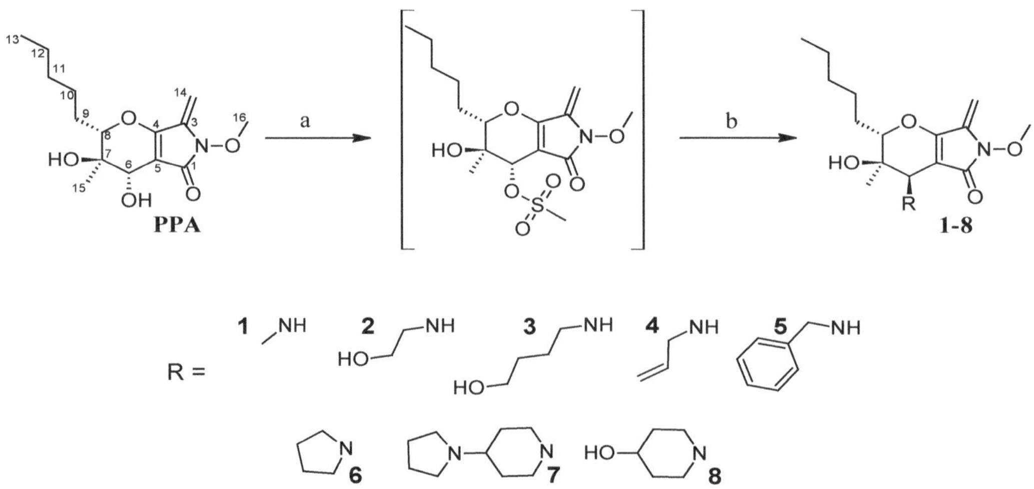

Scheme 1. Synthesis of compounds **1–8**. *Reagents and conditions*: (**a**) MsCl, TEA, CH_2Cl_2, 0 °C, 1 h; (**b**) cyclic or primary amine, with or without TEA, acetonitrile or THF, room temperature or 70–75 °C.

Treatment of the mesylate with cyclic amines and (or without) TEA in acetonitrile (or THF) at room temperature (or at 70–75 °C) or with primary amines in acetonitrile at room temperature gave the corresponding amino derivatives in 11–27% yield with inversion occurring on the C-6 atom. The ROESY spectra of the products showed a correlation between the methyl protons (H-15) and the H-6 proton confirming the inversion of configuration of the C-6 atom (see Supplementary Material). Product **6** was synthesized by our research group in 2017 with the present method doubling the total yield [16]. Previously it was impossible to obtain the desired derivatives through chloroacetyl PPA derivative from primary amines as those reactions proceeded solely at the exocyclic double bond (unpublished data) [17].

2.2. Biological Evaluation

2.2.1. Cytotoxicity Assay Using 9 Tumor Cell Lines and HEF Cell Line

All newly synthesized PPA derivatives **1–8** were evaluated for their anti-proliferative activity against human breast cancer MCF-7, human prostate adenocarcinoma PC-3, human colorectal cancer HCT-116, human lung cancer A549, human chronic myelogenous leukemia K562, human acute monocytic leukemia THP-1, human multiple myeloma RPMI8226, human acute T-cell leukemia Jurkat, human multiple myeloma NCI-H929, and human embryonic fibroblasts HEF cell lines by MTT assays. All cells were incubated with different concentrations of PPA derivatives for 72 h, with etoposide and PPA used as reference compounds. The anticancer activity of the tested compounds was described as the concentration of drug inhibiting 50% cell growth IC_{50} (Tables 1 and 2).

Table 1. IC_{50} values for the respective compounds when studied on the adhesive cell lines. Data was expressed as the inhibitory ratio ± SD based on three independent experiments (n = 3).

Compound	Adhesive Cell Cultures, IC_{50} (μM)				
	HCT-116	PC-3	MCF-7	A549	HEF
PPA	24.21 ± 0.75	32.14 ± 0.77	20.30 ± 0.8	41.10 ± 2.6	19.05 ± 0.25
1	3.68 ± 0.81	3.35 ± 0.92	4.10 ± 0.44	12.73 ± 0.40	22.30 ± 0.44
2	4.63 ± 0.04	5.55 ± 1.48	3.23 ± 1.07	15.14 ± 0.45	16.20 ± 0.26
3	2.90 ± 0.98	4.50 ± 1.56	3.05 ± 1.20	11.41 ± 0,19	15.19 ± 1.02
4	8.40 ± 0.24	6.37 ± 0.18	4.13 ± 0.23	12.65 ± 0.27	5.03 ± 0.15
5	12.93 ± 0.30	24.67 ± 1.24	35.71 ± 0.65	37.51 ± 1.33	53.11 ± 1.06
6	0.47 ± 0.01	0.20 ± 0.07	3.25 ± 0.64	10.11 ± 0.5	4.00 ± 0.17
7	1.65 ± 0.63	3.65 ± 0.64	1.80 ± 0.44	12.22 ± 0.2	22.30 ± 0.33
8	2.64 ± 0.05	4.53 ± 0.40	3.20 ± 0.52	9.40 ± 0.14	6.70 ± 0.23
Etoposide	22.00 ± 1.10	2.70 ± 0.05	9.60 ± 0.27	>100	>100

Table 2. IC_{50} values for the respective compounds when studied on the suspension cell lines. Data were expressed as inhibitory ratio ± SD based on three independent experiments (n = 3).

Compound	Suspension Cell Cultures, IC_{50} (μM)				
	K562	NCI-H929	Jurkat	THP-1	RPMI8228
PPA	20.47 ± 1.46	6.50 ± 0.30	9.70 ± 0.42	19.10 ± 0.45	9.15 ± 0.64
1	3.25 ± 0.64	**1.35 ± 0.69**	2.75 ± 0.21	2.25 ± 0.21	3.97 ± 0.68
2	5.50 ± 0.57	2.05 ± 0.35	2.60 ± 0.99	2.30 ± 0.57	3.50 ± 0.82
3	6.70 ± 0.28	1.95 ± 0.21	3.15 ± 1.77	2.60 ± 0.57	2.70 ± 0.28
4	10.48 ± 0.41	2.35 ± 0.09	3.27 ± 0.07	3.32 ± 0.10	6.00 ± 0.13
5	14.13 ± 0.48	7.73 ± 0,25	10.10 ± 0.44	15.11 ± 0.36	16 ± 0.16
6	**0.54 ± 0.03**	**0.23 ± 0.02**	**0.55 ± 0.29**	2.05 ± 0.21	**0.63 ± 0.23**
7	6.03 ± 0.91	**2.00 ± 0.26**	2.73 ± 1.53	3.45 ± 0.21	3.35 ± 1.48
8	4.90 ± 2.40	1.87 ± 0.25	2.60 ± 1.13	2.10 ± 0.28	1.40 ± 0.28
Etoposide	8.47 ± 0.95	0.92 ± 0.03	0.88 ± 0.74	0.83 ± 0.21	4.60 ± 0.28

Compound **6** was found to be the most potent against six cancer cell lines (0.47 μM for HCT-116, 0.2 μM for PC-3, 0.54 μM for K562, 0.23 μM for NCI-H929, 0.55 μM for Jurkat and 0.63 μM for

RPMI8226), which was 51, 160, 37, 28, 17.5, and 14.5-fold stronger than those of the reference compound PPA, respectively (Figure 1).

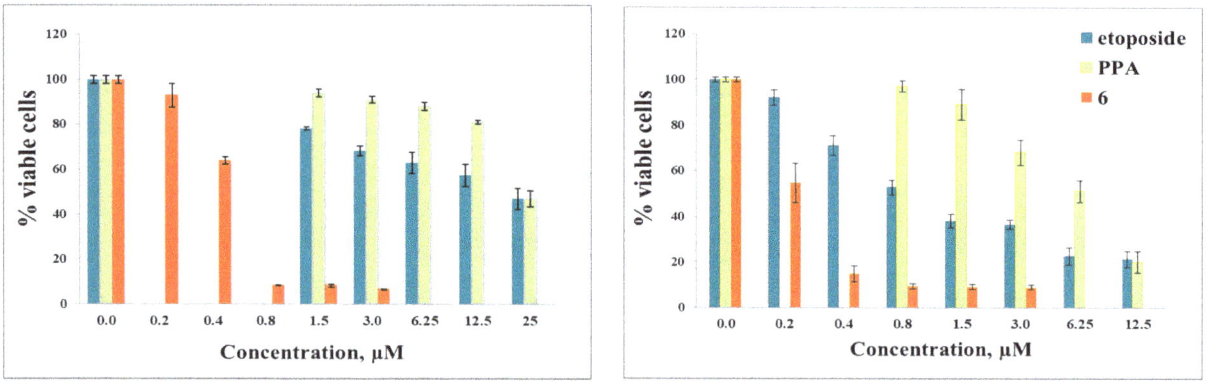

(a) (b)

Figure 1. (**a**) The in vitro effects of compound **6** on the cell viability of human HCT-116 cell line; (**b**) The in vitro effects of compound **6** on the cell viability of human NCI-H929 cell line.

Compound **1** showed selectivity toward the NCI-H929 cell line (IC_{50} = 1.35 ± 0.69 µM) while product **7** was selective against three cancer cell lines (IC_{50} was 1.65 µM, 1.80 µM and 2.00 µM towards HCT-116, MCF-7 and NCI-H929, respectively). The results obtained indicate product **6** to be more toxic than the positive control, etoposide, against HCT-116 (47-fold), PC-3 (13.5-fold), K562 (16-fold), NCI-H929 (4-fold), Jurkat (1.5-fold) and RPMI8226 (7-fold) cancer cell lines. Human embryonic fibroblasts were used as a control.

2.2.2. Acute Intraperitoneal Toxicity Study

No adverse effects were found from compound **6** on body weight and food consumption. There was no indication of morbidity, mortality, or lethal effects during the 14 days after i.p. administration (intraperiotenal) in mice of two low doses (8.25 and 82.5 mg/kg). LD50 was not reached in all experiments. Mortality (two of eight mice) was observed in the highest dose group (one was found deceased on Day 2 and one on Day 3). No effect was observed on mean body weight or mass coefficients (spleen, liver, heart, kidney, lung, thymus, and adrenal). No gross abnormalities were observed in the organs tested. Maximum tolerated dose of **6** after i.p. injection in mice was equal to or more than 82.5 mg/kg. Median lethal dose (LD50) of **6** has not been determined but is believed to be more than 200 mg/kg. It can be concluded that compound **6** is less toxic comparative to etoposide. Intraperitoneal LD50 of etoposide for mice is 64 mg/kg (RTECS # KC0190000).

3. Materials and Methods

3.1. Materials and Instruments

^{1}H-NMR spectra were acquired on an AVANCE III 400 MHz NMR spectrometer (Bruker, Rheinstetten, Germany) in $CDCl_3$. Optical rotations were acquired on a Polaar 3005 Polarimeter (Optical Activity, Huntingdon, Great Britain) using a 2.5 cm cell with a Na 589 nm filter and the concentration of samples was denoted as *c*. Mass spectra data were acquired on a TSQ Quantum Access Max Mass spectrometer (Thermo Fisher Scientific, Waltham, MA, USA). High-resolution mass spectra (HRMS) were acquired on a LTQ Orbitrap Velos spectrometer (Thermo Scientific) and on a Bruker MicrOTOF. FTIR spectra were acquired on an IR Affinity-1 spectrometer (Shimadzu, Thermo Scientific). Organic solvents used were dried by standard methods when necessary. Commercially available reagents were used without further purification. All reactions were monitored by TLC with silica gel coated plates (EMD/Merck KGaA, Darmstadt, Germany), with visualization by UV light and by charring with 0.1% ninhydrin in EtOH. Column chromatography was performed using Merck 60 Å

70–230 mesh silica gel. The optical density was determined using a Multiskan FC spectrophotometer (Thermo Scientific) at a wavelength of 540 nm when using the MTT assay.

3.2. Chemical Syntheses

3.2.1. Synthesis of (2*S*,3*S*,4*S*)-3-Hydroxy-6-methoxy-3-methyl-7-methylene-5-oxo-2-pentyl-2,3,4,5,6,7-hexahydropyrano[2,3-*c*]pyrrol-4-yl methanesulfonate

PPA (1 mmol) was dissolved in CH_2Cl_2 (2 mL) and cooled to 0 °C. Triethylamine (3.5 mmol) was added followed by the dropwise addition of methanesulfonyl chloride (2.5 mmol). The mixture was stirred at 0 °C for 1 h. The reaction was quenched by the addition of saturated $NaHCO_3$ solution and the mixture was extracted with dichloromethane (3 × 20 mL). The organic layer was washed with water and brine, dried over magnesium sulfate, and concentrated in vacuo after filtration. Mesylate was used in the next step without further purification. HRMS revealed an $[M + H]^+$ion with exact mass 376.14219, corresponding to the molecular formula $C_{16}H_{26}NO_7S$.

3.2.2. General Procedure for the Synthesis of Compounds **1**–**5**

A mixture of the crude (2*S*,3*S*,4*S*)-3-hydroxy-6-methoxy-3-methyl-7-methylene-5-oxo-2-pentyl-2,3,4,5,6,7-hexahydropyrano[2,3-*c*]pyrrol-4-yl methanesulfonate (1 mmol) and an appropriate primary amine (2 mmol) was stirred in dry acetonitrile (2 mL) at room temperature until consumption of the starting material was complete as judged by TLC analysis (24–48 h). The reaction mixture was diluted with ether (20 mL) and transferred to a separatory funnel. The layers were separated and the aqueous layer was extracted with ether (3 × 20 mL). The organic extracts were combined, washed with brine (2 × 20 mL), dried over magnesium sulfate, and concentrated in vacuo. The crude product was purified by flash chromatography (DCM:methanol = 60:1).

(2S,3R,4R)-3-Hydroxy-6-methoxy-3-methyl-4-(methylamino)-7-methylene-2-pentyl-3,4,6,7-tetrahydro-pyrano [2,3-c]pyrrol-5(2H)-one (**1**): Yield 17%, yellow oil. $[\alpha]_D^{20.0} = -120.36$ (c 0.28, CH_2Cl_2). ^{1}H-NMR ($CDCl_3$) δ 5.56 (m, 2H), 5.12 (s, 1H), 5.07 (s, 1H), 4.05 (m, 1H), 3.93 (s, 3H), 3.41 (m, 1H), 2.75 (s, 3H), 1.93 (m, 1H), 1.63 (m, 2H), 1.43–1.33 (m, 5H), 1.15 (s, 3H), 0.90 (m, 3H). ^{13}C-NMR ($CDCl_3$) δ 165.87 (s), 159.47 (s), 136.05 (s), 99.07 (s), 93.27 (s), 81.54 (s), 68.97 (s), 64.70 (s), 57.32 (s), 33.50 (s), 31.58 (s), 27.62 (s), 25.99 (s), 22.53 (s), 19.45 (s), 14.05 (s). IR (KBr) 3319, 2955, 2930, 2859, 1721, 1667, 1633, 1438, 1379, 1266, 1196, 1166, 1085, 979, 915 cm^{-1}. HRMS $[M + H]^+$ calcd for $C_{16}H_{27}N_2O_4$ 311.19653, found 311.1953.

(2S,3R,4R)-3-Hydroxy-4-[(2-hydroxyethyl)amino]-6-methoxy-3-methyl-7-methylene-2-pentyl-3,4,6,7-tetra-hydropyrano[2,3-c]pyrrol-5(2H)-one (**2**): Yield 25%, yellow oil. $[\alpha]_D^{20.0} = -99.54$ (c 0.22, CH_2Cl_2). ^{1}H-NMR ($CDCl_3$) δ 5.09 (s, 1H), 5.04 (s, 1H), 3.93 (m, 4H), 3.61 (m, 2H), 3.12 (s, 1H), 3.06–2.91 (m, 2H), 1.94 (m, 1H), 1.65–1.58 (m, 2H), 1.35 (m, 6H), 1.06 (s, 3H), 0.91 (s, 3H). ^{13}C-NMR ($CDCl_3$) δ 167.38 (s), 157.36 (s), 136.27 (s), 104.10 (s), 92.86 (s), 82.53 (s), 69.28 (s), 64.71 (s), 61.07 (s), 54.14 (s), 52.07 (s), 31.66 (s), 27.47 (s), 26.28 (s), 22.57 (s), 18.58 (s), 14.08 (s). IR (KBr) 3322, 2954, 2927, 2857, 1718, 1633, 1547, 1458, 1437, 1378, 1263, 1191, 1117, 1081, 978, 914 cm^{-1}. HRMS $[M + H]^+$ calcd for $C_{17}H_{29}N_2O_5$ 341.20710, found 341.2060.

(2S,3R,4R)-3-Hydroxy-4-[(4-hydroxybutyl)amino]-6-methoxy-3-methyl-7-methylene-2-pentyl-3,4,6,7-tetra-hydropyrano[2,3-c]pyrrol-5(2H)-one (**3**): Yield 20%, yellow oil. $[\alpha]_D^{20.0} = -89.80$ (c 0.51, CH_2Cl_2). ^{1}H-NMR ($CDCl_3$) δ 5.11 (d, *J* = 1.2 Hz, 1H), 5.05 (d, *J* = 1.3 Hz, 1H), 4.94 (m, 3H), 4.05 (m, 1H), 3.93 (s, 3H), 3.80–3.50 (m, 2H), 3.36 (s, 1H), 3.27–3.12 (m, 1H), 3.06–2.87 (m, 1H), 1.95 (m, 1H), 1.78 (m, 2H), 1.69–1.55 (m, 4H), 1.45–1.33 (m, 5H), 1.12 (s, 3H), 0.90 (m, 3H). ^{13}C-NMR ($CDCl_3$) δ 166.37 (s), 158.18 (s), 136.38 (s), 102.16 (s), 92.59 (s), 82.14 (s), 68.78 (s), 64.64 (s), 62.26 (s), 55.97 (s), 48.77 (s), 31.64 (s), 30.14 (s), 27.61 (s), 26.12 (s), 22.57 (s), 19.15 (s), 14.08 (s). IR (KBr) 3292, 2927, 2858, 1712, 1632, 1548, 1438, 1379, 1191, 1083, 989, 914 cm^{-1}. HRMS $[M + H]^+$ calcd for $C_{19}H_{33}N_2O_5$ 369.23840, found 369.2373.

(2S,3R,4R)-4-(Allylamino)-3-hydroxy-6-methoxy-3-methyl-7-methylene-2-pentyl-3,4,6,7-tetrahydropyrano-[2,3-c]pyrrol-5(2H)-one (**4**): Yield 14%, yellow oil. $[\alpha]_D^{20.0} = -157.50$ (c 0.31, CH_2Cl_2). ^{1}H-NMR ($CDCl_3$) δ

5.89 (ddt, *J* = 12.2, 10.1, 6.1 Hz, 1H), 5.25 (dd, *J* = 17.2, 1.3 Hz, 1H), 5.12 (m, 1H), 5.03 (d, *J* = 1.3 Hz, 1H), 4.99 (d, *J* = 1.3 Hz, 1H), 3.93 (s, 3H), 3.78–3.66 (m, 1H), 3.58–3.49 (m, 1H), 3.44 (ddd, *J* = 13.8, 4.6, 1.2 Hz, 1H), 3.03 (s, 1H), 1.94 (m, 1H), 1.60 (m, 2H), 1.43–1.35 (m, 5H), 1.06 (s, 3H), 0.91 (m, 3H). ^{13}C-NMR ($CDCl_3$) δ 166.68 (s), 156.86 (s), 136.78 (s), 136.06 (s), 117.05 (s), 105.17 (s), 91.79 (s), 82.65 (s), 68.23 (s), 64.59 (s), 54.92 (s), 52.14 (s), 31.69 (s), 27.63 (s), 26.29 (s), 22.57 (s), 18.72 (s), 14.09 (s). IR (KBr) 3314, 2955, 2928, 2858, 1720, 1668, 1634, 1437, 1367, 1232, 1192, 1087, 992, 919 cm^{-1}. HRMS [M + H]$^+$ calcd for $C_{18}H_{29}N_2O_4$ 337.21218, found 337.2111.

(2S,3R,4R)-4-(benzylamino)-3-hydroxy-6-methoxy-3-methyl-7-methylene-2-pentyl-3,4,6,7-tetrahydro-pyrano [2,3-c]pyrrol-5(2H)-one (**5**): Yield 17%, yellow oil. $[\alpha]_D^{20.0} = -137.81$ (c 0.43, CH_2Cl_2). ^{1}H-NMR ($CDCl_3$) δ 7.39–7.26 (m, 5H), 5.04 (d, *J* = 1.4 Hz, 1H), 5.00 (d, *J* = 1.4 Hz, 1H), 4.30 (d, *J* = 12.3 Hz, 1H), 3.94 (m, 4H), 3.53 (m, 1H), 3.12 (s, 1H), 1.93 (m, 1H), 1.61 (m, 2H), 1.34 (m, 5H), 1.06 (s, 3H), 0.90 (m, 3H). ^{13}C-NMR ($CDCl_3$) δ 166.78 (s), 156.89 (s), 139.35 (s), 136.81 (s), 128.61 (d, *J* = 8.7 Hz), 127.47 (s), 105.30 (s), 91.89 (s), 82.70 (s), 68.26 (s), 64.63 (s), 55.37 (s), 53.62 (s), 31.68 (s), 27.63 (s), 26.27 (s), 22.56 (s), 18.82 (s), 14.07 (s). IR (KBr) 3309, 2955, 2927, 2858, 1720, 1633, 1454, 1436, 1378, 1232, 1192, 1086, 978, 914 cm^{-1}. HRMS [M + H]$^+$ calcd for $C_{22}H_{31}N_2O_4$ 387.22783, found 387.2262.

3.2.3. General Procedure for the Synthesis of Compounds **6–8**

A mixture of the crude (2*S*,3*S*,4*S*)-3-hydroxy-6-methoxy-3-methyl-7-methylene-5-oxo-2-pentyl-2,3,4,5,6,7-hexahydropyrano[2,3-*c*]pyrrol-4-yl methanesulfonate (1 mmol), the corresponding cyclic amine (1.5 mmol) and triethylamine (3 mmol) was stirred in dry acetonitrile (2 mL) at room temperature until consumption of the starting material was complete as judged by TLC analysis (24–48 h). The reaction mixture was quenched with water and extracted with EtOAc (2 × 20 mL). The organic extract was washed with brine, dried over magnesium sulfate, and concentrated in vacuo. The crude product was purified by flash chromatography (DCM/methanol).

3.2.4. Alternative General Procedure for the Synthesis of Compounds **6–8**

A mixture of the crude (2*S*,3*S*,4*S*)-3-hydroxy-6-methoxy-3-methyl-7-methylene-5-oxo-2-pentyl-2,3,4,5,6,7-hexahydropyrano[2,3-*c*]pyrrol-4-yl methanesulfonate (1 mmol) and the corresponding cyclic amine (5 mmol) in dry THF (2 mL) was heated at 70–75 °C in a sealed tube for 18 h. The mixture was cooled to room temperature, filtered, and the THF solution was diluted with saturated sodium bicarbonate solution (20 mL). The resulting mixture was extracted with DCM (3 × 20 mL). The organic extracts were washed with water, dried with magnesium sulfate, and concentrated in vacuo. The crude product was purified by flash chromatography (DCM/methanol).

(2S,3R,4R)-3-Hydroxy-6-methoxy-3-methyl-7-methylene-2-pentyl-4-pyrrolidin-1-yl-3,4,6,7-tetrahydro-pyrano [2,3-c]pyrrol-5(2H)-one (**6**): Yield 27%, yellow oil. $[\alpha]_D^{20.0} = -176.52$ (c 0.40, CH_2Cl_2). ^{1}H-NMR ($CDCl_3$) δ 5.40 (s, 1H), 5.02 (d, *J* = 1.4 Hz, 1H), 4.98 (d, *J* = 1.4 Hz, 1H), 3.92 (s, 3H), 3.64 (d, *J* = 9.9 Hz, 1H), 3.31 (s, 1H), 3.10–2.55 (m, 4H), 2.03–1.89 (m, 1H), 1.84–1.70 (m, 4H), 1.69–1.52 (m, 2H), 1.45–1.29 (m, 5H), 1.05 (s, 3H), 0.91 (t, *J* = 6.7 Hz, 3H). ^{13}C-NMR ($CDCl_3$) δ 167.11 (s), 158.44 (s), 137.00 (s), 101.65 (s), 91.38 (s), 83.60 (s), 68.00 (s), 64.41 (s), 59.55 (s), 31.73 (s), 28.21 (s), 26.43 (s), 23.91 (s), 22.55 (s), 19.66 (s), 14.04 (s). IR (KBr) 3430, 2957, 2930, 2860, 1722, 1633, 1438, 1190, 1144 cm^{-1}. HRMS [M + H]$^+$, calcd. for $C_{19}H_{31}N_2O_4$ 351.227834, found 351.22733.

(2S,3R,4R)-3-Hydroxy-6-methoxy-3-methyl-7-methylene-2-pentyl-4-(4-pyrrolidin-1-ylpiperidin-1-yl)-3,4,6,7-tetrahydropyrano[2,3-c]pyrrol-5(2H)-one (**7**): Yield 11%, yellow oil. $[\alpha]_D^{20.0} = -115.82$ (c 0.41, CH_2Cl_2). ^{1}H-NMR ($CDCl_3$) δ 5.05 (s, 1H), 5.00 (s, 1H), 3.91 (s, 3H), 3.56 (m, 1H), 3.29–2.91 (m, 8H), 2.81 (m, 1H), 2.65 (s, 1H), 2.27 (t, *J* = 10.9 Hz, 1H), 2.11–1.83 (m, 9H), 1.69–1.48 (m, 2H), 1.35 (s, 5H), 1.02 (s, 3H), 0.91 (s, 3H). ^{13}C-NMR ($CDCl_3$) δ 167.08 (s), 158.19 (s), 136.87 (s), 101.35 (s), 91.69 (s), 83.39 (s), 68.22 (s), 64.49 (s), 62.51 (s), 61.35 (s), 55.67 (s), 51.39 (s), 49.52 (s), 32.19 (s), 31.74 (s), 28.29 (s), 26.44 (s), 23.20 (s), 22.57 (s), 19.96 (s), 14.08 (s). IR (KBr) 3213, 2928, 2857, 2782, 1724, 1669, 1635, 1437, 1377, 1354, 1321, 1193, 1150, 1126, 1085, 979 cm^{-1}. HRMS [M + H]$^+$ calcd for $C_{24}H_{40}N_3O_4$ 434.30133, found 434.3009.

(2S,3R,4R)-3-Hydroxy-4-(4-hydroxypiperidin-1-yl)-6-methoxy-3-methyl-7-methylene-2-pentyl-3,4,6,7-tetrahydropyrano[2,3-c]pyrrol-5(2H)-one (**8**): Yield 16%, yellow oil. $[\alpha]_D^{20.0} = -111.11$ (c 0.36, CH_2Cl_2). ^{1}H-NMR ($CDCl_3$) δ 5.17 (s, 1H), 5.03 (d, J = 1.1 Hz, 1H), 5.00 (d, J = 1.1 Hz, 1H), 3.93 (s, 3H), 3.68 (s, 1H), 3.59 (m, 1H), 3.02 (s, 1H), 2.87 (s, 2H), 2.35 (s, 1H), 2.03–1.85 (m, 3H), 1.68–1.50 (m, 6H), 1.35 (m, 5H), 1.05 (s, 3H), 0.91 (m, 3H). ^{13}C-NMR ($CDCl_3$) δ 167.01 (s), 158.15 (s), 136.85 (s), 101.35 (s), 91.75 (s), 83.35 (s), 68.20 (s), 64.53 (s), 62.45 (s), 35.20 (s), 31.79 (s), 28.35 (s), 26.48 (s), 22.58 (s), 20.00 (s), 14.09 (s). IR (KBr) 3213, 2926, 2855, 1720, 1671, 1634, 1547, 1438, 1375, 1139, 1066, 1045 cm^{-1}. HRMS $[M + H]^+$ calcd for $C_{20}H_{33}N_2O_5$ 381.23840, found 381.2377.

3.3. Bio-Evaluation Methods

3.3.1. In-Vitro Cytotoxicity Study (MTT Assay)

MCF-7 (breast cancer), PC-3 (prostate adenocarcinoma), HCT-116 (colorectal cancer cell), A549 (lung cancer), K562 (chronic myelogenous leukemia), THP-1 (acute monocytic leukemia), and RPMI8226 (multiple myeloma), Jurkat (acute T-cell leukemia), HEF (human embryonic fibroblasts) was purchased from the Russian Academy of Sciences Cells Bank (Institute of Cytology of the Russian Academy of Sciences, Saint Petersburg, Russian Federation). Multiple myeloma cell line NCI-H929 was purchased from ATCC (USA). The MCF-7, A549 and HEF (human embryonic fibroblasts) were cultured in DMEM medium. Other cell lines were cultured in RPMI1640 medium, (PanEco, Russia) supplemented with 10% fetal bovine serum (GE Healthcare LifeSciences, São Paulo, Brazil), and gentamicin at a concentration of 40 μg/mL and cultured at 37 °C in a humidified atmosphere containing 5% CO_2. All experiments were performed with cells at passages 3 to 7 in the logarithmic phase of growth.

Cells were seeded into 96-well plates of 5×10^3 for adhesive cultures and 20×10^3 for suspension cultures per well in 90 μL and 135 μL of culture medium, respectively. The test substances were dissolved in DMSO to a concentration of 1×10^{-2} M. For subsequent dilution of the substances, a serum-free culture medium was used as the diluent. Final concentration of DMSO in wells was no more than 1%. It was found that this concentration of DMSO didn't affect the cells. Substances were added to the cells in 3–4 replicates after 24 h for adhesive cultures and immediately for suspension cultures. 10–15 μL of serum-free medium was added to the control wells with non-exposed cells. Cells were cultured for 72 h at 37 °C in an atmosphere of 5% CO_2.

3.3.2. Experimental Animals

Six to eight-week-old outbreed male mice were purchased from the Rappolovo Animal Farm of the Russian Academy of Sciences. Animals were group housed in solid bottom polycarbonate cages (3–5 animals/cage) and provided with sterilized pelleted food and pure water ad libitum.

3.3.3. Ethical Guidelines

Animal care and protocols of the study were conducted in compliance with ethical standards and recommendations for the human treatment of animals used in experimental and other scientific purposes according to the European Convention for the Protection of Vertebrate Animals used for Experimental and other Scientific Purposes (and protocol of amendment ETS No 170), the National Standard of the Russian Federation GOST R-53434-2009, "Principles of Good Laboratory Practice," and by the order of the Ministry of Health of the Russian Federation 01.04.2016, No 199n «On approval of the rules of good laboratory practice».

3.3.4. Acute Intraperitoneal Toxicity Study

Thirty mice were randomly assigned to the acute toxicity study. Animals in experimental groups (8 per/group) received a dose formulation containing compound **6** solution in 5% DMSO at various dosages (8.25, 82.5 and 200 mg/kg) via single i.p. injection. Mice in the control group treated with vehicle (5% DMSO). The location of the i.p. injection was in the lower left abdominal quadrant. Volume of injection did not exceed 250 μL. After treatments, the following parameters and end points were evaluated for 14 days: mortality, clinical signs, body weight, food consumption, locomotion, salivation, diarrhea, and lethargy. The maximum tolerated dose in this study is defined as the highest dose that will be tolerated and not produce major life-threatening toxicity for the study duration [18]. All experimental procedures were performed according to the principles and guidelines for the care and use of laboratory animals. The animals were sacrificed by carbon dioxide asphyxiation and cervical dislocation. All efforts were made to minimize suffering. Post mortem evaluation included gross examination for all animals at terminal necropsy and calculation of organ mass coefficients. No histopathological examinations were performed.

4. Conclusions

In summary, a series of PPA derivatives were synthesized via mesylation and amination. Some of these derivatives represent a promising class of cytotoxic agents with potential therapeutic values. Compound **6** demonstrated the highest cytotoxicity and was less toxic when used in vivo compared with the clinically used etoposide.

Author Contributions: V.A. performed the research, analyzed the data and wrote the paper. S.Z. carried out the synthesis of the target compounds. P.B. and N.M. performed the biological assay of the products. J.M. and A.H. analyzed data and revised the manuscript. Y.T. and V.K. conceived the work, gave critical comments. P.B. performed animal studies. A.B. isolated phaeosphaeride A from a fungal strain.

References

1. Goodman, L.S.; Wintrobe, M.M.; Dameshek, W.; Goodman, M.J.; Gilman, A.Z.; McLennan, M.T. Nitrogen mustard therapy. Use of methyl-bis(beta-chloroethyl)amine hydrochloride and tris(beta-chloroethyl)amine hydrochloride for hodgkin's disease, lymphosarcoma, leukemia and certain allied and miscellaneous disorders. *J. Am. Med. Assoc.* **1946**, *132*, 126–132. [CrossRef] [PubMed]
2. Wilson, A.L.; Plebanski, M.; Stephens, A.N. New trends in anti-cancer therapy: Combining conventional chemotherapeutics with novel immunomodulators. *Curr. Med. Chem.* **2017**. [CrossRef] [PubMed]
3. Bhavana, V.; Sudharshan, S.J.S.; Madhu, D. Natural anticancer compounds and their derivatives in clinical trials. In *Anticancer Plants: Clinical Trials and Nanotechnology*; Akhtar, M., Swamy, M., Eds.; Springer: Singapore, 2017; pp. 51–104.
4. Cragg, G.M.; Newman, D.J. Plants as a source of anti-cancer agents. *J. Ethnopharmacol.* **2005**, *100*, 72–79. [CrossRef] [PubMed]
5. Cragg, G.M.; Newman, D.J. Natural products: A continuing source of novel drug leads. *Biochim. Biophys. Acta.* **2013**, *1830*, 3670–3695. [CrossRef] [PubMed]
6. Newman, D.J.; Cragg, G.M. Natural products as sources of new drugs from 1981 to 2014. *J. Nat. Prod.* **2016**, *79*, 629–661. [CrossRef] [PubMed]
7. Kobayashi, K.; Kobayashi, Y.; Nakamura, M.; Tamura, O.; Kogen, H. Establishment of Relative and Absolute Configurations of Phaeosphaeride A: Total Synthesis of ent-Phaeosphaeride A. *J. Org. Chem.* **2015**, *80*, 1243–1248. [CrossRef] [PubMed]
8. Kobayashi, K.; Tanaka, K., III; Kogen, H. Total Synthesis and Biological Evaluation of Phaeosphaerides. *Catalysts* **2018**, *8*, 206–215. [CrossRef]
9. Abzianidze, V.V.; Poluektova, E.V.; Bolshakova, K.P.; Panikorovskii, T.L.; Bogachenkov, A.S.; Berestetskiy, A.O. Crystal structure of natural phaeosphaeride A. *Acta Crystallogr. E: Crystallogr. Commun.* **2015**, *71*, 625–626. [CrossRef] [PubMed]
10. Wake, M.S.; Watson, C.J. STAT3 the oncogene–still eluding therapy? *FEBS J.* **2015**, *282*, 2600–2611. [CrossRef] [PubMed]
11. Johnston, P.A.; Grandis, J.R. STAT3 signaling: Anticancer strategies and challenges. *Mol. Interv.* **2011**, *11*, 18–26. [CrossRef] [PubMed]

12. Maloney, K.N.; Hao, W.; Xu, J.; Gibbons, J.; Hucul, J.; Roll, D.; Brady, S.F.; Schroeder, F.C.; Clardy, J. Phaeosphaeride A, an inhibitor of STAT3-dependent signaling isolated from an endophytic fungus. *Org. Lett.* **2006**, *8*, 4067–4070. [CrossRef] [PubMed]
13. Shao, H.; Cheng, H.Y.; Cook, R.G.; Tweardy, D.J. Identification and characterization of signal transducer and activator of transcription 3 recruitment sites within the epidermal growth factor receptor. *Cancer Res.* **2003**, *63*, 3923–3930. [PubMed]
14. Chatzimpaloglou, A.; Yavropoulou, M.P.; Rooij, K.E.; Biedermann, R.; Mueller, U.; Kaskel, S.; Sarli, V. Total Synthesis and Biological Activity of the Proposed Structure of Phaeosphaeride A. *J. Org. Chem.* **2012**, *77*, 9659–9667. [CrossRef] [PubMed]
15. Chatzimpaloglou, A.; Kolosov, M.; Eckols, T.K.; Tweardy, D.J.; Sarli, V. Synthetic and Biological Studies of Phaeosphaerides. *J. Org. Chem.* **2014**, *79*, 4043–4054. [CrossRef] [PubMed]
16. Abzianidze, V.V.; Efimova, K.P.; Poluektova, E.V.; Trishin, Y.G.; Kuznetsov, V.A. Synthesis of natural phaeosphaeride A and semi-natural phaeosphaeride B derivatives. *Mendeleev Commun.* **2017**, *27*, 490–492. [CrossRef]
17. Efimova, K.P. Synthesis of Natural Phaeosphaeride A Derivatives with Antitumor and Herbicidal Activity. Master's Thesis, Saint-Petersburg State University of Industrial Technologies and Design, Saint Petersburg, Russia, July 2017.
18. Robinson, S.; Delongeas, J.L.; Donald, E.; Dreher, D.; Festag, M.; Kervyn, S.; Lampo, A.; Nahas, K.; Nogues, V.; Ockert, D.; et al. A European pharmaceutical company initiative challenging the regulatory requirement for acute toxicity studies in pharmaceutical drug development. *Regul. Toxicol. Pharmacol.* **2008**, *50*, 345–352. [CrossRef] [PubMed]

2

Gene Therapy Approaches to Functional Cure and Protection of Hematopoietic Potential in HIV Infection

Tetsuo Tsukamoto

Department of Immunology, Kindai University Faculty of Medicine, Osaka 5898511, Japan; ttsukamoto@med.kindai.ac.jp

Abstract: Although current antiretroviral drug therapy can suppress the replication of human immunodeficiency virus (HIV), a lifelong prescription is necessary to avoid viral rebound. The problem of persistent and ineradicable viral reservoirs in HIV-infected people continues to be a global threat. In addition, some HIV-infected patients do not experience sufficient T-cell immune restoration despite being aviremic during treatment. This is likely due to altered hematopoietic potential. To achieve the global eradication of HIV disease, a cure is needed. To this end, tremendous efforts have been made in the field of anti-HIV gene therapy. This review will discuss the concepts of HIV cure and relative viral attenuation and provide an overview of various gene therapy approaches aimed at a complete or functional HIV cure and protection of hematopoietic functions.

Keywords: human immunodeficiency virus; acquired immunodeficiency syndrome; hematopoietic stem/progenitor cells; gene therapy

1. Introduction

Human immunodeficiency virus (HIV) infects CD4$^+$ T cells and causes acquired immunodeficiency syndrome (AIDS). AIDS remains as a global threat due to multifactorial reasons, including the difficulty in developing an effective vaccine [1]. According to The Joint United Nations Programme on HIV/AIDS (UNAIDS), in 2017, about 36.9 million people were living with AIDS while only 21.7 million patients were receiving antiretroviral therapy (ART), resulting in about 1.8 million newly HIV-infected people per year [2]. Although ART can limit the size and distribution of HIV reservoirs depending on the earliness of its initiation, it cannot eliminate latent HIV infections from the host and thus, a lifelong prescription is required for suppressing viral rebound from the reservoirs [3]. Therefore, further exploration is vital to discover new treatment options and effective vaccines [4].

The depletion of memory CD4$^+$ T cells preceding AIDS manifestation may be mainly due to the infection of these cells. However, HIV may also reduce the production of naïve T cells by infecting CD4$^+$ thymocytes [5–8]. On the other hand, although the dynamics of hematopoietic stem/progenitor cells (HSPCs) in HIV-infected settings is still unclear, it is well established that HIV infections are associated with hematological changes, such as anemia and pancytopenia [9]. These hematological changes are likely due to the modified HSPCs and hematopoietic potential of the host. Therefore, a cure for HIV disease should consider not only the absence of newly HIV-infected CD4$^+$ cells but also the normal production rates of CD4$^+$ T cells and other hematopoietic cells. To achieve an HIV cure in its strict sense, the protection of bone marrow hematopoietic functions is essential (Figure 1).

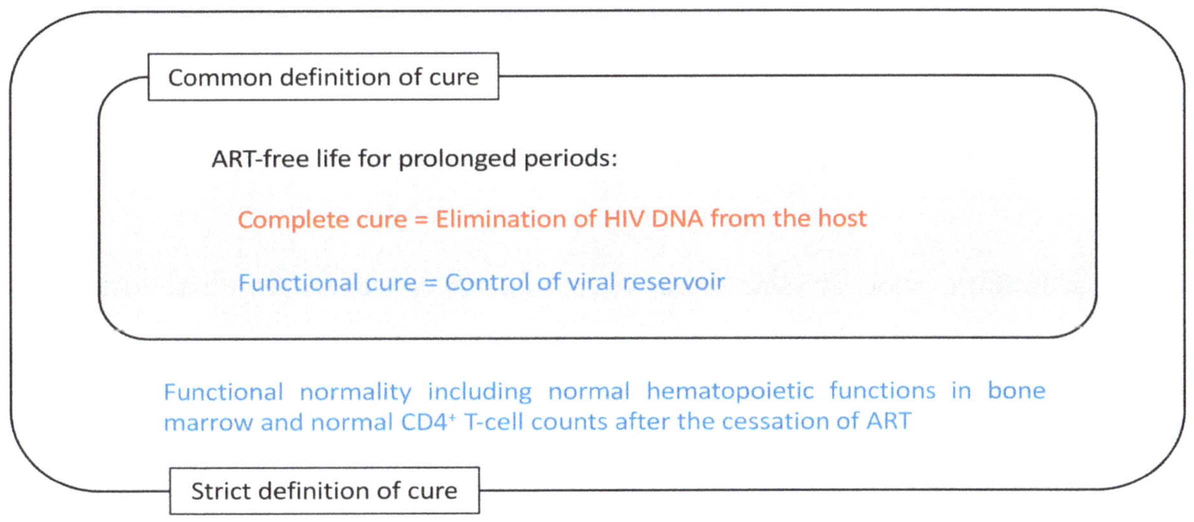

Figure 1. The concepts of human immunodeficiency virus (HIV) cure. A cure for the HIV disease is commonly interpreted as antiretroviral drug therapy (ART)-free life without viral rebound for prolonged periods. In addition, the cure for bone marrow dysfunctionalities observed in HIV-infected patients could be included in a stricter definition of a HIV cure.

This review first describes the current evidence of modified bone marrow hematopoietic potential in HIV infection, leading to the strict definition of an HIV cure. It then explains how anti-HIV gene therapy methods applied to HSPCs can support the preservation of hematopoietic potential and a functional cure. This will be followed by an overview of different potential gene therapy methods for achieving this goal.

2. Evidence of Modified CD34$^+$ Cell Dynamics and Functions in HIV Infection

HIV-1 may cause the loss of primitive hematopoietic progenitors without directly infecting these cells [10]. However, HIV infection does not cause the complete loss of CD34$^+$ stem cells and therefore, it is possible to harvest stem cells from HIV-infected patients suffering from lymphoma [11] albeit with reduced efficiencies in relation to the reduction of peripheral CD4$^+$ T-cell counts [12] or reduced in vitro lymphopoiesis capacities [13]. The recovery of CD4$^+$ T-cell counts after successful antiretroviral drug therapy treatment may depend on the recovery of CD34$^+$ cell counts [14].

A number of potential mechanisms have been suggested for the changes of CD34$^+$ cells in the presence of HIV, such as reduced expression of the proto-oncogene *c-mpl* on CD34$^+$ cells [15] and elevated plasma stromal cell-derived factor 1 (SDF-1) levels [16]. HIV-1 infection causes the upregulation of inflammatory cytokine production that may affect the dynamics and functions [17] or induce Fas-mediated apoptosis [18] of bone marrow CD34$^+$ cells. On the other hand, HSPCs themselves may contribute to inflammation and allergies [19]. This may be partly due to the fact that inflammatory signals are involved in HSPC development [20]. Recent evidence has suggested that CD34$^+$CD226(DNAM-1)^{bright}CXCR4$^+$ cells may represent a subset of common lymphoid progenitors associated with chronic HIV infection and inflammation, reflecting the altered dynamics of natural killer cells and α/β T cells [21].

Humanized mouse models are useful for analyzing bone marrow CD34$^+$ loss or changes after the HIV-1 challenge. In studies with humanized mice infected with CXCR4-tropic HIV-1$_{NL4\text{-}3}$, CD34$^+$ hematopoietic progenitor cells were depleted and showed impaired ex vivo myeloid/erythroid colony forming capacities after the challenge [22,23]. A reduction of bone marrow CD34$^+$ cell counts after CCR5-tropic HIV-1 infection was also detected in another study [24]. Interestingly, the depletion of bone marrow CD34$^+$ cells following CCR5-tropic HIV infection has been reported to depend on plasmacytoid dendritic cells [25] or to be associated with the expression of CXCR4 [26]. The latter implicates a potential role of the SDF-1/CXCR4 axis in the loss of CD34$^+$ cells. Another recent in vitro study suggested that $CD34^+CD7^+CXCR4^+$ lymphoid progenitor cells may be depleted in the presence of CXCR4-tropic HIV-1 in the coculture of HIV-infected cord-derived $CD34^+$ cells with mouse stromal OP9-DL1 cells, which allow the differentiation of T cells [27].

3. The Idea of Intracellular Immunization of HSPCs to Replace the Whole Hematopoietic System

After this, it is important to consider how we could deal with hematopoietic changes in HIV infection. A potential solution is gene therapy. In 1988, David Baltimore presented his idea of intracellular immunization by gene therapy [28] and his concepts are still valid today. First, he suggested expressing inhibitory molecules against HIV in target cells. Second, he proposed using retroviral vectors to transduce cells although lentiviral vectors are widely used today. Third, he conceived the use of gene-modified HSPCs to replace the immune system of the hosts with an HIV-resistant one. These concepts may be summarized as intracellular artificial immune systems designed against HIV and working independently from HIV-specific $CD4^+$ helper T cells, which are the most vulnerable HIV targets [29]. Since his work, a number of candidate gene therapies have been proposed and tested and are described later in this article.

4. The Protection of Bone Marrow $CD34^+$ Cells by an Anti-HIV Gene Therapy Demonstrated In Vivo

However, there have been few reports so far that have tested the protection of $CD34^+$ cells after HIV infection by gene therapy. This may be because viral suppression and $CD4^+$ counts have been widely accepted as measures for the effect of gene therapies against HIV. However, the true goal for any gene therapy against HIV should be the protection of hematopoietic potential because this is another arm of the definition of AIDS, i.e., the loss of cellular immunity (Figure 1).

Regarding this, we have recently reported that a transcriptional gene silencing (TGS) approach using a short hairpin (sh) RNA, which is called shPromA (Figure 2), resulted in limited CXCR4-associated depletion of bone marrow $CD34^+$ cells following CCR5-tropic HIV infection in humanized mice (Figure 3). This suggests that anti-HIV gene therapy can support the preservation of the hematopoietic potential of the hosts [26]. Further characteristics of shPromA and previous studies testing its efficacy as a functional cure gene therapy method is discussed in Section 8.

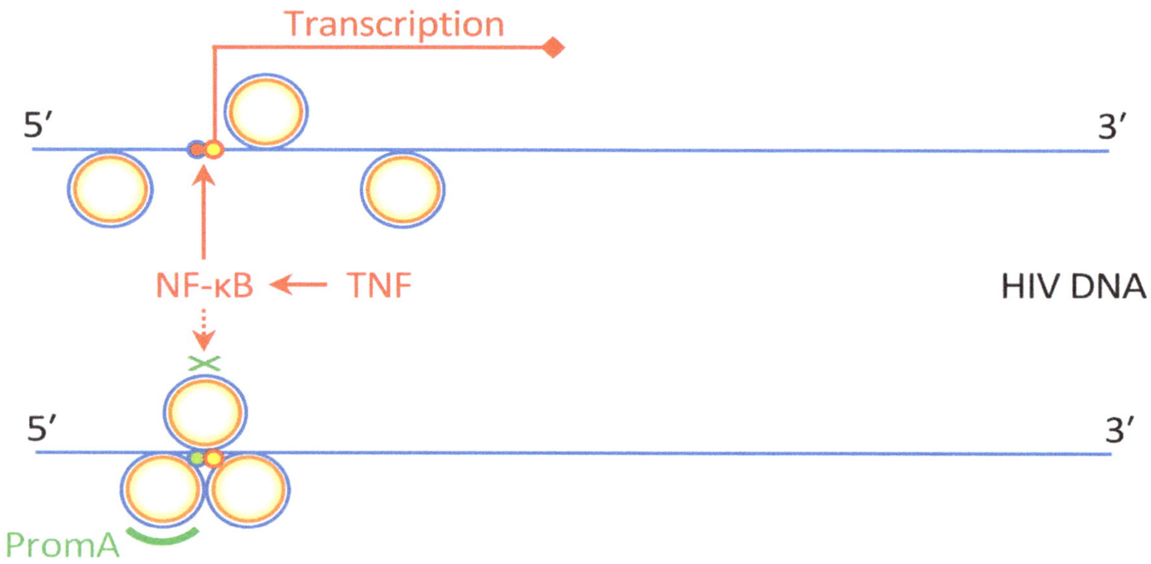

Figure 2. A schematic overview of PromA. PromA induces chromatin compaction in the human immunodeficiency virus (HIV)-1 promoter. This prevents HIV-1 DNA from reactivation, such as NF-κB-mediated reactivation by tissue necrosis factor (TNF). For details on the molecular mechanisms involved in transcriptional gene silencing induced by PromA, see Klemm et al., 2016 [30] and Mendez et al., 2018 [31].

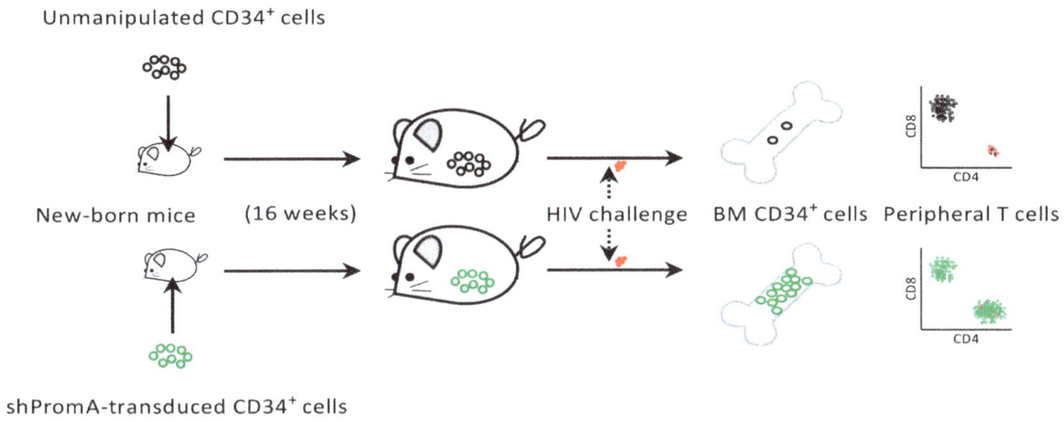

Figure 3. Summary of the humanized mouse study to test the efficacy of shRNA PromA (shPromA) [26]. Newborn NOD/SCID/Jak3^{null} mice were intrahepatically transfused with unmanipulated cord-derived CD34$^+$ cells or CD34$^+$ cells lentivirally transduced with shPromA. Those mice showing engraftment of human cells were challenged with CCR5-tropic HIV-1$_{JRFL}$. Two weeks after the challenge, the mice were sacrificed and their bone marrow (BM) CD34$^+$ cells and peripheral T cells were analyzed. Interestingly, mice transplanted with unmanipulated CD34$^+$ cells showed unexpectedly low BM CD34$^+$ cell counts 2 weeks after HIV infection, with concomitant depletion of peripheral CD4$^+$ T cells. On the other hand, mice engrafted with shPromA-expressing CD34$^+$ cells showed preserved BM CD34$^+$ cell and peripheral CD4$^+$ T-cell populations at 2 weeks post challenge.

5. Target Cells for Anti-HIV Gene Therapies

Recent studies, including the above shPromA study, indicate that ideal anti-HIV gene therapy targets should be hematopoietic stem cells rather than more differentiated cells, such as peripheral CD4$^+$ T cells, because the transduced cells could engraft the host bone marrow and act as a lifelong source of HIV-resistant CD4$^+$ cells [26,32,33]. Potential gene therapies using CD34$^+$ cells have been investigated in vitro using cell culture experiments [26,34–36] or in vivo using humanized mice [26,35,37–40]. Furthermore, the transplantation of macaques with gene-modified autologous CD34$^+$ cells followed by an infection with SIV has also been tested [41,42] although strategies may differ between gene therapies [33]. Based on such basic study results, the clinical trials using the transplantation of retrovirally or lentivirally gene-modified CD34$^+$ cells in HIV-positive patients have been carried out [43–45]. Gene therapies of CD34$^+$ cells have been considered as a cure for monogenic immune diseases. For example, the patients with adenosine deaminase deficiency [46], Wiskott–Aldrich syndrome (WAS) [47] and X-linked severe combined immunodeficiency [48,49] were successfully treated in clinical trials by transplantation of autologous CD34$^+$ cells retrovirally or lentivirally transduced with the wild-type gene. Lentiviral vectors may be more efficient in gene transfer into resting stem cells at the G0/G1 phase compared with murine retroviral vectors [50]. If applied to the gene therapy of HSPCs, both retroviral and lentiviral vectors could have adverse effects, including the deregulation of gene expression [51] and the triggering of the p53 protein [52]. However, lentiviral vectors may be safer than retroviral vectors because the latter may occasionally cause insertional mutagenesis near the active start regions of genes, which could possibly lead to oncogenesis and cancers, such as leukemias [48]. Self-inactivating retroviral or lentiviral vectors lacking the U3 region of 3′ LTRs have further safety advantages [53]. Moreover, recent evidence has shown that the transplantation of WAS patients with autologous CD34$^+$ cells transduced with lentiviral vectors encoding WAS protein results in the long-term survival of genetically engineered hematopoietic stem cells and lymphoid-committed progenitors [54]. Thus, this provides hope for lifelong protection from HIV.

Induced pluripotent stem cells (iPSCs) may also be candidates for anti-HIV gene transfer. iPSCs can be generated from the somatic cells of patients, which can differentiate to any cells in vitro and are expected to be utilized for the treatment of a broad range of genetic diseases [55–58]. Although CD34$^+$ cells can engraft in the bone marrow following transplantation and differentiate to hematopoietic cells in vivo, iPSCs may be more convenient for in vitro hematopoiesis compared to CD34$^+$ cells because of their ease of culture [59]. Interestingly, the impact of shPromA-transduced iPSCs on the suppression of viral replication in vitro has recently been demonstrated, suggesting that the large-scale production of gene-modified monocytes or lymphocytes in vitro for adoptive therapy could be a future option [60]. Additionally, the generation of iPSCs from HIV epitope-specific CD8$^+$ cytotoxic T cells followed by their redifferentiation into the identical epitope-specific CD8$^+$ T cells for adoptive transfer could be an effective immunotherapy [61].

6. Complete Cure vs. Functional Cure for HIV Infection

Before describing individual anti-HIV gene therapy methods, this review looks back on Figure 1 to summarize two major strategies for the treatment of HIV infection. One is to eliminate all the HIV DNA copies within the host, which is termed a complete cure (Figure 1). In pursuing the feasibility of this goal, tremendous efforts have been made to (1) find a method to detect all the latently infected HIV DNAs in viral reservoirs and to (2) eliminate all the detected HIV DNAs so that the host would become sterile in terms of HIV infection [62]. Among the methods to achieve this, the so-called "shock and kill" method, in which the reactivation of the viral reservoir is attempted with a shock-inducing agent followed by the immune-mediated killing of the reactivated cells, has been widely investigated [63–67]. These efforts have been partly successful [62,68]. However, the difficulty of viral eradication in vivo is not limited to HIV but include other viruses that induce long-lasting latent infections, such as herpes simplex viruses, varicella–zoster virus, cytomegalovirus and Epstein–Barr virus, making them ineradicable [69]. HIV may differ from other latently infecting viruses as the viral replication from the latent reservoir can resume quickly even if the host is not considered to be immunocompromised [70]. Moreover, even in the case of the Berlin patient who exhibited no sign of HIV existence following allogeneic transplantation with CCR5-Δ32/Δ32 hematopoietic stem cells, a complete cure was assumed rather than being fully demonstrated [71,72].

Alternatively, some potential gene therapy methods aim at a functional cure that is evidenced by the control of HIV replication below the limit of detection and the immune system being functionally normal despite residual cells harboring HIV proviral DNAs in the host (Figure 1) [68,73]. This approach might be more practical than the complete cure approach, given that many successful vaccines for chronic viral infections so far exert a functional cure rather than achieving the elimination of the targeted viruses [74]. In light of this, it could be stated that for those pathogens where an effective vaccine has not been developed to date, researchers could instead develop gene therapies aimed at a functional cure. In this way, there is an overlap between the concept of functional-cure gene therapy and the concept of vaccines against chronic pathogens [75]. In the next paragraph, the relevance of this is better clarified by looking at a similarity between live-attenuated vaccines and functional-cure gene therapy.

7. Connection between Functional-Cure Gene Therapies and Live-Attenuated Vaccine Approaches

Anti-HIV gene therapy might be compared to some of the vaccine candidates tested so far in order to better foresee its future direction. Live-attenuated vaccines have been tested in macaque AIDS models using simian immunodeficiency virus (SIV) strains [76–82]. After the infection of a host with a live-attenuated SIV or simian-human immunodeficiency virus (SHIV), the vaccine strain is controlled by T-cell response but remains slowly replicating in the infected host. This results in further immunization of the host to prepare for the subsequent superinfections of wild-type SIV or SHIV. Therefore, even if live-attenuated vaccines are powerful, they provide a functional but not a complete cure. This means that there is a scientific connection between live-attenuated vaccines and gene therapy approaches for a functional cure because the latter confer viral attenuation indirectly by rendering the host cells HIV-resistant (Figure 4a). The two distinct strategies can be collectively interpreted as the relative attenuation of the infected virus to the unmanipulated/gene-modified host cells (Figure 4b). Thus, relative viral attenuation might help the host immunity to control the virus [83].

(a)

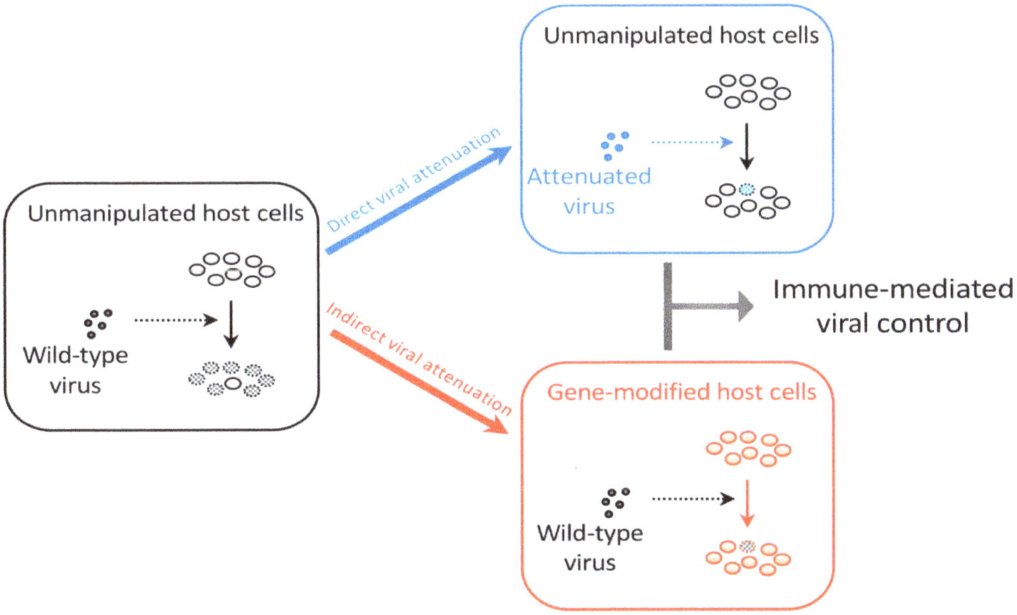

(b)

Given the following parameters:

v_0 ... Virulence of the wild type virus
v_1 ... Virulence of the live-attenuated virus
r_0 ... Viral resistance of the unmanipulated host cells
r_1 ... Viral resistance of the gene-modified host cells

"Relative viral attenuation $f(t_1)$" can be defined as follows, using the direct viral attenuation index (v_0/v_1) and the indirect viral attenuation index (r_1/r_0).

$$f(t_1) = \frac{v_0}{v_1} \times \frac{r_1}{r_0}$$

Direct attenuation of the virus to make a vaccine strain

Gene therapy-mediated increase in viral resistance of the host cells

Figure 4. The concept of relative viral attenuation. (**a**) A schema describing direct and indirect viral attenuation. HIV usually infects host CD4[+] cells efficiently and replicates rapidly. As a result, the host immune system fails to control viral replication (left). However, accumulating evidence in macaque AIDS models suggests that a live-attenuated virus, which infects and replicates slowly because of partial defects in the viral genome, can be controlled by the immune system and helps in further immunization against a potential superinfection with immunodeficiency virus strains that are homologous to the vaccine strain (upper right). The live attenuation method cannot be directly applied to HIV infection in humans because of safety concerns. However, indirect viral attenuation can be achieved by rendering the host cells HIV-resistant by an "intracellular immunization" gene therapy (lower right); (**b**) The definition of relative viral attenuation. This idea can connect live-attenuated vaccine studies and gene therapy approaches to achieve a functional cure. While live-attenuated HIV vaccines are not testable in humans for safety concerns, functional-cure gene therapy could be an alternative.

8. Gene Therapy Strategies against HIV

The Berlin patient, an HIV-positive male United States citizen who was diagnosed with HIV while attending university in Berlin and later suffered from acute myelogenous leukemia, received a transplantation of allogeneic hematopoietic stem cells homozygous for CCR5-Δ32. This resulted in a subsequent functional HIV cure [71,72]. Because CCR5 is critical in HIV infection and transmission, as observed with CCR5-Δ32 homozygous cells resistant to HIV infection [84], the manipulation of CCR5 expression on HIV target cells has been intensively investigated and is considered to be effective [34,35,37,39,40,85–102]. CCR5 can be targeted by zinc finger nucleases [103,104], ribozymes [105], CRISPR/Cas9 methods [106], transcription activator-like effector nucleases [106] and shRNAs [86,107,108]. Among these, several gene therapy methods, including one using lentiviral vector LVsh5/C46 that expresses shRNA against CCR5 and HIV-1 entry inhibitor C46 [109] have been tested in clinical trials [93]. While CCR5 is involved in numerous pathologic states, including inflammatory and infectious diseases [110], a complete knockout of CCR5 can be related to an increased sensitivity to some viral infections [111,112]. Therefore, CCR5 gene editing should only be considered for an HIV cure [110].

The targeting of HIV RNA sequences by ribozymes or RNAs [44,99,113–123] and HIV DNA sequences by the CRISPR/Cas9 system [124] has been investigated and is also considered a major strategy [100,125]. The latter method has recently been of great interest, which is primarily because of its potential for targeting and disrupting integrated HIV DNA sequences to achieve a complete cure. A recent study targeted and inactivated the HIV-1 long terminal repeat (LTR) U3 region in vitro by Cas9 and guide RNAs (gRNAs), with no off-target gene editing to the host cells being detected [126]. Another study also successfully targeted the HIV-1 LTR U3 region using the CRISPR/Cas9 system. However, this study also detected the emergence of escape variant viruses mediated by the error-prone non-homologous end joining (NHEJ) DNA repair following the CRISPR/Cas9 targeting in the host cells [127]. The mutagenesis problem with CRISPR/Cas9 has also been observed in the treatments of other diseases [128] but can be a serious problem when targeting the HIV DNAs because the strategy might require sustained expression of Cas9 and gRNA in the potential HIV target cells, which means a sustained risk of mutagenesis [129]. Therefore, an improved method for disrupting HIV DNA while prohibiting the emergence of replication-competent escape variants caused by the NHEJ repair system might be necessary. Nevertheless, radical approaches can still be tested in cultured cells and animals. For example, a recent study demonstrated that the in vivo gene delivery of multiplex single-gRNAs and *Staphylococcus aureus* Cas9 to transgenic mice bearing HIV DNA using an adeno-associated virus (AAV) vector resulted in an efficient excision of HIV DNA in various tissues and organs [130]. If safety concerns are met, such a gene delivery method can be a powerful tool to achieve the systemic elimination of latent viral reservoirs in hematopoietic cells and nonhematopoietic cells, such as astrocytes [131]. Wang et al. (2018) have written a thorough review of topics regarding the targeting of HIV DNA by CRISPR/Cas9 [124].

An alternative to the CRISPR/Cas9 strategy is the silencing approach, which aims to reduce the production rate of HIV viral particles per integrated HIV DNA copy [68]. Lentiviral gene delivery enables RNA-based gene silencing, including the previously characterized small interfering RNA (siRNA) called PromA [30,132]. PromA is a short RNA sequence specific for the two NF-κB binding sites in the HIV LTR U3 region. While specific mRNA cleavage by post-transcriptional gene silencing is the best-known mechanism for siRNAs, PromA triggers TGS, which is mediated by epigenetic changes, such as DNA methylation and heterochromatin formation [116,133]. In fact, PromA has been shown to induce chromatin compaction in the HIV-1 promoter region [133]. This means that in contrast to methods attempting to eradicate HIV DNA, PromA locks and stabilizes the latently infecting HIV provirus and prevents the reactivation of viral reservoirs from stimuli, such as tissue necrosis factor (Figure 2) [31,134,135]. The efficacy of PromA in suppressing HIV-1 replication in vivo was first demonstrated by an HIV challenge study using humanized NOD/SCID/JAK3^{null} (NOJ) mice transplanted with human peripheral mononuclear cells expressing shPromA [135]. Our recent study to extend the results using NOJ mice engrafted with shPromA-transduced $CD34^+$ cells and their derivatives further demonstrated that PromA could be an effective gene therapy for protecting bone marrow $CD34^+$ cells and the hematopoietic potential of the host from HIV infection (Figure 3) [26].

Other potential gene therapy methods include the secretion of soluble HIV entry inhibitors [38]; the rescue of hematopoiesis, including myelopoiesis, erythropoiesis and megakaryopoiesis using *c-mpl* [136]; the expression of a chimeric human-simian TRIM5α [137]; the expression of p68 kinase [138]; and the expression of HIV Gag mutants [36].

9. Application of Gene Therapy Methods to Immunotherapies

This section sheds lights on a different application of gene therapy methods to fight against HIV. Immunotherapy approaches based on gene therapy methods have been extensively investigated. Chimeric antigen receptor (CAR) T cells are engineered T cells expressing CARs for the recognition and killing of target cells [139,140]. Most typical CARs are engineered to recognize an antigen with a monoclonal antibody-derived extracellular domain that is conjugated to T-cell receptor-derived transmembrane and intracellular domains. Therefore, despite the use of T-cell signaling pathways, such CAR T-cell therapies might be regarded as an enhancement of antibody-based therapies [141,142]. To date, most successful CAR T-cell therapies have been against cancers [143]. For example, the high efficacy of the adoptive transfer of CAR T cells recognizing CD19 has been demonstrated for the treatment of patients with B-cell acute lymphoblastic leukemia [144] and diffuse large B-cell lymphoma [145]. In contrast, CAR T-cell therapies may require the manufacture of autologous CAR T cells for each patient and thus are not yet widely available [145]. Several broadly neutralizing antibodies have been considered for generating CAR T cells against HIV infection [146–148]. Despite the shared concern of escape mutations with antibody-based therapies, CAR T cells are MHC-independent and more potent than the administration of neutralizing antibodies so better outcomes can be expected. A further improvement of HIV CAR gene therapy has been tested to make CAR T cells HIV-resistant by the insertion of the HIV CAR gene expression cassette into the CCR5 locus, which results in the disruption of CCR5 [148]. Finally, an adoptive transfer therapy using autologous $CD34^+$ cells transduced with lentivirus expressing a CD4-based CAR that is able to bind the HIV envelope protein has been tested in humanized mice infected with HIV-1 [149] and pigtail macaques infected with a SHIV [150].

Another exciting gene transfer-based immunotherapy involves programming the production of specific anti-HIV antibodies [151,152]. Compared with vaccination, passive immunization using a set of broadly neutralizing antibodies is customizable, MHC-independent and provides instant and reliable protection against HIV [153,154]. However, neutralizing antibodies need repeated administration to provide prolonged protection [154]. Thus, the concept of antibody gene transfer is to overcome the limitation of passive immunization, which is only transiently effective [155]. It was demonstrated in a humanized mouse model that antibody gene transfer by intramuscular inoculation of an AAV vector encoding a full-length antibody was able to induce the production of the antibody by muscle cells and confer protection against intravenous HIV-1 challenge [156]. In another study, an adenovirus serotype 5 (Ad5) vector encoding an HIV-1-specific broadly neutralizing antibody PGT121 (Ad5.PGT121) afforded a more rapid and robust antibody response than an AAV encoding PGT121 (AAV1.PGT121) in HIV-1-infected bone marrow-liver-thymus humanized mice [157].

10. Biosafety and Bioethics Concerns Regarding the Application of Anti-HIV Gene Therapies to Human Germline Cells for Pregnancy

In the last part of the review, I would like to comment on the recent issue raised against anti-HIV gene therapy. In late 2018, it was reported that a Chinese researcher used the CRISPR/Cas9 technology to create twins bearing CCR5 double knockouts to confer HIV resistance [158]. However, the inheritable gene modification of human germline cells culminating in human pregnancy is currently unacceptable [159]. If applied to germline cells, CRISPR/Cas9 could cause additional inheritable mutations in the host genome DNA [128,160–162] and the influence of this is not entirely predictable at this moment. Therefore, such an investigation on human germline cells should be limited to nonclinical (i.e., in vitro) studies. Regarding the targeted gene, it should be emphasized that CCR5 knockout has not been proven to be safe. Even if a small population of people, mostly of Caucasian origin, is living without functional CCR5 alleles, this does not mean that the loss of CCR5 is universally harmless. This is partly because CCR5 has been reported to play important roles in some viral infections [111,112]. Moreover, there is an unexcluded possibility that the lack of CCR5 function among those carrying the CCR5-Δ32/Δ32 double mutations could be compensated by accompanying genetic variations that do not exist in the majority of human populations with the wild-type CCR5 alleles. Regarding the protection from HIV-1 infection, CCR5-knockout individuals are still susceptible to the infection of CXCR4-tropic HIV-1 strains despite these risks. We refer to the statement published in 2017 by an American Society of Human Genetics workgroup regarding human germline genome editing [163].

11. Conclusions

The evidence suggests that the HIV infection alters the bone marrow hematopoietic potential of the host. This can lead to impaired $CD4^+$ T-cell generation and contributes to the loss of peripheral $CD4^+$ T cells and the manifestation of AIDS. Further investigations on the topics discussed in this review will collectively enhance our understanding of the important role that HIV gene therapy can contribute toward an HIV cure. Intracellular immunization gene therapies, including silencing approaches, are expected to confer relative viral attenuation without interfering with the HIV genome and assist cellular immunity to kill HIV-infected cells. This will ultimately lead to better viral control and a functional cure. In light of this, the long-term preservation of bone marrow $CD34^+$ cells and hematopoietic potential as well as aviremic states and restored peripheral $CD4^+$ T-cell counts may be an appropriate endpoint of future anti-HIV gene therapies. With this regard, our recent in vivo study using humanized mice transplanted with shRNA (shPromA)-transduced $CD34^+$ cells and challenged with HIV-1 has been described to show that the anti-HIV intracellular immunization gene therapy can indeed protect bone marrow HSPCs. Although the efficacy and safety of those novel gene therapy strategies need further improvements for the future applications to autologous HSPC transplantation of HIV-infected patients, a combination of a gene therapy and host immunization based on preserved bone marrow hematopoietic potential and relative viral attenuation will give a hope for a functional cure. Furthermore, the recent advances in gene therapy-based immunotherapy approaches against HIV have also been described in this review.

Acknowledgments: I thank Enago (www.enago.jp) for the English language review.

References

1. McMichael, A.J. Is a Human CD8 T-Cell Vaccine Possible, and if So, What Would It Take? Could a CD8(+) T-Cell Vaccine Prevent Persistent HIV Infection? *Cold Spring Harb. Perspect. Biol.* **2018**, *10*. [CrossRef] [PubMed]
2. UNAIDS. *UNAIDS Data 2018*; UNAIDS: Geneva, Switzerland, 2018.
3. Hong, F.F.; Mellors, J.W. Changes in HIV reservoirs during long-term antiretroviral therapy. *Curr. Opin. HIV AIDS* **2015**, *10*, 43–48. [CrossRef] [PubMed]
4. Ghosn, J.; Taiwo, B.; Seedat, S.; Autran, B.; Katlama, C. HIV. *Lancet* **2018**, *392*, 685–697. [CrossRef]
5. Zou, W.; Denton, P.W.; Watkins, R.L.; Krisko, J.F.; Nochi, T.; Foster, J.L.; Garcia, J.V. Nef functions in BLT mice to enhance HIV-1 replication and deplete CD4+CD8+ thymocytes. *Retrovirology* **2012**, *9*, 44. [CrossRef] [PubMed]
6. Meissner, E.G.; Duus, K.M.; Loomis, R.; D'Agostin, R.; Su, L. HIV-1 replication and pathogenesis in the human thymus. *Curr. HIV Res.* **2003**, *1*, 275–285. [CrossRef] [PubMed]

7. Zaitseva, M.B.; Lee, S.; Rabin, R.L.; Tiffany, H.L.; Farber, J.M.; Peden, K.W.; Murphy, P.M.; Golding, H. CXCR4 and CCR5 on human thymocytes: Biological function and role in HIV-1 infection. *J. Immunol.* **1998**, *161*, 3103–3113. [PubMed]
8. Taylor, J.R., Jr.; Kimbrell, K.C.; Scoggins, R.; Delaney, M.; Wu, L.; Camerini, D. Expression and function of chemokine receptors on human thymocytes: Implications for infection by human immunodeficiency virus type 1. *J. Virol.* **2001**, *75*, 8752–8760. [CrossRef] [PubMed]
9. Parinitha, S.; Kulkarni, M. Haematological changes in HIV infection with correlation to CD4 cell count. *Australas. Med. J.* **2012**, *5*, 157–162. [CrossRef] [PubMed]
10. Marandin, A.; Katz, A.; Oksenhendler, E.; Tulliez, M.; Picard, F.; Vainchenker, W.; Louache, F. Loss of primitive hematopoietic progenitors in patients with human immunodeficiency virus infection. *Blood* **1996**, *88*, 4568–4578. [PubMed]
11. Re, A.; Cattaneo, C.; Skert, C.; Balsalobre, P.; Michieli, M.; Bower, M.; Ferreri, A.J.; Hentrich, M.; Ribera, J.M.; Allione, B.; et al. Stem cell mobilization in HIV seropositive patients with lymphoma. *Haematologica* **2013**, *98*, 1762–1768. [CrossRef] [PubMed]
12. Schooley, R.T.; Mladenovic, J.; Sevin, A.; Chiu, S.; Miles, S.A.; Pomerantz, R.J.; Campbell, T.B.; Bell, D.; Ambruso, D.; Wong, R.; et al. Reduced mobilization of CD34+ stem cells in advanced human immunodeficiency virus type 1 disease. *J. Infect. Dis.* **2000**, *181*, 148–157. [CrossRef] [PubMed]
13. Nielsen, S.D.; Clark, D.R.; Hutchings, M.; Dam-Larsen, S.; Repping, S.; Nielsen, J.O.; Mathiesen, L.; Miedema, F.; Hansen, J.E. Treatment with granulocyte colony-stimulating factor decreases the capacity of hematopoietic progenitor cells for generation of lymphocytes in human immunodeficiency virus-infected persons. *J. Infect. Dis.* **1999**, *180*, 1819–1826. [CrossRef] [PubMed]
14. Sauce, D.; Larsen, M.; Fastenackels, S.; Pauchard, M.; Ait-Mohand, H.; Schneider, L.; Guihot, A.; Boufassa, F.; Zaunders, J.; Iguertsira, M.; et al. HIV disease progression despite suppression of viral replication is associated with exhaustion of lymphopoiesis. *Blood* **2011**, *117*, 5142–5151. [CrossRef] [PubMed]
15. Koka, P.S.; Kitchen, C.M.; Reddy, S.T. Targeting c-Mpl for revival of human immunodeficiency virus type 1-induced hematopoietic inhibition when CD34+ progenitor cells are re-engrafted into a fresh stromal microenvironment in vivo. *J. Virol.* **2004**, *78*, 11385–11392. [CrossRef] [PubMed]
16. Ikegawa, M.; Yuan, J.; Matsumoto, K.; Herrmann, S.; Iwamoto, A.; Nakamura, T.; Matsushita, S.; Kimura, T.; Honjo, T.; Tashiro, K. Elevated plasma stromal cell-derived factor 1 protein level in the progression of HIV type 1 infection/AIDS. *AIDS Res. Hum. Retroviruses* **2001**, *17*, 587–595. [CrossRef] [PubMed]
17. Bordoni, V.; Bibas, M.; Viola, D.; Sacchi, A.; Cimini, E.; Tumino, N.; Casetti, R.; Amendola, A.; Ammassari, A.; Agrati, C.; et al. Bone Marrow CD34(+) Progenitor Cells from HIV-Infected Patients Show an Impaired T Cell Differentiation Potential Related to Proinflammatory Cytokines. *AIDS Res. Hum. Retroviruses* **2017**, *33*, 590–596. [CrossRef] [PubMed]
18. Isgro, A.; Mezzaroma, I.; Aiuti, A.; Fantauzzi, A.; Pinti, M.; Cossarizza, A.; Aiuti, F. Decreased apoptosis of bone marrow progenitor cells in HIV-1-infected patients during highly active antiretroviral therapy. *AIDS* **2004**, *18*, 1335–1337. [CrossRef] [PubMed]
19. Fischer, K.D.; Agrawal, D.K. Hematopoietic stem and progenitor cells in inflammation and allergy. *Front. Immunol.* **2013**, *4*, 428. [CrossRef] [PubMed]
20. Luis, T.C.; Tremblay, C.S.; Manz, M.G.; North, T.E.; King, K.Y.; Challen, G.A. Inflammatory signals in HSPC development and homeostasis: Too much of a good thing? *Exp. Hematol.* **2016**, *44*, 908–912. [CrossRef] [PubMed]
21. Bozzano, F.; Marras, F.; Ascierto, M.L.; Cantoni, C.; Cenderello, G.; Dentone, C.; Di Biagio, A.; Orofino, G.; Mantia, E.; Boni, S.; et al. 'Emergency exit' of bone-marrow-resident CD34(+)DNAM-1(bright)CXCR4(+)-committed lymphoid precursors during chronic infection and inflammation. *Nat. Commun.* **2015**, *6*, 8109. [CrossRef] [PubMed]
22. Koka, P.S.; Fraser, J.K.; Bryson, Y.; Bristol, G.C.; Aldrovandi, G.M.; Daar, E.S.; Zack, J.A. Human immunodeficiency virus inhibits multilineage hematopoiesis in vivo. *J. Virol.* **1998**, *72*, 5121–5127. [PubMed]
23. Jenkins, M.; Hanley, M.B.; Moreno, M.B.; Wieder, E.; McCune, J.M. Human immunodeficiency virus-1 infection interrupts thymopoiesis and multilineage hematopoiesis in vivo. *Blood* **1998**, *91*, 2672–2678. [PubMed]
24. Arainga, M.; Su, H.; Poluektova, L.Y.; Gorantla, S.; Gendelman, H.E. HIV-1 cellular and tissue replication patterns in infected humanized mice. *Sci. Rep.* **2016**, *6*, 23513. [CrossRef] [PubMed]

25. Li, G.; Zhao, J.; Cheng, L.; Jiang, Q.; Kan, S.; Qin, E.; Tu, B.; Zhang, X.; Zhang, L.; Su, L.; et al. HIV-1 infection depletes human CD34+CD38- hematopoietic progenitor cells via pDC-dependent mechanisms. *PLoS Pathog.* **2017**, *13*, e1006505. [CrossRef] [PubMed]
26. Tsukamoto, T. Transcriptional gene silencing limits CXCR4-associated depletion of bone marrow CD34+ cells in HIV-1 infection. *AIDS* **2018**, *32*, 1737–1747; Erratum in **2018**, *32*, 2857–2858. [CrossRef] [PubMed]
27. Tsukamoto, T. HIV Impacts CD34+ Progenitors Involved in T-Cell Differentiation During Coculture With Mouse Stromal OP9-DL1 Cells. *Front. Immunol.* **2019**, *10*, 81. [CrossRef] [PubMed]
28. Baltimore, D. Gene therapy. Intracellular immunization. *Nature* **1988**, *335*, 395–396. [CrossRef] [PubMed]
29. Tsukamoto, T.; Yamamoto, H.; Okada, S.; Matano, T. Recursion-based depletion of human immunodeficiency virus-specific naive CD4(+) T cells may facilitate persistent viral replication and chronic viraemia leading to acquired immunodeficiency syndrome. *Med. Hypotheses* **2016**, *94*, 81–85. [CrossRef] [PubMed]
30. Klemm, V.; Mitchell, J.; Cortez-Jugo, C.; Cavalieri, F.; Symonds, G.; Caruso, F.; Kelleher, A.D.; Ahlenstiel, C. Achieving HIV-1 Control through RNA-Directed Gene Regulation. *Genes* **2016**, *7*, 119. [CrossRef] [PubMed]
31. Mendez, C.; Ledger, S.; Petoumenos, K.; Ahlenstiel, C.; Kelleher, A.D. RNA-induced epigenetic silencing inhibits HIV-1 reactivation from latency. *Retrovirology* **2018**, *15*, 67. [CrossRef] [PubMed]
32. Savkovic, B.; Nichols, J.; Birkett, D.; Applegate, T.; Ledger, S.; Symonds, G.; Murray, J.M. A quantitative comparison of anti-HIV gene therapy delivered to hematopoietic stem cells versus CD4+ T cells. *PLoS Comput. Biol.* **2014**, *10*, e1003681. [CrossRef] [PubMed]
33. Kitchen, S.G.; Shimizu, S.; An, D.S. Stem cell-based anti-HIV gene therapy. *Virology* **2011**, *411*, 260–272. [CrossRef] [PubMed]
34. Chattong, S.; Chaikomon, K.; Chaiya, T.; Tangkosakul, T.; Palavutitotai, N.; Anusornvongchai, T.; Manotham, K. Efficient ZFN-Mediated Stop Codon Integration into the CCR5 Locus in Hematopoietic Stem Cells: A Possible Source for Intrabone Marrow Cell Transplantation. *AIDS Res. Hum. Retroviruses* **2018**. [CrossRef] [PubMed]
35. Li, L.; Krymskaya, L.; Wang, J.; Henley, J.; Rao, A.; Cao, L.F.; Tran, C.A.; Torres-Coronado, M.; Gardner, A.; Gonzalez, N.; et al. Genomic editing of the HIV-1 coreceptor CCR5 in adult hematopoietic stem and progenitor cells using zinc finger nucleases. *Mol. Ther.* **2013**, *21*, 1259–1269. [CrossRef] [PubMed]
36. Joshi, A.; Garg, H.; Ablan, S.; Freed, E.O.; Nagashima, K.; Manjunath, N.; Shankar, P. Targeting the HIV entry, assembly and release pathways for anti-HIV gene therapy. *Virology* **2011**, *415*, 95–106. [CrossRef] [PubMed]
37. Khamaikawin, W.; Shimizu, S.; Kamata, M.; Cortado, R.; Jung, Y.; Lam, J.; Wen, J.; Kim, P.; Xie, Y.; Kim, S.; et al. Modeling Anti-HIV-1 HSPC-Based Gene Therapy in Humanized Mice Previously Infected with HIV-1. *Mol. Ther. Methods Clin. Dev.* **2018**, *9*, 23–32. [CrossRef] [PubMed]
38. Falkenhagen, A.; Singh, J.; Asad, S.; Leontyev, D.; Read, S.; Zuniga-Pflucker, J.C.; Joshi, S. Control of HIV Infection In Vivo Using Gene Therapy with a Secreted Entry Inhibitor. *Mol. Ther. Nucleic Acids* **2017**, *9*, 132–144. [CrossRef] [PubMed]
39. Petit, N.Y.; Baillou, C.; Burlion, A.; Dorgham, K.; Levacher, B.; Amiel, C.; Schneider, V.; Lemoine, F.M.; Gorochov, G.; Marodon, G. Gene transfer of two entry inhibitors protects CD4(+) T cell from HIV-1 infection in humanized mice. *Gene Ther.* **2016**, *23*, 144–150. [CrossRef] [PubMed]
40. Myburgh, R.; Ivic, S.; Pepper, M.S.; Gers-Huber, G.; Li, D.; Audige, A.; Rochat, M.A.; Jaquet, V.; Regenass, S.; Manz, M.G.; et al. Lentivector Knockdown of CCR5 in Hematopoietic Stem and Progenitor Cells Confers Functional and Persistent HIV-1 Resistance in Humanized Mice. *J. Virol.* **2015**, *89*, 6761–6772. [CrossRef] [PubMed]
41. Rosenzweig, M.; Marks, D.F.; Hempel, D.; Heusch, M.; Kraus, G.; Wong-Staal, F.; Johnson, R.P. Intracellular immunization of rhesus CD34+ hematopoietic progenitor cells with a hairpin ribozyme protects T cells and macrophages from simian immunodeficiency virus infection. *Blood* **1997**, *90*, 4822–4831. [PubMed]
42. An, D.S.; Donahue, R.E.; Kamata, M.; Poon, B.; Metzger, M.; Mao, S.H.; Bonifacino, A.; Krouse, A.E.; Darlix, J.L.; Baltimore, D.; et al. Stable reduction of CCR5 by RNAi through hematopoietic stem cell transplant in non-human primates. *Proc. Natl. Acad. Sci. USA* **2007**, *104*, 13110–13115. [CrossRef] [PubMed]
43. DiGiusto, D.L.; Krishnan, A.; Li, L.; Li, H.; Li, S.; Rao, A.; Mi, S.; Yam, P.; Stinson, S.; Kalos, M.; et al. RNA-based gene therapy for HIV with lentiviral vector-modified CD34(+) cells in patients undergoing transplantation for AIDS-related lymphoma. *Sci. Transl. Med.* **2010**, *2*, 36ra43. [CrossRef] [PubMed]

44. Mitsuyasu, R.T.; Merigan, T.C.; Carr, A.; Zack, J.A.; Winters, M.A.; Workman, C.; Bloch, M.; Lalezari, J.; Becker, S.; Thornton, L.; et al. Phase 2 gene therapy trial of an anti-HIV ribozyme in autologous CD34+ cells. *Nat. Med.* **2009**, *15*, 285–292. [CrossRef] [PubMed]
45. Podsakoff, G.M.; Engel, B.C.; Carbonaro, D.A.; Choi, C.; Smogorzewska, E.M.; Bauer, G.; Selander, D.; Csik, S.; Wilson, K.; Betts, M.R.; et al. Selective survival of peripheral blood lymphocytes in children with HIV-1 following delivery of an anti-HIV gene to bone marrow CD34(+) cells. *Mol. Ther.* **2005**, *12*, 77–86. [CrossRef] [PubMed]
46. Aiuti, A.; Cattaneo, F.; Galimberti, S.; Benninghoff, U.; Cassani, B.; Callegaro, L.; Scaramuzza, S.; Andolfi, G.; Mirolo, M.; Brigida, I.; et al. Gene therapy for immunodeficiency due to adenosine deaminase deficiency. *N. Engl. J. Med.* **2009**, *360*, 447–458. [CrossRef] [PubMed]
47. Boztug, K.; Schmidt, M.; Schwarzer, A.; Banerjee, P.P.; Diez, I.A.; Dewey, R.A.; Bohm, M.; Nowrouzi, A.; Ball, C.R.; Glimm, H.; et al. Stem-cell gene therapy for the Wiskott-Aldrich syndrome. *N. Engl. J. Med.* **2010**, *363*, 1918–1927. [CrossRef] [PubMed]
48. Hacein-Bey-Abina, S.; Hauer, J.; Lim, A.; Picard, C.; Wang, G.P.; Berry, C.C.; Martinache, C.; Rieux-Laucat, F.; Latour, S.; Belohradsky, B.H.; et al. Efficacy of gene therapy for X-linked severe combined immunodeficiency. *N. Engl. J. Med.* **2010**, *363*, 355–364. [CrossRef] [PubMed]
49. De Ravin, S.S.; Wu, X.; Moir, S.; Anaya-O'Brien, S.; Kwatemaa, N.; Littel, P.; Theobald, N.; Choi, U.; Su, L.; Marquesen, M.; et al. Lentiviral hematopoietic stem cell gene therapy for X-linked severe combined immunodeficiency. *Sci. Transl. Med.* **2016**, *8*, 335ra357. [CrossRef] [PubMed]
50. Uchida, N.; Sutton, R.E.; Friera, A.M.; He, D.; Reitsma, M.J.; Chang, W.C.; Veres, G.; Scollay, R.; Weissman, I.L. HIV, but not murine leukemia virus, vectors mediate high efficiency gene transfer into freshly isolated G0/G1 human hematopoietic stem cells. *Proc. Natl. Acad. Sci. USA* **1998**, *95*, 11939–11944. [CrossRef] [PubMed]
51. Cattoglio, C.; Pellin, D.; Rizzi, E.; Maruggi, G.; Corti, G.; Miselli, F.; Sartori, D.; Guffanti, A.; Di Serio, C.; Ambrosi, A.; et al. High-definition mapping of retroviral integration sites identifies active regulatory elements in human multipotent hematopoietic progenitors. *Blood* **2010**, *116*, 5507–5517. [CrossRef] [PubMed]
52. Piras, F.; Riba, M.; Petrillo, C.; Lazarevic, D.; Cuccovillo, I.; Bartolaccini, S.; Stupka, E.; Gentner, B.; Cittaro, D.; Naldini, L.; et al. Lentiviral vectors escape innate sensing but trigger p53 in human hematopoietic stem and progenitor cells. *EMBO Mol. Med.* **2017**, *9*, 1198–1211. [CrossRef] [PubMed]
53. Yu, S.F.; von Ruden, T.; Kantoff, P.W.; Garber, C.; Seiberg, M.; Ruther, U.; Anderson, W.F.; Wagner, E.F.; Gilboa, E. Self-inactivating retroviral vectors designed for transfer of whole genes into mammalian cells. *Proc. Natl. Acad. Sci. USA* **1986**, *83*, 3194–3198. [CrossRef] [PubMed]
54. Scala, S.; Basso-Ricci, L.; Dionisio, F.; Pellin, D.; Giannelli, S.; Salerio, F.A.; Leonardelli, L.; Cicalese, M.P.; Ferrua, F.; Aiuti, A.; et al. Dynamics of genetically engineered hematopoietic stem and progenitor cells after autologous transplantation in humans. *Nat. Med.* **2018**, *24*, 1683–1690. [CrossRef] [PubMed]
55. Nasimuzzaman, M.; Lynn, D.; Ernst, R.; Beuerlein, M.; Smith, R.H.; Shrestha, A.; Cross, S.; Link, K.; Lutzko, C.; Nordling, D.; et al. Production and purification of high-titer foamy virus vector for the treatment of leukocyte adhesion deficiency. *Mol. Ther. Methods Clin. Dev.* **2016**, *3*, 16004. [CrossRef] [PubMed]
56. Vanhee, S.; Vandekerckhove, B. Pluripotent stem cell based gene therapy for hematological diseases. *Crit. Rev. Oncol. Hematol.* **2016**, *97*, 238–246. [CrossRef] [PubMed]
57. Li, Y.; Chan, L.; Nguyen, H.V.; Tsang, S.H. Personalized Medicine: Cell and Gene Therapy Based on Patient-Specific iPSC-Derived Retinal Pigment Epithelium Cells. *Adv. Exp. Med. Biol.* **2016**, *854*, 549–555. [CrossRef] [PubMed]
58. Ou, Z.; Niu, X.; He, W.; Chen, Y.; Song, B.; Xian, Y.; Fan, D.; Tang, D.; Sun, X. The Combination of CRISPR/Cas9 and iPSC Technologies in the Gene Therapy of Human beta-thalassemia in Mice. *Sci. Rep.* **2016**, *6*, 32463. [CrossRef] [PubMed]
59. Carpenter, L.; Malladi, R.; Yang, C.T.; French, A.; Pilkington, K.J.; Forsey, R.W.; Sloane-Stanley, J.; Silk, K.M.; Davies, T.J.; Fairchild, P.J.; et al. Human induced pluripotent stem cells are capable of B-cell lymphopoiesis. *Blood* **2011**, *117*, 4008–4011. [CrossRef] [PubMed]
60. Higaki, K.; Hirao, M.; Kawana-Tachikawa, A.; Iriguchi, S.; Kumagai, A.; Ueda, N.; Bo, W.; Kamibayashi, S.; Watanabe, A.; Nakauchi, H.; et al. Generation of HIV-Resistant Macrophages from IPSCs by Using Transcriptional Gene Silencing and Promoter-Targeted RNA. *Mol. Ther. Nucleic Acids* **2018**, *12*, 793–804. [CrossRef] [PubMed]

61. Nishimura, T.; Kaneko, S.; Kawana-Tachikawa, A.; Tajima, Y.; Goto, H.; Zhu, D.; Nakayama-Hosoya, K.; Iriguchi, S.; Uemura, Y.; Shimizu, T.; et al. Generation of rejuvenated antigen-specific T cells by reprogramming to pluripotency and redifferentiation. *Cell Stem Cell* **2013**, *12*, 114–126. [CrossRef] [PubMed]
62. Huyghe, J.; Magdalena, S.; Vandekerckhove, L. Fight fire with fire: Gene therapy strategies to cure HIV. *Expert Rev. Anti Infect. Ther.* **2017**, *15*, 747–758. [CrossRef] [PubMed]
63. Deeks, S.G. HIV: Shock and kill. *Nature* **2012**, *487*, 439–440. [CrossRef] [PubMed]
64. Darcis, G.; Kula, A.; Bouchat, S.; Fujinaga, K.; Corazza, F.; Ait-Ammar, A.; Delacourt, N.; Melard, A.; Kabeya, K.; Vanhulle, C.; et al. An In-Depth Comparison of Latency-Reversing Agent Combinations in Various In Vitro and Ex Vivo HIV-1 Latency Models Identified Bryostatin-1+JQ1 and Ingenol-B+JQ1 to Potently Reactivate Viral Gene Expression. *PLoS Pathog.* **2015**, *11*, e1005063. [CrossRef] [PubMed]
65. Archin, N.M.; Liberty, A.L.; Kashuba, A.D.; Choudhary, S.K.; Kuruc, J.D.; Crooks, A.M.; Parker, D.C.; Anderson, E.M.; Kearney, M.F.; Strain, M.C.; et al. Administration of vorinostat disrupts HIV-1 latency in patients on antiretroviral therapy. *Nature* **2012**, *487*, 482–485. [CrossRef] [PubMed]
66. Elliott, J.H.; Wightman, F.; Solomon, A.; Ghneim, K.; Ahlers, J.; Cameron, M.J.; Smith, M.Z.; Spelman, T.; McMahon, J.; Velayudham, P.; et al. Activation of HIV transcription with short-course vorinostat in HIV-infected patients on suppressive antiretroviral therapy. *PLoS Pathog.* **2014**, *10*, e1004473. [CrossRef] [PubMed]
67. Rasmussen, T.A.; Tolstrup, M.; Brinkmann, C.R.; Olesen, R.; Erikstrup, C.; Solomon, A.; Winckelmann, A.; Palmer, S.; Dinarello, C.; Buzon, M.; et al. Panobinostat, a histone deacetylase inhibitor, for latent-virus reactivation in HIV-infected patients on suppressive antiretroviral therapy: A phase 1/2, single group, clinical trial. *Lancet HIV* **2014**, *1*, e13–e21. [CrossRef]
68. Cary, D.C.; Peterlin, B.M. Targeting the latent reservoir to achieve functional HIV cure. *F1000Research* **2016**, *5*, F1000. [CrossRef] [PubMed]
69. Chen, T.; Hudnall, S.D. Anatomical mapping of human herpesvirus reservoirs of infection. *Mod. Pathol.* **2006**, *19*, 726–737. [CrossRef] [PubMed]
70. Sengupta, S.; Siliciano, R.F. Targeting the Latent Reservoir for HIV-1. *Immunity* **2018**, *48*, 872–895. [CrossRef] [PubMed]
71. Hutter, G.; Nowak, D.; Mossner, M.; Ganepola, S.; Mussig, A.; Allers, K.; Schneider, T.; Hofmann, J.; Kucherer, C.; Blau, O.; et al. Long-term control of HIV by CCR5 Delta32/Delta32 stem-cell transplantation. *N. Engl. J. Med.* **2009**, *360*, 692–698. [CrossRef] [PubMed]
72. Allers, K.; Hutter, G.; Hofmann, J.; Loddenkemper, C.; Rieger, K.; Thiel, E.; Schneider, T. Evidence for the cure of HIV infection by CCR5Delta32/Delta32 stem cell transplantation. *Blood* **2011**, *117*, 2791–2799. [CrossRef] [PubMed]
73. Archin, N.M.; Margolis, D.M. Emerging strategies to deplete the HIV reservoir. *Curr. Opin. Infect. Dis.* **2014**, *27*, 29–35. [CrossRef] [PubMed]
74. Berzofsky, J.A.; Ahlers, J.D.; Janik, J.; Morris, J.; Oh, S.; Terabe, M.; Belyakov, I.M. Progress on new vaccine strategies against chronic viral infections. *J. Clin. Invest.* **2004**, *114*, 450–462. [CrossRef] [PubMed]
75. Noto, A.; Trautmann, L. Developing Combined HIV Vaccine Strategies for a Functional Cure. *Vaccines* **2013**, *1*, 481–496. [CrossRef] [PubMed]
76. Reeves, R.K.; Gillis, J.; Wong, F.E.; Johnson, R.P. Vaccination with SIVmac239Deltanef activates CD4+ T cells in the absence of CD4 T-cell loss. *J. Med. Primatol.* **2009**, *38* (Suppl. 1), 8–16. [CrossRef]
77. Whitney, J.B.; Ruprecht, R.M. Live attenuated HIV vaccines: Pitfalls and prospects. *Curr. Opin. Infect. Dis.* **2004**, *17*, 17–26. [CrossRef] [PubMed]
78. Sutton, M.S.; Burns, C.M.; Weiler, A.M.; Balgeman, A.J.; Braasch, A.; Lehrer-Brey, G.; Friedrich, T.C.; O'Connor, S.L. Vaccination with Live Attenuated Simian Immunodeficiency Virus (SIV) Protects from Mucosal, but Not Necessarily Intravenous, Challenge with a Minimally Heterologous SIV. *J. Virol.* **2016**, *90*, 5541–5548. [CrossRef] [PubMed]
79. Abel, K.; Compton, L.; Rourke, T.; Montefiori, D.; Lu, D.; Rothaeusler, K.; Fritts, L.; Bost, K.; Miller, C.J. Simian-human immunodeficiency virus SHIV89.6-induced protection against intravaginal challenge with pathogenic SIVmac239 is independent of the route of immunization and is associated with a combination of cytotoxic T-lymphocyte and alpha interferon responses. *J. Virol.* **2003**, *77*, 3099–3118. [PubMed]

80. Nilsson, C.; Makitalo, B.; Thorstensson, R.; Norley, S.; Binninger-Schinzel, D.; Cranage, M.; Rud, E.; Biberfeld, G.; Putkonen, P. Live attenuated simian immunodeficiency virus (SIV)mac in macaques can induce protection against mucosal infection with SIVsm. *AIDS* **1998**, *12*, 2261–2270. [CrossRef] [PubMed]
81. Connor, R.I.; Montefiori, D.C.; Binley, J.M.; Moore, J.P.; Bonhoeffer, S.; Gettie, A.; Fenamore, E.A.; Sheridan, K.E.; Ho, D.D.; Dailey, P.J.; et al. Temporal analyses of virus replication, immune responses, and efficacy in rhesus macaques immunized with a live, attenuated simian immunodeficiency virus vaccine. *J. Virol.* **1998**, *72*, 7501–7509. [PubMed]
82. Sugimoto, C.; Watanabe, S.; Naruse, T.; Kajiwara, E.; Shiino, T.; Umano, N.; Ueda, K.; Sato, H.; Ohgimoto, S.; Hirsch, V.; et al. Protection of macaques with diverse MHC genotypes against a heterologous SIV by vaccination with a deglycosylated live-attenuated SIV. *PLoS ONE* **2010**, *5*, e11678. [CrossRef] [PubMed]
83. Tsukamoto, T.; Yamamoto, H.; Matano, T. CD8(+) Cytotoxic-T-Lymphocyte Breadth Could Facilitate Early Immune Detection of Immunodeficiency Virus-Derived Epitopes with Limited Expression Levels. *mSphere* **2019**, *4*. [CrossRef] [PubMed]
84. Duarte, R.F.; Salgado, M.; Sanchez-Ortega, I.; Arnan, M.; Canals, C.; Domingo-Domenech, E.; Fernandez-de-Sevilla, A.; Gonzalez-Barca, E.; Moron-Lopez, S.; Nogues, N.; et al. CCR5 Delta32 homozygous cord blood allogeneic transplantation in a patient with HIV: A case report. *Lancet HIV* **2015**, *2*, e236–e242. [CrossRef]
85. Xu, L.; Yang, H.; Gao, Y.; Chen, Z.; Xie, L.; Liu, Y.; Liu, Y.; Wang, X.; Li, H.; Lai, W.; et al. CRISPR/Cas9-Mediated CCR5 Ablation in Human Hematopoietic Stem/Progenitor Cells Confers HIV-1 Resistance In Vivo. *Mol. Ther.* **2017**, *25*, 1782–1789. [CrossRef] [PubMed]
86. Symonds, G.; Bartlett, J.S.; Kiem, H.P.; Tsie, M.; Breton, L. Cell-Delivered Entry Inhibitors for HIV-1: CCR5 Downregulation and Blocking Virus/Membrane Fusion in Defending the Host Cell Population. *AIDS Patient Care STDS* **2016**, *30*, 545–550. [CrossRef] [PubMed]
87. Shi, B.; Li, J.; Shi, X.; Jia, W.; Wen, Y.; Hu, X.; Zhuang, F.; Xi, J.; Zhang, L. TALEN-Mediated Knockout of CCR5 Confers Protection Against Infection of Human Immunodeficiency Virus. *J. Acquir. Immune Defic. Syndr.* **2017**, *74*, 229–241. [CrossRef] [PubMed]
88. Shimizu, S.; Yadav, S.S.; An, D.S. Stable Delivery of CCR5-Directed shRNA into Human Primary Peripheral Blood Mononuclear Cells and Hematopoietic Stem/Progenitor Cells via a Lentiviral Vector. *Methods Mol. Biol.* **2016**, *1364*, 235–248. [CrossRef] [PubMed]
89. Sather, B.D.; Romano Ibarra, G.S.; Sommer, K.; Curinga, G.; Hale, M.; Khan, I.F.; Singh, S.; Song, Y.; Gwiazda, K.; Sahni, J.; et al. Efficient modification of CCR5 in primary human hematopoietic cells using a megaTAL nuclease and AAV donor template. *Sci. Transl. Med.* **2015**, *7*, 307ra156. [CrossRef] [PubMed]
90. Saydaminova, K.; Ye, X.; Wang, H.; Richter, M.; Ho, M.; Chen, H.; Xu, N.; Kim, J.S.; Papapetrou, E.; Holmes, M.C.; et al. Efficient genome editing in hematopoietic stem cells with helper-dependent Ad5/35 vectors expressing site-specific endonucleases under microRNA regulation. *Mol. Ther. Methods Clin. Dev.* **2015**, *1*, 14057. [CrossRef] [PubMed]
91. Manotham, K.; Chattong, S.; Setpakdee, A. Generation of CCR5-defective CD34 cells from ZFN-driven stop codon-integrated mesenchymal stem cell clones. *J. Biomed. Sci.* **2015**, *22*, 25. [CrossRef] [PubMed]
92. Burke, B.P.; Levin, B.R.; Zhang, J.; Sahakyan, A.; Boyer, J.; Carroll, M.V.; Colon, J.C.; Keech, N.; Rezek, V.; Bristol, G.; et al. Engineering Cellular Resistance to HIV-1 Infection In Vivo Using a Dual Therapeutic Lentiviral Vector. *Mol. Ther. Nucleic Acids* **2015**, *4*, e236. [CrossRef] [PubMed]
93. Wolstein, O.; Boyd, M.; Millington, M.; Impey, H.; Boyer, J.; Howe, A.; Delebecque, F.; Cornetta, K.; Rothe, M.; Baum, C.; et al. Preclinical safety and efficacy of an anti-HIV-1 lentiviral vector containing a short hairpin RNA to CCR5 and the C46 fusion inhibitor. *Mol. Ther. Methods Clin. Dev.* **2014**, *1*, 11. [CrossRef] [PubMed]
94. Holt, N.; Wang, J.; Kim, K.; Friedman, G.; Wang, X.; Taupin, V.; Crooks, G.M.; Kohn, D.B.; Gregory, P.D.; Holmes, M.C.; et al. Human hematopoietic stem/progenitor cells modified by zinc-finger nucleases targeted to CCR5 control HIV-1 in vivo. *Nat. Biotechnol.* **2010**, *28*, 839–847. [CrossRef] [PubMed]
95. Liang, M.; Kamata, M.; Chen, K.N.; Pariente, N.; An, D.S.; Chen, I.S. Inhibition of HIV-1 infection by a unique short hairpin RNA to chemokine receptor 5 delivered into macrophages through hematopoietic progenitor cell transduction. *J. Gene Med.* **2010**, *12*, 255–265. [CrossRef] [PubMed]
96. Shimizu, S.; Hong, P.; Arumugam, B.; Pokomo, L.; Boyer, J.; Koizumi, N.; Kittipongdaja, P.; Chen, A.; Bristol, G.; Galic, Z.; et al. A highly efficient short hairpin RNA potently down-regulates CCR5 expression in systemic lymphoid organs in the hu-BLT mouse model. *Blood* **2010**, *115*, 1534–1544. [CrossRef] [PubMed]

97. Anderson, J.S.; Javien, J.; Nolta, J.A.; Bauer, G. Preintegration HIV-1 inhibition by a combination lentiviral vector containing a chimeric TRIM5 alpha protein, a CCR5 shRNA, and a TAR decoy. *Mol. Ther.* **2009**, *17*, 2103–2114. [CrossRef] [PubMed]
98. Anderson, J.; Akkina, R. Complete knockdown of CCR5 by lentiviral vector-expressed siRNAs and protection of transgenic macrophages against HIV-1 infection. *Gene Ther.* **2007**, *14*, 1287–1297. [CrossRef] [PubMed]
99. Anderson, J.; Li, M.J.; Palmer, B.; Remling, L.; Li, S.; Yam, P.; Yee, J.K.; Rossi, J.; Zaia, J.; Akkina, R. Safety and Efficacy of a Lentiviral Vector Containing Three Anti-HIV Genes-CCR5 Ribozyme, Tat-rev siRNA, and TAR Decoy-in SCID-hu Mouse-Derived T Cells. *Mol. Ther.* **2007**, *15*, 1182–1188. [CrossRef] [PubMed]
100. Li, M.J.; Kim, J.; Li, S.; Zaia, J.; Yee, J.K.; Anderson, J.; Akkina, R.; Rossi, J.J. Long-term inhibition of HIV-1 infection in primary hematopoietic cells by lentiviral vector delivery of a triple combination of anti-HIV shRNA, anti-CCR5 ribozyme, and a nucleolar-localizing TAR decoy. *Mol. Ther.* **2005**, *12*, 900–909. [CrossRef] [PubMed]
101. Bai, J.; Rossi, J.; Akkina, R. Multivalent anti-CCR ribozymes for stem cell-based HIV type 1 gene therapy. *AIDS Res. Hum. Retroviruses* **2001**, *17*, 385–399. [CrossRef] [PubMed]
102. Bai, J.; Gorantla, S.; Banda, N.; Cagnon, L.; Rossi, J.; Akkina, R. Characterization of anti-CCR5 ribozyme-transduced CD34+ hematopoietic progenitor cells in vitro and in a SCID-hu mouse model in vivo. *Mol. Ther.* **2000**, *1*, 244–254. [CrossRef] [PubMed]
103. Jamieson, A.C.; Miller, J.C.; Pabo, C.O. Drug discovery with engineered zinc-finger proteins. *Nat. Rev. Drug Discov.* **2003**, *2*, 361–368. [CrossRef] [PubMed]
104. Tebas, P.; Stein, D.; Tang, W.W.; Frank, I.; Wang, S.Q.; Lee, G.; Spratt, S.K.; Surosky, R.T.; Giedlin, M.A.; Nichol, G.; et al. Gene editing of CCR5 in autologous CD4 T cells of persons infected with HIV. *N. Engl. J. Med.* **2014**, *370*, 901–910. [CrossRef] [PubMed]
105. Scarborough, R.J.; Gatignol, A. HIV and Ribozymes. *Adv. Exp. Med. Biol.* **2015**, *848*, 97–116. [CrossRef] [PubMed]
106. Cornu, T.I.; Mussolino, C.; Cathomen, T. Refining strategies to translate genome editing to the clinic. *Nat. Med.* **2017**, *23*, 415–423. [CrossRef] [PubMed]
107. Swamy, M.N.; Wu, H.; Shankar, P. Recent advances in RNAi-based strategies for therapy and prevention of HIV-1/AIDS. *Adv. Drug Deliv. Rev.* **2016**, *103*, 174–186. [CrossRef] [PubMed]
108. Symonds, G.P.; Johnstone, H.A.; Millington, M.L.; Boyd, M.P.; Burke, B.P.; Breton, L.R. The use of cell-delivered gene therapy for the treatment of HIV/AIDS. *Immunol. Res.* **2010**, *48*, 84–98. [CrossRef] [PubMed]
109. Ledger, S.; Howe, A.; Turville, S.; Aggarwal, A.; Savkovic, B.; Ong, A.; Wolstein, O.; Boyd, M.; Millington, M.; Gorry, P.R.; et al. Analysis and dissociation of anti-HIV effects of shRNA to CCR5 and the fusion inhibitor C46. *J. Gene Med.* **2018**, *20*, e3006. [CrossRef] [PubMed]
110. Vangelista, L.; Vento, S. The Expanding Therapeutic Perspective of CCR5 Blockade. *Front. Immunol.* **2017**, *8*, 1981. [CrossRef] [PubMed]
111. Lim, J.K.; Louie, C.Y.; Glaser, C.; Jean, C.; Johnson, B.; Johnson, H.; McDermott, D.H.; Murphy, P.M. Genetic deficiency of chemokine receptor CCR5 is a strong risk factor for symptomatic West Nile virus infection: A meta-analysis of 4 cohorts in the US epidemic. *J. Infect. Dis.* **2008**, *197*, 262–265. [CrossRef] [PubMed]
112. Glass, W.G.; McDermott, D.H.; Lim, J.K.; Lekhong, S.; Yu, S.F.; Frank, W.A.; Pape, J.; Cheshier, R.C.; Murphy, P.M. CCR5 deficiency increases risk of symptomatic West Nile virus infection. *J. Exp. Med.* **2006**, *203*, 35–40. [CrossRef] [PubMed]
113. Liu, Y.P.; Westerink, J.T.; ter Brake, O.; Berkhout, B. RNAi-inducing lentiviral vectors for anti-HIV-1 gene therapy. *Methods Mol. Biol.* **2011**, *721*, 293–311. [CrossRef] [PubMed]
114. Kumar, P.; Ban, H.S.; Kim, S.S.; Wu, H.; Pearson, T.; Greiner, D.L.; Laouar, A.; Yao, J.; Haridas, V.; Habiro, K.; et al. T cell-specific siRNA delivery suppresses HIV-1 infection in humanized mice. *Cell* **2008**, *134*, 577–586. [CrossRef] [PubMed]
115. ter Brake, O.; Legrand, N.; von Eije, K.J.; Centlivre, M.; Spits, H.; Weijer, K.; Blom, B.; Berkhout, B. Evaluation of safety and efficacy of RNAi against HIV-1 in the human immune system (Rag-2(-/-)gammac(-/-)) mouse model. *Gene Ther.* **2009**, *16*, 148–153. [CrossRef] [PubMed]
116. Suzuki, K.; Shijuuku, T.; Fukamachi, T.; Zaunders, J.; Guillemin, G.; Cooper, D.; Kelleher, A. Prolonged transcriptional silencing and CpG methylation induced by siRNAs targeted to the HIV-1 promoter region. *J. RNAi Gene Silenc.* **2005**, *1*, 66–78. [PubMed]

117. Santat, L.; Paz, H.; Wong, C.; Li, L.; Macer, J.; Forman, S.; Wong, K.K.; Chatterjee, S. Recombinant AAV2 transduction of primitive human hematopoietic stem cells capable of serial engraftment in immune-deficient mice. *Proc. Natl. Acad. Sci. USA* **2005**, *102*, 11053–11058. [CrossRef] [PubMed]
118. Li, M.J.; Bauer, G.; Michienzi, A.; Yee, J.K.; Lee, N.S.; Kim, J.; Li, S.; Castanotto, D.; Zaia, J.; Rossi, J.J. Inhibition of HIV-1 infection by lentiviral vectors expressing Pol III-promoted anti-HIV RNAs. *Mol. Ther.* **2003**, *8*, 196–206. [CrossRef]
119. Akkina, R.; Banerjea, A.; Bai, J.; Anderson, J.; Li, M.J.; Rossi, J. siRNAs, ribozymes and RNA decoys in modeling stem cell-based gene therapy for HIV/AIDS. *Anticancer Res.* **2003**, *23*, 1997–2005. [PubMed]
120. Banerjea, A.; Li, M.J.; Bauer, G.; Remling, L.; Lee, N.S.; Rossi, J.; Akkina, R. Inhibition of HIV-1 by lentiviral vector-transduced siRNAs in T lymphocytes differentiated in SCID-hu mice and CD34+ progenitor cell-derived macrophages. *Mol. Ther.* **2003**, *8*, 62–71. [CrossRef]
121. Bauer, G.; Valdez, P.; Kearns, K.; Bahner, I.; Wen, S.F.; Zaia, J.A.; Kohn, D.B. Inhibition of human immunodeficiency virus-1 (HIV-1) replication after transduction of granulocyte colony-stimulating factor-mobilized CD34+ cells from HIV-1-infected donors using retroviral vectors containing anti-HIV-1 genes. *Blood* **1997**, *89*, 2259–2267. [PubMed]
122. Rosenzweig, M.; Marks, D.F.; Hempel, D.; Lisziewicz, J.; Johnson, R.P. Transduction of CD34+ hematopoietic progenitor cells with an antitat gene protects T-cell and macrophage progeny from AIDS virus infection. *J. Virol.* **1997**, *71*, 2740–2746. [PubMed]
123. Yu, M.; Leavitt, M.C.; Maruyama, M.; Yamada, O.; Young, D.; Ho, A.D.; Wong-Staal, F. Intracellular immunization of human fetal cord blood stem/progenitor cells with a ribozyme against human immunodeficiency virus type 1. *Proc. Natl. Acad. Sci. USA* **1995**, *92*, 699–703. [CrossRef] [PubMed]
124. Wang, G.; Zhao, N.; Berkhout, B.; Das, A.T. CRISPR-Cas based antiviral strategies against HIV-1. *Virus Res.* **2018**, *244*, 321–332. [CrossRef] [PubMed]
125. Herrera-Carrillo, E.; Berkhout, B. Attacking HIV-1 RNA versus DNA by sequence-specific approaches: RNAi versus CRISPR-Cas. *Biochem. Soc. Trans.* **2016**, *44*, 1355–1365. [CrossRef] [PubMed]
126. Hu, W.; Kaminski, R.; Yang, F.; Zhang, Y.; Cosentino, L.; Li, F.; Luo, B.; Alvarez-Carbonell, D.; Garcia-Mesa, Y.; Karn, J.; et al. RNA-directed gene editing specifically eradicates latent and prevents new HIV-1 infection. *Proc. Natl. Acad. Sci. USA* **2014**, *111*, 11461–11466. [CrossRef] [PubMed]
127. Wang, Z.; Pan, Q.; Gendron, P.; Zhu, W.; Guo, F.; Cen, S.; Wainberg, M.A.; Liang, C. CRISPR/Cas9-Derived Mutations Both Inhibit HIV-1 Replication and Accelerate Viral Escape. *Cell Rep.* **2016**, *15*, 481–489. [CrossRef] [PubMed]
128. Man, D.; Sansbury, B.; Bialk, P.; Bloh, K.; Kolb, E.A.; Kmiec, E.B. Target Site Mutagenesis during Crispr/ Cas 9/Single-Stranded- Oligonucleotide Directed Gene Editing for Sickle Cell Anemia. *Blood* **2016**, *128*, 4706.
129. White, M.K.; Kaminski, R.; Young, W.B.; Roehm, P.C.; Khalili, K. CRISPR Editing Technology in Biological and Biomedical Investigation. *J. Cell. Biochem.* **2017**, *118*, 3586–3594. [CrossRef] [PubMed]
130. Yin, C.; Zhang, T.; Qu, X.; Zhang, Y.; Putatunda, R.; Xiao, X.; Li, F.; Xiao, W.; Zhao, H.; Dai, S.; et al. In Vivo Excision of HIV-1 Provirus by saCas9 and Multiplex Single-Guide RNAs in Animal Models. *Mol. Ther.* **2017**, *25*, 1168–1186. [CrossRef] [PubMed]
131. Kunze, C.; Borner, K.; Kienle, E.; Orschmann, T.; Rusha, E.; Schneider, M.; Radivojkov-Blagojevic, M.; Drukker, M.; Desbordes, S.; Grimm, D.; et al. Synthetic AAV/CRISPR vectors for blocking HIV-1 expression in persistently infected astrocytes. *Glia* **2018**, *66*, 413–427. [CrossRef] [PubMed]
132. Ahlenstiel, C.L.; Suzuki, K.; Marks, K.; Symonds, G.P.; Kelleher, A.D. Controlling HIV-1: Non-Coding RNA Gene Therapy Approaches to a Functional Cure. *Front. Immunol.* **2015**, *6*, 474. [CrossRef] [PubMed]
133. Suzuki, K.; Juelich, T.; Lim, H.; Ishida, T.; Watanebe, T.; Cooper, D.A.; Rao, S.; Kelleher, A.D. Closed chromatin architecture is induced by an RNA duplex targeting the HIV-1 promoter region. *J. Biol. Chem.* **2008**, *283*, 23353–23363. [CrossRef] [PubMed]
134. Ahlenstiel, C.; Mendez, C.; Lim, S.T.; Marks, K.; Turville, S.; Cooper, D.A.; Kelleher, A.D.; Suzuki, K. Novel RNA Duplex Locks HIV-1 in a Latent State via Chromatin-mediated Transcriptional Silencing. *Mol. Ther. Nucleic Acids* **2015**, *4*, e261. [CrossRef] [PubMed]
135. Suzuki, K.; Hattori, S.; Marks, K.; Ahlenstiel, C.; Maeda, Y.; Ishida, T.; Millington, M.; Boyd, M.; Symonds, G.; Cooper, D.A.; et al. Promoter Targeting shRNA Suppresses HIV-1 Infection In vivo Through Transcriptional Gene Silencing. *Mol. Ther. Nucleic Acids* **2013**, *2*, e137. [CrossRef] [PubMed]

136. Zhang, M.; Poh, T.Y.; Louache, F.; Sundell, I.B.; Yuan, J.; Evans, S.; Koka, P.S. Rescue of multi-lineage hematopoiesis during HIV-1 infection by human c-mpl gene transfer and reconstitution of CD34+ progenitor cells in vivo. *J. Stem Cells* **2009**, *4*, 161–177. [PubMed]
137. Anderson, J.; Akkina, R. Human immunodeficiency virus type 1 restriction by human-rhesus chimeric tripartite motif 5alpha (TRIM 5alpha) in CD34(+) cell-derived macrophages in vitro and in T cells in vivo in severe combined immunodeficient (SCID-hu) mice transplanted with human fetal tissue. *Hum. Gene Ther.* **2008**, *19*, 217–228. [CrossRef] [PubMed]
138. Dimitrova, D.I.; Yang, X.; Reichenbach, N.L.; Karakasidis, S.; Sutton, R.E.; Henderson, E.E.; Rogers, T.J.; Suhadolnik, R.J. Lentivirus-mediated transduction of PKR into CD34(+) hematopoietic stem cells inhibits HIV-1 replication in differentiated T cell progeny. *J. Interferon Cytokine Res.* **2005**, *25*, 345–360. [CrossRef] [PubMed]
139. Leibman, R.S.; Richardson, M.W.; Ellebrecht, C.T.; Maldini, C.R.; Glover, J.A.; Secreto, A.J.; Kulikovskaya, I.; Lacey, S.F.; Akkina, S.R.; Yi, Y.; et al. Supraphysiologic control over HIV-1 replication mediated by CD8 T cells expressing a re-engineered CD4-based chimeric antigen receptor. *PLoS Pathog.* **2017**, *13*, e1006613. [CrossRef] [PubMed]
140. Liu, L.; Patel, B.; Ghanem, M.H.; Bundoc, V.; Zheng, Z.; Morgan, R.A.; Rosenberg, S.A.; Dey, B.; Berger, E.A. Novel CD4-Based Bispecific Chimeric Antigen Receptor Designed for Enhanced Anti-HIV Potency and Absence of HIV Entry Receptor Activity. *J. Virol.* **2015**, *89*, 6685–6694. [CrossRef] [PubMed]
141. Hammer, O. CD19 as an attractive target for antibody-based therapy. *MAbs* **2012**, *4*, 571–577. [CrossRef] [PubMed]
142. Pulsipher, M.A. Are CAR T cells better than antibody or HCT therapy in B-ALL? *Hematol. Am. Soc. Hematol. Educ. Program* **2018**, *2018*, 16–24. [CrossRef] [PubMed]
143. Miliotou, A.N.; Papadopoulou, L.C. CAR T-cell Therapy: A New Era in Cancer Immunotherapy. *Curr. Pharm. Biotechnol.* **2018**, *19*, 5–18. [CrossRef] [PubMed]
144. Davila, M.L.; Brentjens, R.J. CD19-Targeted CAR T cells as novel cancer immunotherapy for relapsed or refractory B-cell acute lymphoblastic leukemia. *Clin. Adv. Hematol. Oncol.* **2016**, *14*, 802–808. [PubMed]
145. Quintas-Cardama, A. CD19 directed CAR T cell therapy in diffuse large B-cell lymphoma. *Oncotarget* **2018**, *9*, 29843–29844. [CrossRef] [PubMed]
146. Ali, A.; Kitchen, S.G.; Chen, I.S.Y.; Ng, H.L.; Zack, J.A.; Yang, O.O. HIV-1-Specific Chimeric Antigen Receptors Based on Broadly Neutralizing Antibodies. *J. Virol.* **2016**, *90*, 6999–7006. [CrossRef] [PubMed]
147. Liu, B.; Zou, F.; Lu, L.; Chen, C.; He, D.; Zhang, X.; Tang, X.; Liu, C.; Li, L.; Zhang, H. Chimeric Antigen Receptor T Cells Guided by the Single-Chain Fv of a Broadly Neutralizing Antibody Specifically and Effectively Eradicate Virus Reactivated from Latency in CD4+ T Lymphocytes Isolated from HIV-1-Infected Individuals Receiving Suppressive Combined Antiretroviral Therapy. *J. Virol.* **2016**, *90*, 9712–9724. [CrossRef] [PubMed]
148. Hale, M.; Mesojednik, T.; Romano Ibarra, G.S.; Sahni, J.; Bernard, A.; Sommer, K.; Scharenberg, A.M.; Rawlings, D.J.; Wagner, T.A. Engineering HIV-Resistant, Anti-HIV Chimeric Antigen Receptor T Cells. *Mol. Ther.* **2017**, *25*, 570–579. [CrossRef] [PubMed]
149. Zhen, A.; Kamata, M.; Rezek, V.; Rick, J.; Levin, B.; Kasparian, S.; Chen, I.S.; Yang, O.O.; Zack, J.A.; Kitchen, S.G. HIV-specific Immunity Derived From Chimeric Antigen Receptor-engineered Stem Cells. *Mol. Ther.* **2015**, *23*, 1358–1367. [CrossRef] [PubMed]
150. Zhen, A.; Peterson, C.W.; Carrillo, M.A.; Reddy, S.S.; Youn, C.S.; Lam, B.B.; Chang, N.Y.; Martin, H.A.; Rick, J.W.; Kim, J.; et al. Long-term persistence and function of hematopoietic stem cell-derived chimeric antigen receptor T cells in a nonhuman primate model of HIV/AIDS. *PLoS Pathog.* **2017**, *13*, e1006753. [CrossRef] [PubMed]
151. Luo, X.M.; Maarschalk, E.; O'Connell, R.M.; Wang, P.; Yang, L.; Baltimore, D. Engineering human hematopoietic stem/progenitor cells to produce a broadly neutralizing anti-HIV antibody after in vitro maturation to human B lymphocytes. *Blood* **2009**, *113*, 1422–1431. [CrossRef] [PubMed]
152. Poznansky, M.C.; La Vecchio, J.; Silva-Arietta, S.; Porter-Brooks, J.; Brody, K.; Olszak, I.T.; Adams, G.B.; Ramstedt, U.; Marasco, W.A.; Scadden, D.T. Inhibition of human immunodeficiency virus replication and growth advantage of CD4+ T cells and monocytes derived from CD34+ cells transduced with an intracellular antibody directed against human immunodeficiency virus type 1 Tat. *Hum. Gene Ther.* **1999**, *10*, 2505–2514. [CrossRef] [PubMed]

153. Prince, A.M.; Reesink, H.; Pascual, D.; Horowitz, B.; Hewlett, I.; Murthy, K.K.; Cobb, K.E.; Eichberg, J.W. Prevention of HIV infection by passive immunization with HIV immunoglobulin. *AIDS Res. Hum. Retroviruses* **1991**, *7*, 971–973. [CrossRef] [PubMed]
154. Morris, L.; Mkhize, N.N. Prospects for passive immunity to prevent HIV infection. *PLoS Med.* **2017**, *14*, e1002436. [CrossRef] [PubMed]
155. Balazs, A.B.; West, A.P., Jr. Antibody gene transfer for HIV immunoprophylaxis. *Nat. Immunol.* **2013**, *14*, 1–5. [CrossRef] [PubMed]
156. Balazs, A.B.; Chen, J.; Hong, C.M.; Rao, D.S.; Yang, L.; Baltimore, D. Antibody-based protection against HIV infection by vectored immunoprophylaxis. *Nature* **2011**, *481*, 81–84. [CrossRef] [PubMed]
157. Badamchi-Zadeh, A.; Tartaglia, L.J.; Abbink, P.; Bricault, C.A.; Liu, P.T.; Boyd, M.; Kirilova, M.; Mercado, N.B.; Nanayakkara, O.S.; Vrbanac, V.D.; et al. Therapeutic Efficacy of Vectored PGT121 Gene Delivery in HIV-1-Infected Humanized Mice. *J. Virol.* **2018**, *92*. [CrossRef] [PubMed]
158. Cyranoski, D.; Ledford, H. Genome-edited baby claim provokes international outcry. *Nature* **2018**, *563*, 607–608. [CrossRef] [PubMed]
159. Frankel, M.S.; Chapman, A.R. Genetic technologies. Facing inheritable genetic modifications. *Science* **2001**, *292*, 1303. [CrossRef] [PubMed]
160. Zhang, X.H.; Tee, L.Y.; Wang, X.G.; Huang, Q.S.; Yang, S.H. Off-target Effects in CRISPR/Cas9-mediated Genome Engineering. *Mol. Ther. Nucleic Acids* **2015**, *4*, e264. [CrossRef] [PubMed]
161. Keep off-target effects in focus. *Nat. Med.* **2018**, *24*, 1081. [CrossRef] [PubMed]
162. Aryal, N.K.; Wasylishen, A.R.; Lozano, G. CRISPR/Cas9 can mediate high-efficiency off-target mutations in mice in vivo. *Cell Death Dis.* **2018**, *9*, 1099. [CrossRef] [PubMed]
163. Ormond, K.E.; Mortlock, D.P.; Scholes, D.T.; Bombard, Y.; Brody, L.C.; Faucett, W.A.; Garrison, N.A.; Hercher, L.; Isasi, R.; Middleton, A.; et al. Human Germline Genome Editing. *Am. J. Hum. Genet.* **2017**, *101*, 167–176. [CrossRef] [PubMed]

3

Novel Antiretroviral Structures from Marine Organisms

Karlo Wittine, Lara Saftić, Željka Peršurić and Sandra Kraljević Pavelić *

University of Rijeka, Department of Biotechnology, Centre for high-throughput technologies, Radmile Matejčić 2, 51000 Rijeka, Croatia
* Correspondence: sandrakp@biotech.uniri.hr

Academic Editor: Kyoko Nakagawa-Goto

Abstract: In spite of significant advancements and success in antiretroviral therapies directed against HIV infection, there is no cure for HIV, which scan persist in a human body in its latent form and become reactivated under favorable conditions. Therefore, novel antiretroviral drugs with different modes of actions are still a major focus for researchers. In particular, novel lead structures are being sought from natural sources. So far, a number of compounds from marine organisms have been identified as promising therapeutics for HIV infection. Therefore, in this paper, we provide an overview of marine natural products that were first identified in the period between 2013 and 2018 that could be potentially used, or further optimized, as novel antiretroviral agents. This pipeline includes the systematization of antiretroviral activities for several categories of marine structures including chitosan and its derivatives, sulfated polysaccharides, lectins, bromotyrosine derivatives, peptides, alkaloids, diterpenes, phlorotannins, and xanthones as well as adjuvants to the HAART therapy such as fish oil. We critically discuss the structures and activities of the most promising new marine anti-HIV compounds.

Keywords: antiretroviral agents; anti-HIV; marine metabolites; natural products; drug development

---

1. Introduction

Human immunodeficiency virus (HIV) infections pose a global challenge given that in 2017, according to the World Health Organization data, 36.9 million people were living with HIV and additional 1.8 million people were becoming newly infected globally (Table 1). HIV targets immune cells and impairs the human defense against pneumonia, tuberculosis, and shingles as well as certain types of cancer [1]. The most advanced stage of HIV infection is the Acquired Immunodeficiency Syndrome (AIDS), which can take from two to 15 years to develop, depending on the individual [2].

Table 1. Summary of the global human immunodeficiency virus (HIV) epidemic (2017) according to World Health Organization (WHO) data.

	People Living with HIV in 2017	People Newly Infected with HIV in 2017	HIV-Related Deaths in 2017
total	36.9 million (31.3–43.9 million)	1.8 million (1.4–2.4 million)	940,000 (670,000–1.3 million)
adults	35 million (29.6–41.7 million)	1.6 million (1.3–2.1 million)	830 000 (590,000–1.2 million)
women	18.2 million (15.6–21.4 million)		
men	16.8 million (13.9–20.4 million)		
children (<15 years)	1.8 million (1.3–2.4 million)	180,000 (110,000–260,000)	110,000 (63,000–160,000)

HIV has two viral forms: HIV-1 (the most common form that accounts for around 95% of all infections worldwide) and HIV-2 (relatively uncommon and less infectious). HIV-1 consists of groups M, N, O, and P with at least nine genetically distinct subtypes of HIV-1 within group M (A, B, C, D, F, G, H, J, and K). Additionally, different subtypes can combine genetic material to form a hybrid virus known as the 'circulating recombinant form' (CRFs) (Figure 1). HIV-2 consists of eight known groups (A to H). Of these, only groups A and B are pandemic. The HIV-2 mechanism is not clearly defined and neither is its difference from HIV-1. However, the transmission rate is much lower in HIV-2 than in HIV-1. HIV-2 is estimated to be more than 55% genetically distinct from HIV-1.

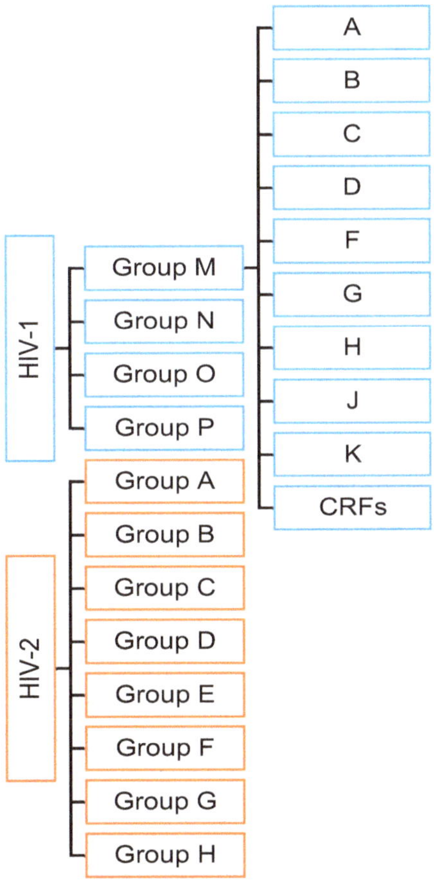

Figure 1. HIV types and strains classification.

The HIV-1 genome has reading frames coding for structural and regulatory proteins. The *gag* gene encodes the Pr55Gag precursor of inner structural proteins p24 (capsid protein, CA), p17 (matrix protein, MA), p7 (nucleoprotein, NC), and p6 involved in the virus particle release. The *pol* gene encodes the Pr160GagPol precursor of the viral enzymes p10 (protease, PR), p51 (reverse transcriptase, RT), p15 (RNase H), and p32 (integrase, IN). The *env* gene encodes the PrGp160 precursor of the gp120 (surface glycoprotein, SU) and gp41 (transmembrane protein, TM). Other genes include *tat*, encoding p14 (transactivator protein), *rev*, encoding p19 (RNA splicing regulator), *nef*, encoding p27 (negative regulating factor), *vif*, encoding p23 (viral infectivity protein), *vpr*, encoding p15 (virus protein r), *vpu*, encoding p16 (virus protein unique), *vpx* in HIV2, encoding p15 (virus protein x), and *tev*, encoding p26 (tat/rev protein) [3].

The HIV infections are extremely problematic as the virus targets the CD4+ memory T-cells population, which is essential for organism immunity. HIV can attach itself to the host cell through 1) a relatively nonspecific interaction with negatively charged cell-surface heparan sulfate proteoglycans [4], 2) specific interactions between the Env and $\alpha 4\beta 7$ integrin [5,6], and/or 3) the interaction with pattern-recognition receptors, such as the dendritic cell-specific intercellular adhesion molecular 3-grabbing non-integrin (DC-SIGN) [7]. The attachment of HIV in any of the abovementioned ways can increase the efficacy of infection because it brings Env, a heavily glycosylated trimer of gp120 and gp41 heterodimers, into close proximity with the viral receptor CD4 and co-receptor [8]. Finally, in order for the viral entry to occur, Env needs to bind itself to the host protein CD4 [9,10].

The binding of the HIV glycoprotein gp120 to the host cell CD4 receptor causes conformational changes of the gp120 glycoprotein, which uncover additional binding sites that interact with distinct proteins on the host cell membrane, known as β-chemokine co-receptors (mainly CCR5 and CXCR4), which facilitate the virus entry into the cell [11].

After the infection, a progressive decline of CD4 + cells consequently leads to the failure of the immune system function and the development of opportunistic infections that usually lead to death [1]. In HIV-infected patients, immunodeficiency develops both as a result of the viral replication and the failure of the patients' homeostatic mechanisms. The continuous viral presence in the patients after the application of therapy is attributed to the CD4 + T-cell homeostasis owing to a pool of latently infected and resting CD4 + T-cells, macrophages, and follicular dendritic cells that remain in the organism. Indeed, the complex interactions of the patient's immune system with the virus, and vice versa after the viral suppression, are thought to be crucial for the control of disease progression [12,13].

Current therapeutic approaches mainly target proteins that are vital for the viral cycle. One of the prominent examples is the linear 36-amino acid synthetic peptide enfuviritide (T20, Fuzeon), developed by Hoffmann-La Roche, and the first FDA approved fusion inhibitor for the treatment of HIV-1/AIDS acting through the binding to the gp41 subunit of the HIV-1 envelope glycoprotein. This induces a conformational change that brings the viral and cellular membranes into close enough proximity for the fusion and the subsequent viral entry into the host-cell to occur. Nevertheless, several restrictions, such as a low genetic barrier for drug resistance and a short in vivo half-life, limit its clinical use [14–17].

Other various FDA-approved antiretroviral drugs from seven mechanistic classes of inhibitors of the HIV replication are also available for the treatment of infected patients, namely, the nucleoside reverse-transcriptase inhibitors NRTIs, non-nucleoside reverse-transcriptase (RT) inhibitors NNRTIs, protein inhibitors PIs, fusion inhibitors, entry inhibitors—CCR5 co-receptor antagonists, HIV integrase strand transfer inhibitors, and multi-class combinations. None of the mentioned drug classes alone or in combination, the latter being known as the highly active antiretroviral therapy (HAART), can eradicate the HIV infection, and effective vaccines remain unavailable.

The difficulties of HIV-1 vaccine research are, in part, a result of 1) the unavailability of a model for natural immunity related to HIV; 2) the existence of genetically distinct subtypes of HIV and frequent mutations; 3) unidentified correlates of specific immune response to HIV; 4) lack of a reliable, non-human animal model for HIV infection (SIV in monkeys vs. HIV in humans).

The established latent pro-viral reservoirs in the patient's body can stochastically begin to reproduce viral particles, which makes the HIV disease practically incurable. From over 160 compounds identified so far as latency-reversing agents (LRAs), none have led to a promising cure [18].

Several rare and long-term remissions of HIV cases are described in the literature. For example, Berlin, London, and Düsseldorf's patients underwent bone marrow transplantation with stem cells from a donor with a rare genetic mutation of the CCR5. The Mississippi baby received a very early antiretroviral therapy that extended the time of the viral rebound for more than 27 months. There undoubtedly remains a lot to be learned from these cases, and further investigation of stem-cell transplantation in people living with HIV is required [19–21].

The currently used antiretroviral treatment, alone or in combination, extends the quality and life expectancy of HIV-infected individuals but does not cure them. Drug resistance, along with the emergence of drug-resistant virus strains, a high-cost of the lifetime treatment regimen, cell toxicity, and serious side effects of currently used anti-HIV drugs [2] underlie the need for a synthetic development of new drugs or the search for active anti-HIV molecules in natural sources. Mother Nature has been perfecting its chemistry for three billion years, and most of it has been done in water. Intense competition and feeding pressure as well as non-static marine environmental conditions yield compounds with chemical and structural features generally not found in terrestrial natural products.

New efficient molecules directed against HIV should demonstrate better performance in comparison with the currently approved drugs and suppress the HIV virus and/or eliminate the latent HIV reservoirs present in the human body.

Around 60% of drugs currently available on the market are derived or inspired by nature [22]. Turning to nature for drug development holds great potential, especially when it comes to marine organisms. Only few marine-derived drugs have been approved on the market so far but many are in the preclinical or clinical stage of development [23]. Marine organisms make up to two-thirds of Earth's species and produce, as a consequence of living in a highly competitive environment, unique and structurally diverse metabolites. Over the last 40 years, bioprospecting efforts have resulted in over 20,000 compounds of marine origin. The highest share of marine metabolites (up to 70%) are obtained from marine sponges, corals, and microorganisms, while mollusks, ascidians, and algae metabolites form only a minor part [24]. Oceans are, indeed, still a rather underexploited habitat, and biodiversity appears to be higher in the oceans than on land, which might be relevant when focusing on the marine environment as an untapped reservoir of novel antiretroviral candidates. In the discovery of new antiviral marine-derived drugs, researchers usually implement two strategies. They either screen the extracts from different strains (e.g., cyanobacteria, microalgae) or search directly for bioactive molecules in organisms—extract and purify them for evaluation within the drug development pipeline. It is thought that the marine environment might yield more potent anti-HIV candidates characterized by a higher efficiency (lower effective dose) and a better selectivity and which do not induce resistance development. This could, of course, only be speculation based on some of the previous success stories in the discovery of drugs from natural sources such as, e.g., lovastatin and paclitaxel. However, nature generally does create more sophisticated and perfected systems with a complex mode of action.

An excellent example is protein lectin, derived from marine red algae *Griffithsia* sp. named Griffithsin with mid-picomolar activities, which groups it among the most potent HIV entry inhibitors reported so far [25]. It inhibits the HIV infection by binding itself to high mannose glycan structures on the surface of gp120, altering the gp120 structure or its oligomeric state [26]. This interaction relies on the specific trimeric "sugar tower," including N295 and N448 [27]. Griffitshin can also prevent infections caused by other glycoprotein-enveloped viruses such as the Ebola virus, hepatitis C virus, and the severe acute respiratory syndrome coronavirus. It has been shown that the dimerization of Griffithsin is necessary for a high potency inhibition of HIV-1 [28]. However, the discrepancy between the HIV gp120 binding activity and the HIV inhibitory activity points to the presence of mechanism unrelated to a merely simple HIV gp120 binding [26]. The most promising application of Griffithsin would be its incorporation into vaginal and rectal gels, creams, or suppositories acting as an antiviral microbicide to prevent the transmission of HIV.

Despite the vast number of structurally diverse and unique bioactive molecules from the marine environment, the global marine pharmaceutical pipeline includes only eight approved drugs: Adcetris®, Cytosar-U®, Halaven®, Yondelis®, Carragelose®, Vira-A®, Lovaza®, and Prialt® [29]. Overall, it has taken 20 to 30 years from their discovery to their entry into the market. A sustainable supply, structural complexity, optimization of formulation, and ADMET properties, and a scale-up issue have prevented further development of several highly promising marine compounds. It is by no means an easy task to identify a marine candidate that may be considered as a potential drug. Initial high costs of developing a natural product into a drug could be balanced out with careful long-term considerations (biodiversity, supply, and technical, market) [30].

This paper provides an overview of natural marine metabolites that were first identified in the period between 2013 and 2018 or the previously identified marine constituents with a recently confirmed anti-HIV activity that could be potentially used or further optimized as novel ant-HIV agents. We also comprehensively summarize anti-HIV activities for several categories of marine structures including chitosan and its derivatives, sulfated polysaccharides, lectins, bromotyrosine derivatives, peptides, alkaloids, diterpenes, phlorotannins, and xanthones as well as fish oil as an auxiliary to HAART therapy.

2. Marine Compounds in the Treatment of HIV/AIDS

2.1. *Chitosan and Its Derivatives*

Chitosan (**2**, Figure 2), a natural marine byproduct, is a poly-cationic linear polysaccharide derived from chitin (**1**, Figure 2) after partial deacetylation. Chitin is a structural element in the exoskeleton of mainly shrimps and crabs and is mainly composed of the randomly distributed β-(1-4)-linked D-glucosamine and *N*-acetyl-D-glucosamine. It has been previously shown that this compound can exhibit a large scale of different bioactivities and can also be used as a carrier for anti-HIV drugs [31]. Chitosan is loaded with saquinavir, an anti-HIV drug with a protease inhibitory activity, which showed better cell targeting efficiency than saquinavir alone [32]. Furthermore, trimethyl chitosan has improved Atripla, an anti-HIV drug consisting of efavirenz, emtricitabine, and tenofovir disoproxil fumarate, anti-HIV 1 activity, and has allowed it to be used in lower concentrations [33]. The antiretroviral activity is manifested in the chitosan-specific cationic nature that allows the formation of electrostatic complexes or multilayer structures with other negatively charged polymers [34]. Karagozlu et al. reported about new QMW-COS and WMQ-COS oligomers with anti-HIV activities. These oligomers are conjugates of chitosan and the Gln-Met-Trp peptide, which were constructed as a continuation of the authors' previous research, in which a high potency of synthetically constructed chitosan oligomers was confirmed in anti-HIV therapy. More specifically, it was shown that these oligomers suppress syncytium formation, which occurs as a fusion of infected cells with neighboring cells, induced by HIV in a dose-dependent manner. However, the authors also noticed that after a certain period, the number of syncytia once again increased, suggesting that the cells should be re-treated with QMW-COS and WMQ-COS oligomers to maintain the primary therapeutically-relevant effect. The inhibition of the HIV-1 induced lytic effect, determined by the cell viability assay, showed that IC_{50} for QMW-COS was 48.14 µg/mL and was almost identical for WMQ-COS, 48.01 µg/mL. These oligomers effectively reduced the HIV load but showed no effects on HIV-1 RT and protease in vitro. Higher dosages were also required for the reduction in the HIV-1IIIB p24 antigen production assessed by the ELISA assay and the HIV-1_{RTMDR} p24 antigen production. The highest difference between the compounds was reflected in IC_{50} values obtained from studies on the virus-induced luciferase activity in infected cells, where QMW-COS had a higher potency in comparison with WMQ-COS. Lastly, the authors determined the effects of oligomers on the interaction between gp41 and CD4 by using the CD4-gp41 ELISA assay, whereby both oligomers showed high potency. The effect of these oligomers was highest when they were applied immediately upon the HIV-1 infection of cells, indicating that they should be used as a potential treatment in the early stages of HIV infection, probably at the entry stage [31].

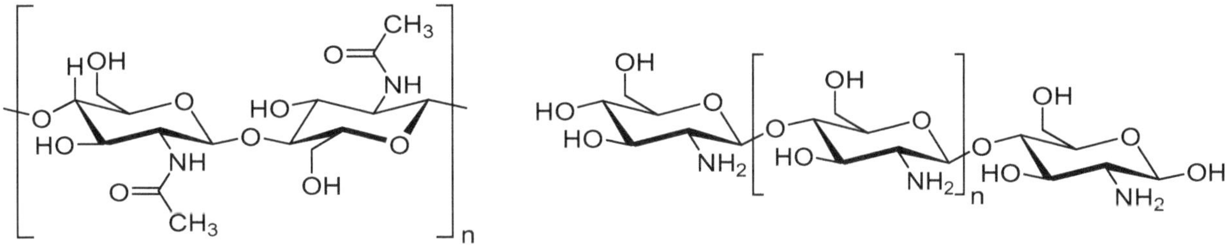

1 2

Figure 2. Chemical structures of chitin (**1**) and chitosan (**2**).

2.2. *Sulfated Polysaccharides*

Sulfated polysaccharides (SP) are the most studied class of antiviral polysaccharides that are structural components of the alga cell wall where they play both the storage and structural role. They are an important source of galactans, commercially known as agar and carrageenan in red alga (Rhodophyta), fucans (fucoidan, sargassan, ascophyllan, and glucuronoxylofucan) in brown alga (Phaeophyta), and ulvans-sulfated heteropolysaccharides that contain galactose, xylose, arabinose, mannose, glucuronic acid, or glucose [35–37]. Many studies indicate that, in marine algae, sulfated polysaccharides facilitate water and ion retention in extracellular matrices, which is an important mechanism for coping with desiccation and osmotic stress in a highly salted environment [38–40]. The antiviral activity of this group of compounds is mainly connected to the degree of sulfation, constituent sugars, molecular weight, conformation, and dynamic stereochemistry [41,42]. The effect of counter cation should also be considered as an important factor in observed biological activity.

The antagonizing effect of the negatively charged sulfated polysaccharides on the HIV-1 entry into cells may be due to 1) their binding onto the positively charged V3 domain of gp120, thereby preventing the virus attachment to the cell surface [43–45] or 2) the masking of the docking sites of gp120 for sCD4 on the surface of T lymphocytes, thereby disrupting the CD4-gp120 interaction [46–48] and subsequently inhibiting the expression of the viral antigen and the activity of the viral reverse transcriptase [49,50].

2.2.1. Heparan Sulfate

Heparinoid polysaccharides can interact with the positive-charge regions of cell-surface glycoproteins, leading to a shielding effect on these regions, which prevents the binding of viruses to the cell surface [51]. The sulfated polysaccharides content in marine mollusks is high in comparison with the bovine mucosal heparin (73.5%) and the porcine mucosal heparin (72.8%) [52]. The acidic sulfate groups on heparin (**3**, Figure 3), or heparin-like compounds, can inhibit HIV through electrostatic interactions with basic amino-acid residues of the transcriptional activator Tat protein [53].

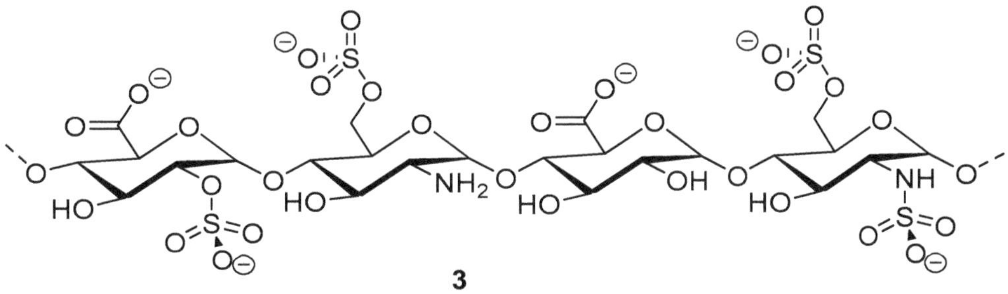

3

Figure 3. Structure of heparan sulfate (**3**).

2.2.2. Fucose Containing SP

So far, the main anti-infectious activities documented for the fucose-containing SP are those against viruses [54]. More importantly, these polysaccharides are selective inhibitors of various enveloped viruses, including HIV [54–56]. FCSP acts during the early phase of infection by blocking the virus attachment and entry into the host cells, but may also inhibit subsequent replication stages in vitro [57].

2.2.3. Fucoidans

Three fucoidans extracted from three brown seaweeds (*Sargassum mcclurei, Sargassum polycystum, Turbinara ornata*) inhibit the early stages of HIV-1 entry into target cells, with IC_{50} ranging from 0.33 to 0.7 μM. Neither the sulfate content nor the position of sulfate groups are related to the anti-HIV activity of fucoidans, suggesting the involvement of other structural parameters such as the molecular weight, the type of glycosidic linkage, or even a unique fucoidan sequence [56]. Although the presence of sulfo-groups seems to be necessary for anti-HIV activity [58], these data do not support random sulfation as the main antiviral factor.

Sulfated fucan polysaccharides, ascophyllan (**4**, Figure 4), and two fucoidans (S and A) (**5** and **6**, Table 2), derived from different sources, significantly inhibit (IC_{50} 1.3; 0.3; 0.6 μg/mL) the early step of HIV-1 (R9 and JR-Fl) infection. They also inhibit the VSV-G-pseudotype HIV-1 infection in HeLa cells [59].

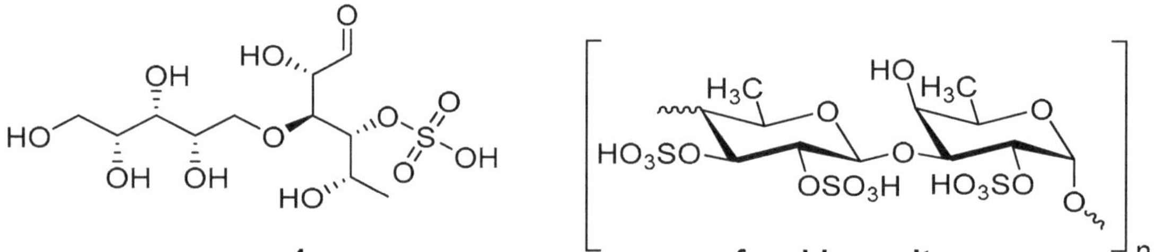

Figure 4. Structure of ascophyllan (**4**) and fucoidan unit.

Table 2. Chemical composition of polysccharides (Fuc, Fucose; Xyl, Xylose; Glu, Glucose; Man, Mannose; Gal, Galactose) in ascophyllan, S- and A-fucoidan.

	Neutral Sugars						
	Fuc	**Xyl**	**Glu**	**Man**	**Gal**	**Uronic Acid**	**SO_3^-**
ascophyllan (**4**)	15.5	13.4	0.3	3.4	0.6	21.4	9.6
S-fucoidan (**5**)	24.8	1.9	0.8	1	3.1	9.6	22.6
A-fucoidan (**6**)	28.4	4.3	2.0	0.8	5.1	5.8	19.4

Chondroitin sulfate with fucosylated branches (FuCS) (**7**, Figure 5) has also attracted attention as an HIV antiviral compound. Depolymerized fucosylated CS, extracted from the sea cucumber, has shown in vitro activity against a range of viral strains, including the resistant ones [60]. FuCS is effective in blocking the laboratory strain HIV-1IIIB entry and replication by inhibiting the p24 antigen production (4.26 and 0.73 μg/mL, respectively) and the infection of the clinic isolate HIV-1KM018 and HIV-1TC-2 (23.75 and 31.86 μg/mL, respectively) as well as suppressing the HIV-1 drug-resistant virus. Additionally, FuCS is also effective in T-20-resistant strains (EC50 values ranging from 0.76 to 1.13 μg/mL). The depolymerized fragments seem to maintain a similar anti-HIV action at the early stages of infection, apparently through interaction with an HIV envelope glycoprotein gp120. The sulfated fucose branches appear necessary for antiviral activity, which is also affected by molecular weight and carboxylation [61]. While the in vitro results of the fucosylated CS against HIV are promising, it is questionable whether the antiviral activity would be maintained in vivo. Other polyanionic HIV entry inhibitors, which advanced into clinical trials, failed to prove effective against the heterosexual HIV-1 transmission. This was related to factors not considered in previous development stages, such as the presence of seminal plasma and the concentration and retention of polyanionic inhibitors [62].

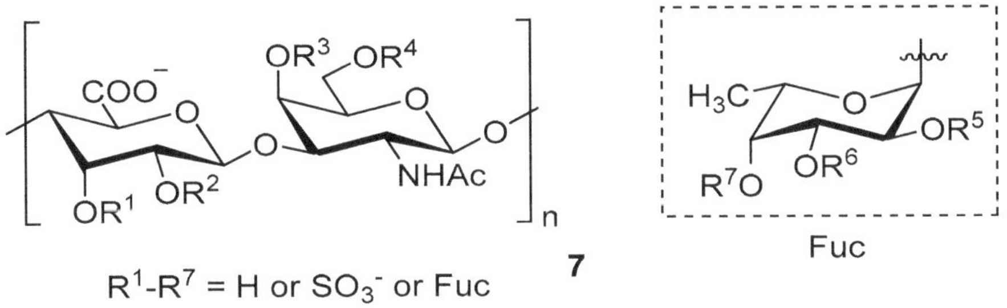

Figure 5. General chemical structure of fucosylated chondroitin sulfate (**7**).

The complex chemical architecture and the sulfate patterning of marine polysaccharides depends on numerous factors (species, tidal cycles, environmental variations (e.g., salinity), harvesting season, plant age, geographical location etc.) [39,63–69], making isolation, purification, and comprehensive chemical characterization a highly challenging task [70]. The development of many polysaccharides into clinical application is hindered by the still limited view of their sophisticated and diverse nature. Despite having good antiviral effects, the use of carbohydrate drugs is still in its infancy, and intensive structure-activity and in vivo studies are needed in the future.

A relatively new strategy in inducing immunity and developing an HIV vaccine is to use carbohydrates. The major difficulty of such an approach lies in mimicking the specific glycan protective epitope. Gp120 of HIV is a highly glycosylated envelope surface glycoprotein responsible for the receptor and co-receptor binding, which, together with gp41, comprises the heterodimeric envelope trimer spikes of HIV. *N*-linked glycans, mainly mannose and complex-type, cover much of the gp120 surface-accessible face of the HIV envelope spike forming the glycan shield. Inadequate mimicry of the glycan shield, tolerance mechanisms, and/or the inability to induce a domain-exchange are reflecting difficulties in creating the proper specificity of Abs [71]. Most of the vaccines for HIV-1 in preclinical trials are based on a Manα1-2Man oligomannosyl epitope (various conjugates, engineered yeast strains, and modified glycoproteins) [72–79]. Better specificity could potentially be gained using carbohydrates of marine origin.

2.3. *Lectins*

Lectins are a group of proteins that specifically, but reversibly, bind glycosylated molecules on the cell surface. Precisely, this group of molecules can affect cell-cell interactions, protect cells from pathogens, influence cell adhesion, and affect the intracellular glycoprotein translocation [80]. Recently, lectins have become promising agents for antiretroviral therapy, and different researches have confirmed their anti-HIV properties. Their antiretroviral activity is manifested through an alteration of the interaction between HIV gp120 or gp41 and the corresponding receptors [81], which, in the end, inhibit the HIV cell function, HIV infectivity, and the formation of the syncytium, multi-nucleated cells [82–84].

Several published review papers describe the previously found marine lectins with antiretroviral action [85,86]. For example, Gogineni et al. reported about some new, unusual lectins, such as the β-galactose specific lectin (CVL), CGL, DTL, DTL-A, SVL-1, and SVL-2 [86]. Additionally, Akkouh et al. reported about some new algal lectins, such as *Boodlea Coacta* Lectin, Griffithsin and *Oscillatoria Agardhii* Agglutinin (OAA), and some cyanobacterial lectins, such as Cyanovirin-N, Scytovirin, Microcystis Viridis Lectin, and Microvirin.

However, in the last few years, there has not been as much research focused on anti-HIV lectins from marine sources. Only Hirayama et al. (2016) reported about the new high-mannose specific lectin and its recombinants that possess anti-HIV activity [87]. In their research performed on the red alga *Kappaphycus alvarezii*, authors confirmed KAA-1 and KAA-2, two KAA mannose-binding lectin isomers, as potent anti-HIV agents. The anti-HIV role of action of these two compounds includes a strong binding to the virus envelope glycoprotein gp120 and, consequently, the inhibition of HIV entry into the host cells. These KAA recombinants, as well as the native one, inhibited the HIV-1 entry at IC_{50}s (neutralization assay in Jurkat cells) of 7.3–12.9 nM. Authors concluded in the end that KAAs, besides their strong inhibitory effect on HIV entry into the cells, have a potential as agents in treatments against other viruses possessing high mannose glycans on their envelope as well.

2.4. Peptides

It has been shown that the majority of marine peptides have strong anti-HIV activity. They are usually isolated from marine organisms through the process of enzymatic hydrolysis [88]. The most common source of such constituents is marine sponges that are known for their unique metabolome [89] and are a source of more than 36% of all marine bioactive compounds [90]. Their bioactive peptides can be found in cyclic or linear forms and contain unusual amino acids that form unique structures rarely found in other species. Antiretroviral activity of such structures works on several different levels: blocking of virus entry, inhibition of the cytopathic viral activity, neutralization of viral particles, or inhibition of viral fusion and entry [89,91].

Recently, Shin et al. discovered two new depsipeptides from marine sponges *Stelletta sp.*, stellettapeptin A (**8**, Figure 6), and stellettapeptin B (**9**, Figure 6), with the inhibition of the cytopathic effect of HIV-1 infection [92]. Confirming the mentioned theory about the unique metabolome of marine sponges, the authors revealed that these two compounds have previously undescribed nonproteinogenic amino-acid parts on peptides that are rarely found in nature. Namely, stellettapeptin A and stellettapeptin B have an unexpected polyketide subunit, 3-hydroxy-6,8-dimethylnon-4-enoic acid, 3-OHGln, and 3-OHAsn residues. Their high potency is witnessed through low EC_{50} values (inhibition of the cytotoxic effect upon HIV infection)—values of 23 nM for stellettapeptin A and 27 nM for stellettapeptin B.

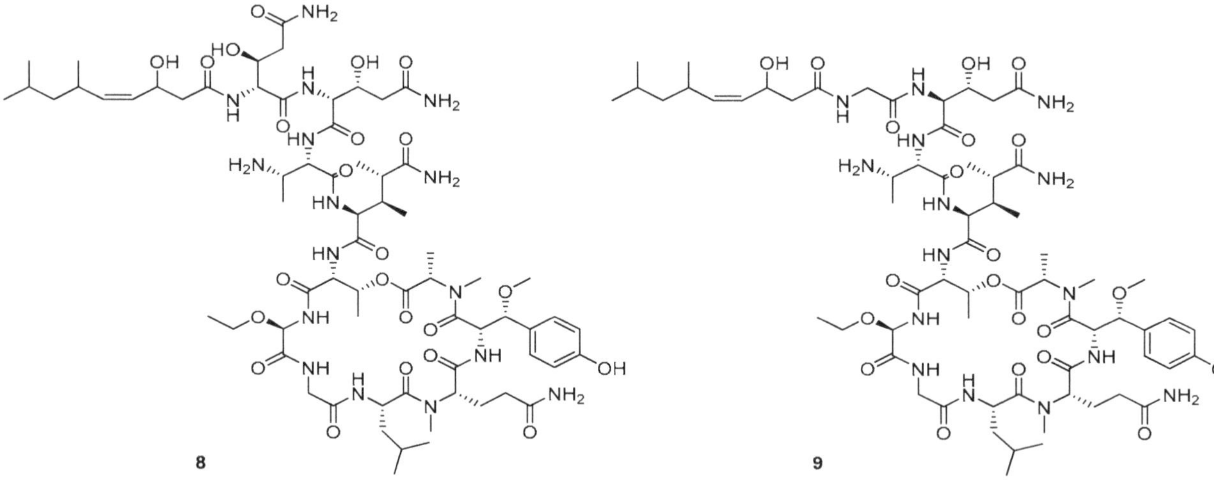

8 9

Figure 6. Structures of stelletapeptin (**8**) A and stelletapeptin B (**9**).

Furthermore, newly discovered anti-HIV constituents derived from marine sponges *Verongula rigida* and *Aiolochoria crassa* with amino-acid structure were published by Gomez-Archila et al. (2014) [93]. In their paper, they evaluated and confirmed the anti-HIV effect of 11 bromotyrosine derivatives (Table 3), whereby aeroplysinin-1 (**10**), 19-deoxyfistularin 3 (**15**), purealidin B (**16**), fistularin 3 (**17**) and 3-bromo-5-hydroxy-O-methyltyrosine (**18**, Figure 7) were the most potent in their anti-HIV activity. Aeroplysinin 1 (**15**) and purealidin B (**16**), compounds found in *V. rigida* species inhibited the HIV-1 replication in a dose-dependent manner by more than 50%. Specifically, for aeroplysinin 1, HIV-a replication was inhibited by 74% at a concentration of 20 μM, whereas purealidin was less potent with inhibitory power of 57% at a concentration of 80 μM. These two compounds had been previously isolated; however, their anti-HIV activity was proven in this research. The same was with 3-bromo-5-hydroxy-*O*-methyltyrosine (**18**) that has a relatively high percentage of inhibition of HIV activity (47%) in a dose-dependent manner. However, the exact mechanism of action remains unclear. In the same study, additional tests with these compounds on the HIV RT inhibition (qPCR of the early and late transcripts), nuclear import (qPCR analysis of 2-LTR transcript), and HIV entry inhibition (viral infectivity assay) were performed. The results showed that aeroplysinin-1 (**10**), 19-deoxyfistularin 3 (**15**), purealidin B (**16**), fistularin 3 (**17**), and 3-bromo-5-hydroxy-*O*-methyltyrosine (**18**) influenced the nuclear import of the HIV virus with around or more than 50% of inhibition: aeroplysinin-1 (**10**) showed 67% of inhibition at 10 μM, 19-deoxyfistularin 3 62% inhibition at 20 μM, purealidin B 66% of inhibition at 20 μM, fistularin 3 47% of inhibition at 10 μM, and 3-bromo-5-hydroxy-*O*-methyltyrosine 73% of inhibition at 80 μM. Viral RT inhibition was not high for all compounds, whereby the highest results were around 50% of inhibition. For example, purealidin B had 58% of inhibition at 20 μM in the qPCR analysis of early transcripts. As for the HIV entry inhibition, all compounds were active in a dose-depended manner, with the highest results of inhibition obtained for 3,5-dibromo-*N,N,N,O*-tetramethyltyraminium (**13**), from 14% to 30%. Finally, the authors stressed the structural similarity of these compounds with the HIV integrase and protease inhibitors, suggesting that these compounds can have a broader mode of antiviral action.

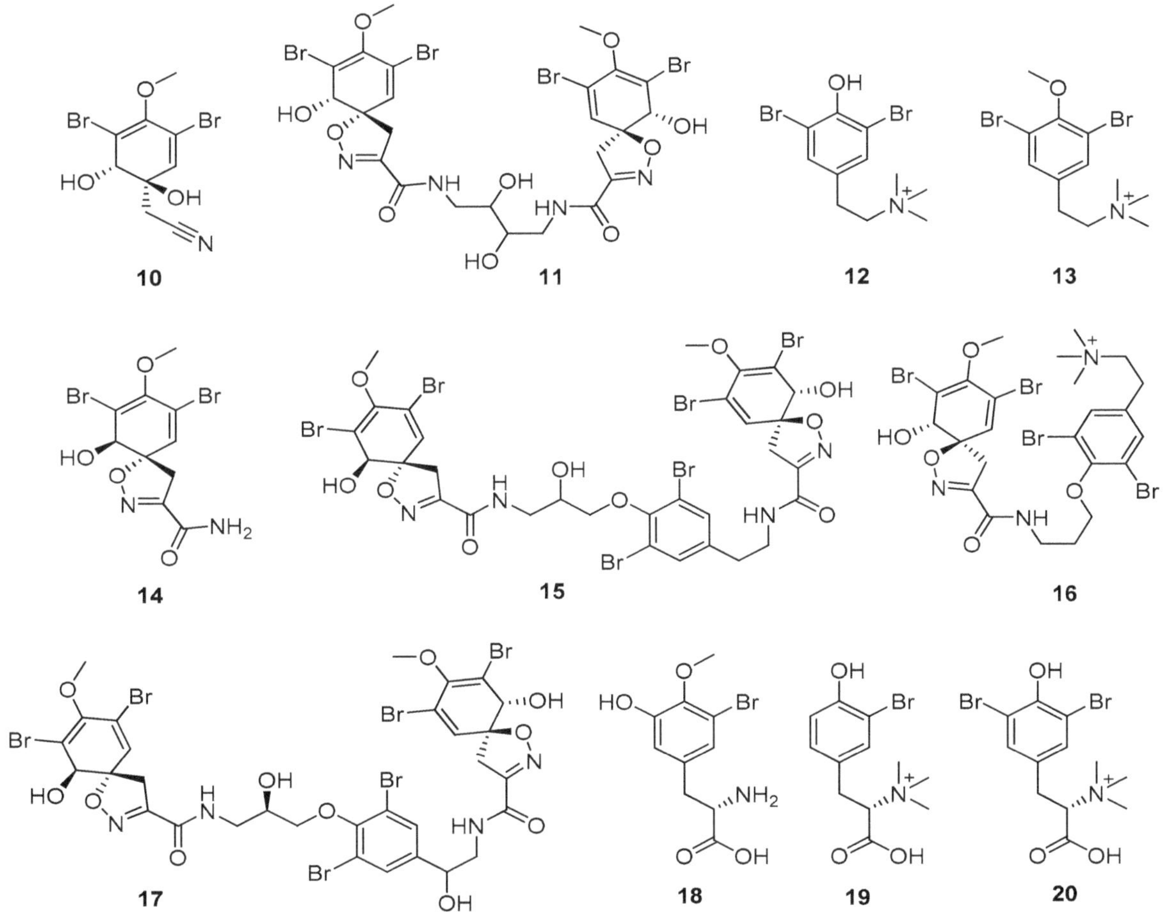

Figure 7. Structures of aeroplysinin-1 (**10**), dihydroxyaerothionin (**11**), 3,4-dibromo-*N,N,N*-trimethyltyraminium (**12**), 3,5-dibromo-*N,N,N,O*-tetramethyltyraminium (**13**), purealidin R (**14**), 19-deohxyfistularin 3 (**15**), purealidin B (**16**), fistularin-3 (**17**), 3-bromo-5-hydroxy-*O*-methyltyrosine (**18**), 3-bromo-*N,N,N*-trimethyltyrosinium (**19**), and 3,5-dibromo-*N,N,N*-trimethyltyrosinium (**20**).

Table 3. Summary of anti-HIV compounds from marine organisms.

Group	Compound	Location	Organism	Assay	Dose	Activity	Structure	Reference
Peptide + chitosan oligomer	QMW-COS	not disclosed [a]	marine byproduct	IC_{50}—inhibition of HIV-1 induced lytic effects (cell viability assay) IC_{50}—inhibition of HIV-1_{IIIB} p24 antigen production (ELISA) IC_{50}—inhibition of HIV-1_{RTMDR} p24 antigen production (ELISA) IC_{50}—inhibition of virus-induced luciferase activity in infected TZM-bl cells IC_{50}—inhibition of the interaction between gp41 and CD4 (CD4-gp41 ELISA)	48.14 μg/mL 67.35 μg/mL 81.03 μg/mL 68.13 μg/mL 39.13 μg/mL	**anti-HIV-1**; inhibition of the HIV entry at an early stage, blocking the fusion of HIV-1 infected cells, interference of gp41-CD4 binding	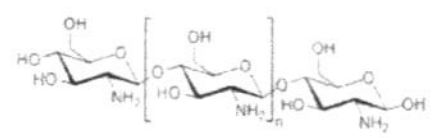 + glutamine (Q), methionine (M), tryptophan (W)	[31]
	WMQ-COS	not disclosed[a]	marine byproduct	IC_{50}—Inhibition of HIV-1 induced lytic effects (cell viability assay) IC_{50}—inhibition of HIV-1IIIB p24 antigen production (ELISA) IC_{50}—inhibition of HIV-1_{RTMDR} p24 antigen production (ELISA) IC_{50}—inhibition of virus-induced luciferase activity in infected TZM-bl cells IC_{50}—inhibition of interaction between gp41 and CD4 (CD4-gp41 ELISA)	48.01 μg/mL 98.73 μg/mL 144.02 μg/mL 250 μg/mL 51.48 μg/ml	**anti-HIV-1**; inhibition of the HIV entry at an early stage	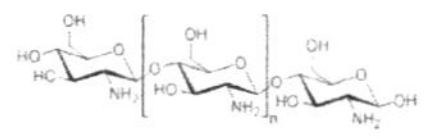 + tryptophan (W) methionine (M), glutamine (Q),	[31]
Sulfated polysaccharides	heparan sulfate (**3**)	not disclosed	-	EC_{50}—inhibition of HIV-1_{IIIB} strain (syncytia assay) EC_{50}—inhibition of HIV-1_{IIIB} strain (p24 assay) EC_{50}—inhibition of HIV-1_{IIIB}/H9 strain (co-cultivation assay) EC_{50}—inhibition of HIV-1_{RF} strain (p24 assay) EC_{50}—inhibition of HIV-1_{KM018} strain (p24 assay) EC_{50}—inhibition of HIV-$1_{TC\text{-}2}$ strain (p24 assay) EC_{50}—inhibition of HIV-1_{A17} strain (p24 assay) EC_{50}—inhibition of HIV-$1_{RF/V82F/184V}$ strain (p24 assay) EC_{50}—inhibition of HIV-$1_{L10R/M461/L63P/V82T/184V}$ strain (p24 assay) EC_{50}—inhibition of HIV-$1_{CBL\text{-}20}$ strain (syncytia assay) EC_{50}—inhibition of HIV-1_{ROD} strain (syncytia assay)	0.24 μg/mL 0.73 μg/mL 4.26 μg/mL 1.14 μg/mL 23.75 μg/mL 31.86 μg/mL 1.09 μg/mL 0.95 μg/mL 1.12 μg/mL 71.76 μg/mL 97.63 μg/ml	**anti-HIV-1**; electrostatic interactions with basic amino acid residues of Tat	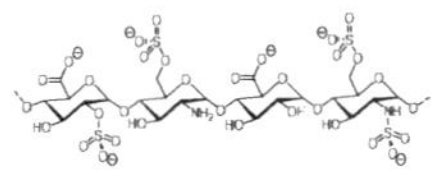	[53]

Table 3. *Cont.*

Group	Compound	Location	Organism	Assay	Dose	Activity	Structure	Reference
	fucose containing	Nha Trang bay, Vietnam	*Sargassum mcclurei*, *Sargassum polycystum*, and *Turbinara Ornate* brown seaweeds	U373-CD4-CXCR4 cells 211 infected with pseudotype viral IC_{50}—inhibition (F_{SP} crude extract)-(p24 ELISA) IC_{50}—inhibition (F_{TO} crude extract)-(p24 ELISA) IC_{50}—inhibition (F_{SM} crude extract)-(p24 ELISA)	 0.34 μg/mL 0.39 μg/mL 0.96 μg/mL	**anti-HIV-1**; inhibition of the early phase of infection, by blocking the virus attachment and entry into the host cells		[56]
	ascophyllan **(4)**	not disclosed	different sources	IC_{50}—inhibition of HIV-1_{R9}-real-time PCR	1.3 μg/mL	**anti-HIV-1**; early step of HIV-1 (R9 and JR-Fl) infection; inhibition of VSV-G-pseudotyped HIV-1 infection in HeLa cells	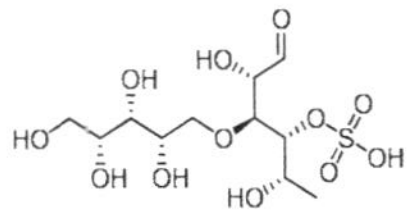	[59]
	fucoidan S **(5)** fucoidan A **(6)**	not disclosed	different sources	IC_{50}—inhibition of HIV-1_{R9}-real-time PCR (fucoidan S) IC_{50}—inhibition of HIV-1_{R9}-real-time PCR (fucoidan A)	0.3 μg/mL 0.6 μg/ml	**anti-HIV-1**; early step of HIV-1 (R9 and JR-Fl) infection; inhibition of VSV-G-pseudotyped HIV-1 infection in HeLa cells	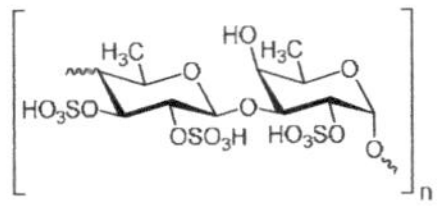	[59]
	chondroitin sulfate (7)	not disclosed		EC_{50}—HIV-1 p24 detection-PBMC assay-inhibition of HIV-1_{IIIB}, HIV-$1_{L10R/M46I/L63P/V82T/I84V}$, HIV-$1_{A17}$, HIV-$1_{RF}$, and HIV-$1_{RF/V82F/184V}$ strains	0.01–0.08 μM	**anti-HIV-1**; inhibition of HIV-1 replication; inhibition of the HIV-1 entry	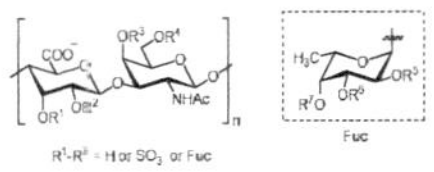	[61]
Lectins	KAA-1	not disclosed	red alga *Kappaphycus alvarezii*	IC_{50}—neutralization assay in Jurkat cells (median tissue culture infectious dose (TCID50) method using Jurkat cells)	9.2 nM	**anti-HIV-1**; inhibition of the HIV-1 entry		[87]
	KAA-2	not disclosed	red alga *Kappaphycus alvarezii*	IC_{50}—neutralization assay in Jurkat cells (median tissue culture infectious dose (TCID50) method using Jurkat cells)	7.3 nM	**anti-HIV-1**; inhibition of the HIV-1 entry		[87]

Table 3. *Cont.*

Group	Compound	Location	Organism	Assay	Dose	Activity	Structure	Reference
Peptides	stellettapeptin A (**8**)	north-western Australia	marine sponge *Stelletta sp.*	EC_{50}—inhibition of the cytotoxic effect upon HIV-1 infection	23 nm	**anti-HIV-1**; cytopathic effect of HIV-1 infection	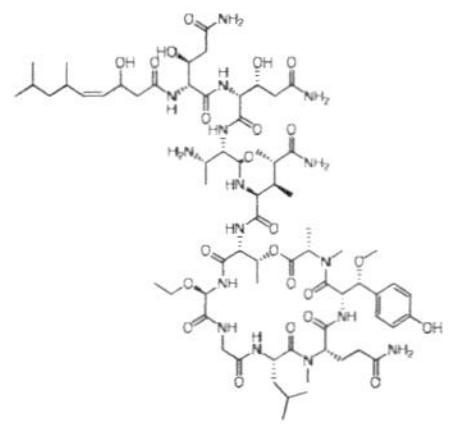	[92]
	stellettapeptin B (**9**)	north-western Australia	marine sponge *Stelletta sp.*	EC_{50}—inhibition of the cytotoxic effect upon HIV-1 infection	27 nm	**anti-HIV-1**; cytopathic effect of HIV-1 infection	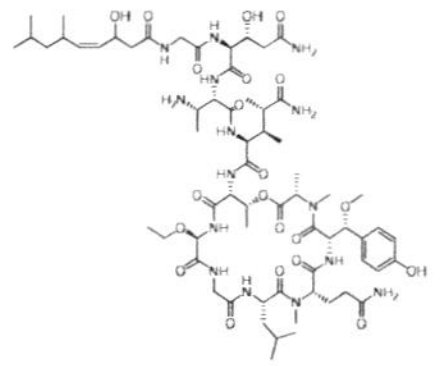	[92]
Bromotyrosine derivatives	aeroplysinin-1 (**10**)	Colombia	marine sponge *Verongula rigida*	% of inhibition of HIV-1 replication by flow cytometry % of reverse transcription inhibition (qPCR analysis of late transcripts) % of nuclear import inhibition (qPCR analysis of 2-LTR transcript) % of HIV entry inhibition (viral infectivity assay)	74% of inhibition at 20 µM 48% of inhibition at 10 µM 67% of inhibition at 10 µM dose dependent manner 2–20%	**anti-HIV-1**; inhibition of HIV-1 replication, RT, nuclear import and entry	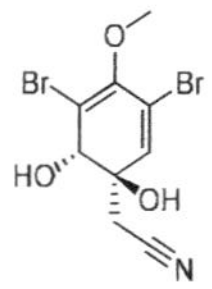	[93]
	3,5-dibromo -*N,N,N,O*-tetramethyl Tyraminium (**13**)	Colombia	marine sponge *Verongula rigida*	% of HIV entry inhibition (viral infectivity assay)	dose depended manner 14–30%	**anti-HIV-1**; inhibition of HIV-1 entry	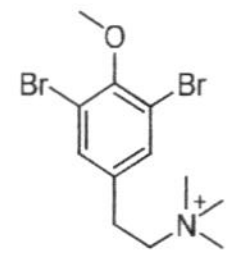	[93]
	19-deoxy fistularin 3 (**15**)	Colombia	marine sponge *Verongula rigida*	% of reverse transcription inhibition (qPCR analysis of early transcripts) % of reverse transcription inhibition (qPCR analysis of late transcripts) % of nuclear import inhibition (qPCR analysis of 2-LTR transcript)	35% inhibition at 20 µM 11% inhibition at 20 µM 62% inhibition at 20 µM	**anti-HIV-1**; inhibition of HIV-1 replication, RT, nuclear import	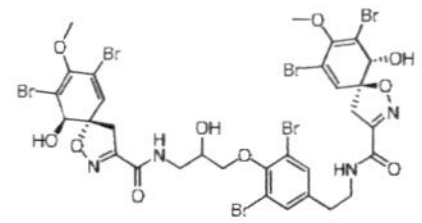	[93]

Table 3. *Cont.*

Group	Compound	Location	Organism	Assay	Dose	Activity	Structure	Reference
	purealidin B (**16**)	Colombia	marine sponge *Verongula rigida*	% of inhibition of HIV-1 replication by flow cytometry % of reverse transcription inhibition (qPCR analysis of early transcripts) % of reverse transcription inhibition (qPCR analysis of late transcripts) % of nuclear import inhibition (qPCR analysis of 2-LTR transcript) % of HIV entry inhibition (viral infectivity assay)	57% of inhibition at 80 μM58% of inhibition at 20 μM 34% of inhibition at 20 μM 66% of inhibition at 20 μM dose depended manner 2–11%	**anti-HIV-1**; inhibition of HIV-1 replication, RT, nuclear import and entry	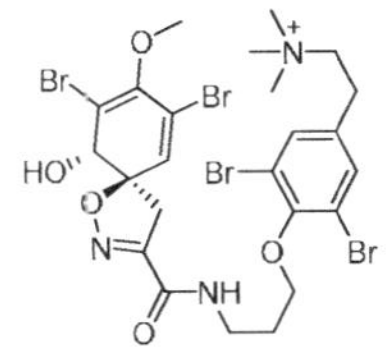	[93]
	fistularin 3 (**17**)	Colombia	marine sponge *Verongula rigida*	% of reverse transcription inhibition (qPCR analysis of late transcripts) % of nuclear import inhibition (qPCR analysis of 2-LTR transcript) % of HIV entry inhibition (viral infectivity assay)	24% of inhibition at 5 μM, 47% of inhibition at 10 μM, dose depended manner 11–13%	**anti-HIV-1**; inhibition of, HIV-1 RT, nuclear import and HIV-1 entry	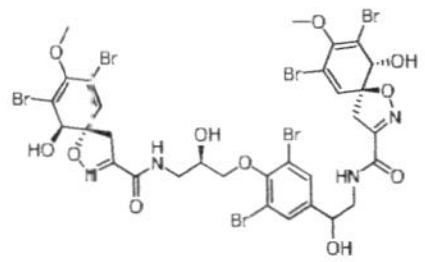	[93]
	3-bromo-5-hydroxy-O-methyltyrosine (**18**)	Colombia	marine sponge *Aiolochroia crassa*	% of inhibition of HIV-1 replication by flow cytometry % of reverse transcription inhibition (qPCR analysis of early transcripts) % of reverse transcription inhibition (qPCR analysis of late transcripts) % of nuclear import inhibition (qPCR analysis of 2-LTR transcript) % of HIV entry inhibition (viral infectivity assay)	47% of inhibition at 80 μM, 54% of inhibition at 160 μM, 50% of inhibition at 40 μM, 73% of inhibition at 80 μM, dose depended manner 2–12%	**anti-HIV-1**; inhibition of HIV-1 replication, RT, nuclear import and entry	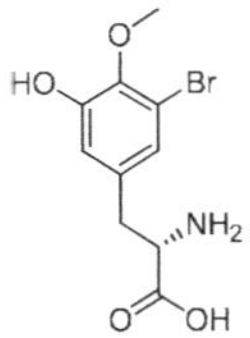	[93]

Table 3. *Cont.*

Group	Compound	Location	Organism	Assay	Dose	Activity	Structure	Reference
Peptides	APCHP (**21**)	not disclosed	Alaska pollack	EC_{50}—against anti-HIV-1 induced cell lysis (MTT assay) EC_{50}—HIV-1-induced RT activation in MT-4 cells EC_{50}—against p24 production (western blot)	459 µM (0.403 mg/mL) 374 µM (0.327 mg/mL) 405 µM (**0.356 mg/mL**)	**anti-HIV-1**; inhibition of induced syncytia formation by interference of HIV fusion inhibition of cell lysis, RT activity and production of p24 antigen	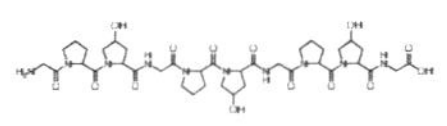	[94]
	SM-peptide	not disclosed	*Spirulina maxima*	IC_{50}—protective activity on HIV-1-induced cell lysis-MTT assay % of RT Inhibition in HIV-1-infected cells (reverse transcriptase assay kit) % of HIV-1 p24 antigen production (p24 antigen production assay)	0.691 mM (0.475 mg/mL) 90% inhibition at 1.093 mM (0.75 mg/mL) 95% of inhibition at 1.093 mM (0.75 mg/mL)	**anti-HIV-1**; inhibition of the HIV-1 RT activity and p24 antigen production	Leu-Asp-Ala-Val-Asn-Arg	[95]
Alkaloids	aspernigrin C (**22**)	Yongxing Island, South China Sea Yongxing Island, South China Sea	marine fungus *Aspergillus niger* SCSIO Jcw6F30 isolated from marine alga *Sargassum sp.*	IC_{50}—inhibitory effects on infection by CCR5-tropic HIV-1 SF162 in TZM-bl cells	4.7 µM	**anti-HIV-1**	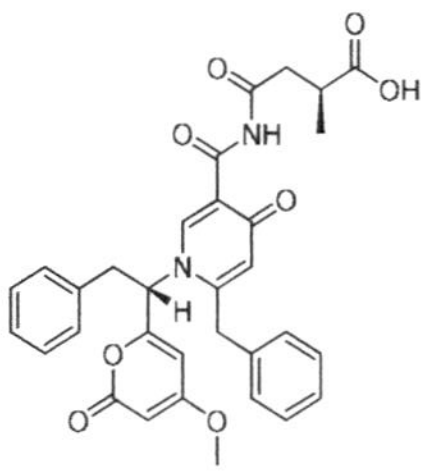	[96]
	malformin C (**23**)	Yongxing Island, South China Sea Yongxing Island, South China Sea	marine fungus *Aspergillus niger* SCSIO Jcw6F30 isolated from marine alga *Sargassum sp.*	IC_{50}—inhibitory effects on infection by CCR5-tropic HIV-1 SF162 in TZM-bl cells	1.4 µM	**anti-HIV-1**	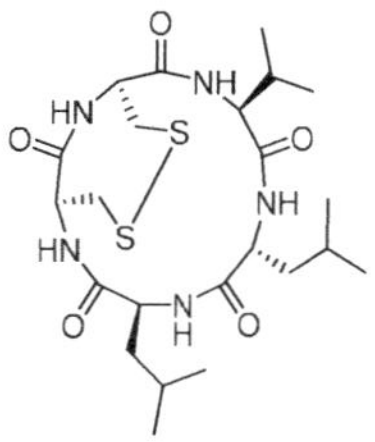	[96]

Table 3. *Cont.*

Group	Compound	Location	Organism	Assay	Dose	Activity	Structure	Reference
	eutypellazine E **(24)**	South Atlantic Ocean	deep-sea sediment fungus *Eutypella sp.* MCCC 3A00281	IC_{50}—anti-HIV bioassay-pNL4.3.Env-.Luc co-transfected 293T cells	3.2 µM	**anti-HIV-1**; inhibitory effects against HIV-1 replication	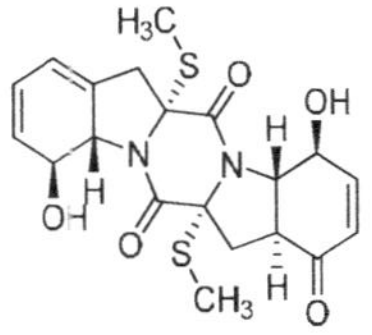	[97]
	eutypellazine J **(25)**	South Atlantic Ocean	deep-sea sediment fungus *Eutypella sp.* MCCC 3A00281	IC_{50}—anti-HIV bioassay-pNL4.3.Env-.Luc co-transfected 293T cells reactivation activity-In vitro latent HIV reactivating assay-flow cytometry-based screening	4.9 µM 80 µM	**anti-HIV-1**; inhibitory effects against HIV-1 replication, latency reactivating agent	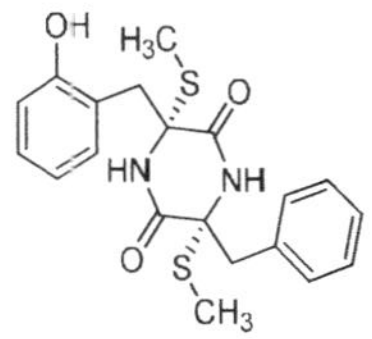	[97]
	debromo-hymenialdisine **(26)**	Coral reefs in the Red Sea	*S. carteri* sponge extract	% of reduction of HIV-1 replication-cell-based assay	30% of inhibition at 13 µM	**anti-HIV 1**; decrease the transcription of the HIV-1, abrogate the G2-checkpoint of the cell cycle	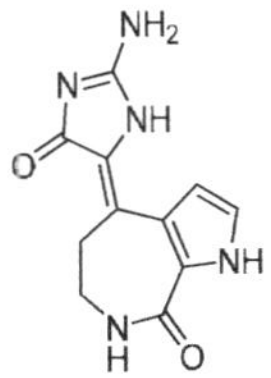	[98]
	Hymenialdisine **(27)**	Coral reefs in the Red Sea	*S. carteri* sponge extract	% of reduction of HIV-1 replication-cell-based assay	<40% of inhibition at 3.1 µM	**anti-HIV 1**; decrease the transcription of the HIV-1, abrogate the G2-checkpoint of the cell cycle	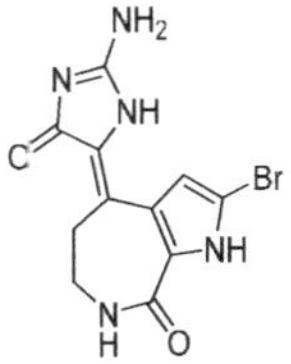	[98]

Table 3. *Cont.*

Group	Compound	Location	Organism	Assay	Dose	Activity	Structure	Reference
	Oroidin (**28**)	Coral reefs in the Red Sea	*S. carteri* sponge extract	% of inhibition - HIV-1 RT biochemical assay % of reduction of HIV-1 replication-cell-based assay	90% of inhibition at >25 μM 50% of inhibition at 50 μM	**anti-HIV-1**; inhibition of HIV-1 RT, reduction of HIV-1 replication	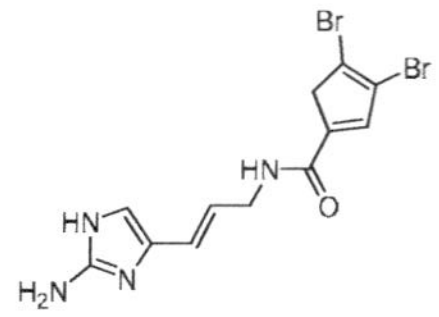	[98]
	3-(phenetyl amino) demethyl(oxy) aaptamine (**29**)	Woody Island (Yongxing, Hainan, China) and Seven Connected Islets in the South China Sea	*A. aptos* sponge extract	% of inhibition against HIV-1 replication-anti-HIV-1 activity assay-cell-based VSVG/HIV-1 pseudotyping system	88% of inhibition at 10 μM	**anti-HIV-1**; inhibitory effects against HIV-1 replication	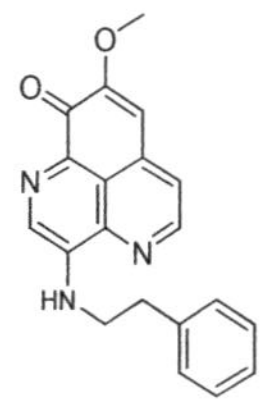	[99]
	3-(isopentyl amino) demethyl(oxy) aaptamine (**30**)	Woody Island (Yongxing, Hainan, China) and Seven Connected Islets in the South China Sea	*A. aptos* sponge extract	% of inhibition against HIV-1 replication-anti-HIV-1 activity assay-cell-based VSVG/HIV-1 pseudotyping system	72.3% of inhibition at 10 μM	**anti-HIV-1**; inhibitory effects against HIV-1 replication	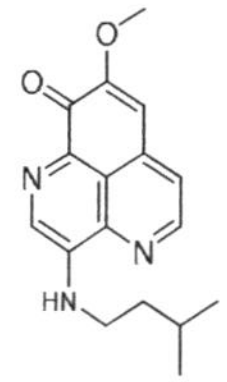	[99]
	bengamide A (**31**)	not disclosed	screening of previously isolated compounds (originally isolated from the sponge *Jaspis* cf. *coriacea*)	EC_{50}—multi-cycle viral replication assay % inhibition of p24^{Gag} production-of PBMC assay-p24^{Gag} was quantified by ELISA EC_{50}—inhibition of LTR promoter-driven gene expression-LTR-based reporter assays	0.015 μM >90% of inhibition at 0.3 μM 0.17 μM	**anti-HIV-1**; inhibition of NF-κB-mediated retroviral gene expression	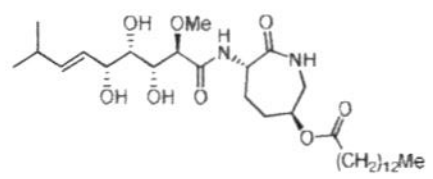	[100]
	haliclony-cyclamine A + B (**32**)	not disclosed	screening of previously isolated compounds	EC_{50}—multi-cycle viral replication assay	3.8 μM	**anti-HIV-1**; inhibitory effects against HIV-1 replication	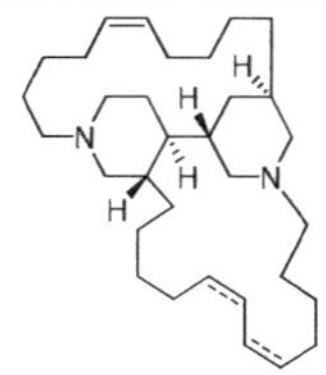	[100]

Table 3. *Cont.*

Group	Compound	Location	Organism	Assay	Dose	Activity	Structure	Reference
	keramamine C **(33)**	not disclosed	screening of previously isolated compounds	EC_5—multi-cycle viral replication assay	3.4 µM	**anti-HIV-1**; inhibitory effects against HIV-1 replication	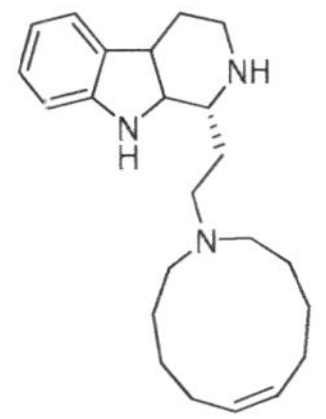	[100]
	stachybotrin D **(34)**	Xisha Island, China	sponge *Xestospongia testudinaris*	EC_{50}—inhibitory Effects on Wild-Type and NNRTI-Resistant HIV-1 Replication: EC_{50}—inhibition of VSVG/HIV-1_{wt} EC_{50}—inhibition of VSVG/HIV-$1_{RT-K103N}$ EC_{50}—inhibition of VSVG/HIV-$1_{RT-L100I,K103N}$ EC_{50}—inhibition of VSVG/HIV-$1_{RT-K103N,V108I}$ EC_{50}—inhibition of VSVG/HIV-$1_{RT-K103N,G190A}$ EC_{50}—inhibition of VSVG/HIV-$1_{RT-K103N,P225H}$	 8.4 µM 7.0 µM 23.8 µM 13.3 µM 14.2 µM 6.2 µM	**anti-HIV-1**; HIV-1 RT inhibition (inhibitory effects on wild type and five NNRTI-resistant HIV-1 strains)	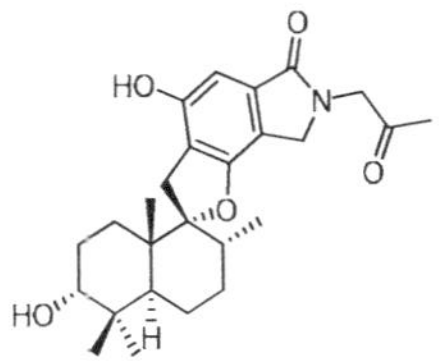	[101]
Diterpenes	dolabelladienol A **(35)**	Atol das Rocas, in Northeast Brazil	brown alga *Dictyota pfaffii*	EC_{50}—inhibition of the cytopathic effect of HIV-1-MT-2 cells—MTT method	2.9 µM	**anti-HIV-1**; -inhibition of the cytopathic effect of HIV-1	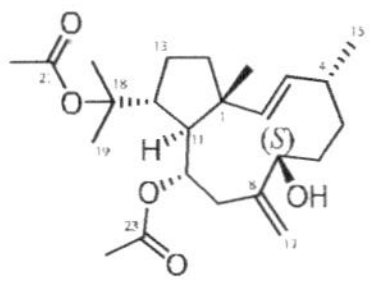	[102]
	dolabelladienol B **(36)**	Atol das Rocas, in Northeast Brazil	brown alga *Dictyota pfaffii*	EC_{50}—inhibition of the cytopathic effect of HIV-1-MT-2 cells—MTT method	4.1 µM	**anti-HIV-1**; -inhibition of the cytopathic effect of HIV-1	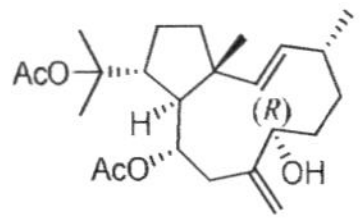	[102]
	dolastane **(38)**	Praia do Velho, Angra dos Reis, in the south of Rio de Janeiro State, Brazil	brown alga *Canistrocarpus cervicornis*	EC_{50}—inhibition of HIV-1 replication-CXCR4-tropic HIV-1–MTT method	0.35 µM	**anti-HIV-1**; inhibition of HIV-1 replication, potent effect on HIV-1 infectivity	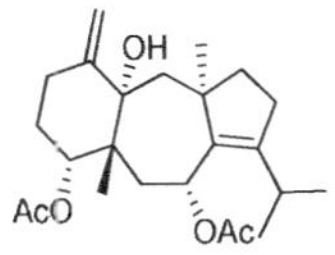	[103]

Table 3. *Cont.*

Group	Compound	Location	Organism	Assay	Dose	Activity	Structure	Reference
	dolastane **(39)**	Praia do Velho, Angra dos Reis, in the south of Rio de Janeiro State, Brazil	brown alga *Canistrocarpus cervicornis*	EC_{50}—inhibition of HIV-1 replication-CXCR4-tropic HIV-1–MTT method	0.794 µM	**anti-HIV-1**; inhibition of HIV-1 replication, potent effect on HIV-1 infectivity	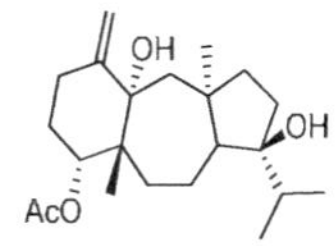	[103]
	secodolastane diterpene **(40)**	Praia do Velho, Angra dos Reis, in the south of Rio de Janeiro State, Brazil	brown alga Canistrocarpus cervicornis	EC_{50}—inhibition of HIV-1 replication-CXCR4-tropic HIV-1–MTT method	3.67 µM	**anti-HIV-1**; inhibition of HIV-1 replication	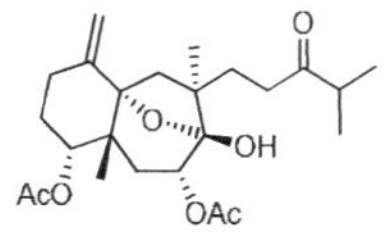	[103]
	8,10,18-trihydroxy-2,6-dolabelladiene **(41)**	Atol das Rocas reef, Brazil	brown alga *Dictyota friabilis*	EC_{50}—inhibition of the cytopathic effect of HIV-1-MT-2 cells—MTT method	6.16 µM	**anti-HIV-1**; inhibition of the cytopathic effect of HIV-1	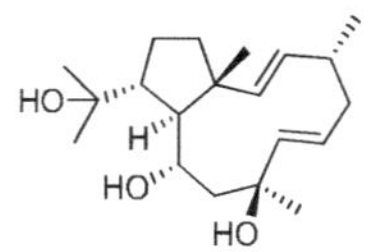	[104,105]
	oxygenated dolabellane **(42)**	Santa Marta Bay (Colombian Caribbean Sea	octocoral *Eunicea laciniata*	EC_{50}—inhibition of HIV-1-Inhibition of the cytopathic effect of HIV-1-MT-2 cells—MTT method	3.9 µM	**anti-HIV-1**; inhibition of the cytopathic effect of HIV-1	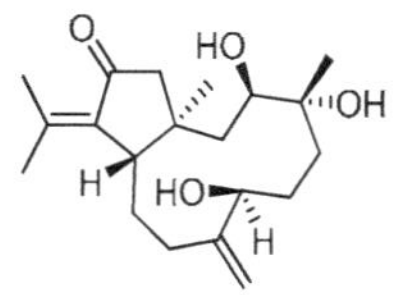	[106]
	oxygenated dolabellane **(43)**	Santa Marta Bay (Colombian Caribbean Sea	octocoral *Eunicea laciniata*	EC_{50}—inhibition of the cytopathic effect of HIV-1-MT-2 cells—MTT method	0.73 µM	**anti-HIV-1**; inhibition of the cytopathic effect of HIV-1	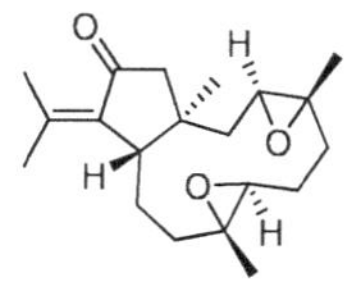	[106]
	oxygenated dolabellane **(44)**	Santa Marta Bay (Colombian Caribbean Sea	octocoral *Eunicea laciniata*	EC_{50}—inhibition of HIV-1-Inhibition of the cytopathic effect of HIV-1-MT-2 cells–MTT method	0.69 µM	**anti-HIV-1**; inhibition of the cytopathic effect of HIV-1	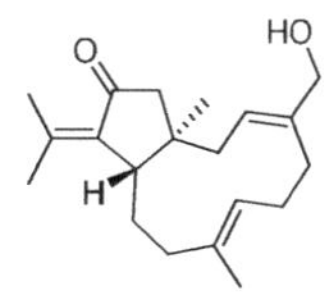	[106]

Table 3. *Cont.*

Group	Compound	Location	Organism	Assay	Dose	Activity	Structure	Reference
	8,4′′′-dieckol (**45**)	not disclosed	brown alga, *Ecklonia cava*	Inhibition of syncytia formation on C8166 cells ($HIV\text{-}1_{IIIB}$, $HIV\text{-}1_{RF}$ and $HIV\text{-}1_{LAI}$)-inverted microscope Inhibition of the cytopathic effect of HIV-1-C8166 cells—MTT method Effect on p24 antigen production-p24 antigen capture ELISA and immunoblast analysis RT activity assay—commercial fluorescence RT assay kit Inhibition of HIV-1 replication-Luciferase gene reporter assay	Inhibition in dose-depended manner * Cell viability was more than 90% dose-dependent inhibition Inhibited 91% activity of $HIV\text{-}1_{IIIB}$ RT and approximat ely 80% for rest of the HIV-1 strains tested, $HIV\text{-}1_{RTMDR1}$ strain was inhibited at a ratio of 76.1% At the highest concentration, inhibition was more than 80% for all viral strains except for RTMDR1 (76.33%)	**anti-HIV-1**; inhibition of the cytopathic effects of HIV-1: inhibition of syncytia formation, lytic effects, inhibition of viral p24 antigen production, HIV-1 entry inhibition and RT inhibition	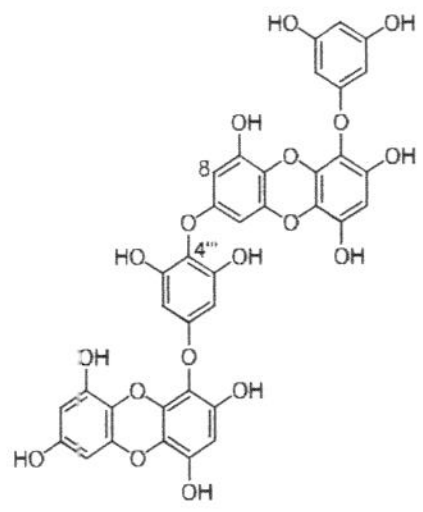	[107]
	penicilli-xanthone A (**46**)	not disclosed	from the jellyfish-derived fungus *Aspergillus fumigates*	IC_{50}—inhibition of PXA on infection by CCR5-tropic HIV-1 in TZM-bl cells IC_{50}—inhibition of PXA on infection by CXCR4-tropic HIV-1 in TZM-bl cells	0.36 μM 0.26 μM	**anti-HIV-1**; inhibition of infection against CCR5-tropic HIV-1 SF162 and CXCR4-tropic HIV-1 NL4-3	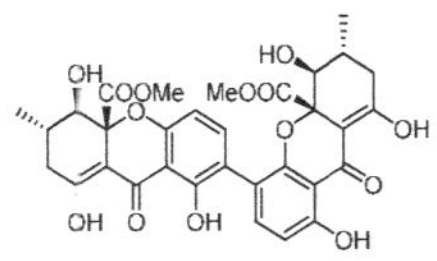	[108]
	docosahexanoic acid (**48**)	not disclosed		In vivo study on male rat models-Male F344 (control) and HIV-1Tg rats		**anti-HIV-1**; neuroprotective effect on neuroinflammations induced by ethanol (in the presence of HIV viral proteins)	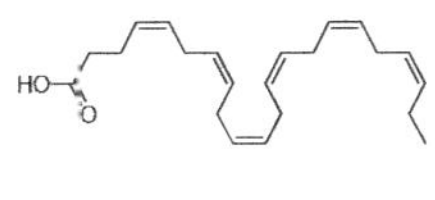	[109]

Table 3. *Cont.*

Group	Compound	Location	Organism	Assay	Dose	Activity	Structure	Reference
	radicicol (**49**)	Tutuila, American Samoa	*H. fuscoatra*	EC_{50}—In Vitro Model of HIV-1 Latency-high-throughput primary cell-based HIV-1 latency assay	9.1 µM	**anti-HIV-1**; reactivation of latent viral loads in CD4+ T-cells	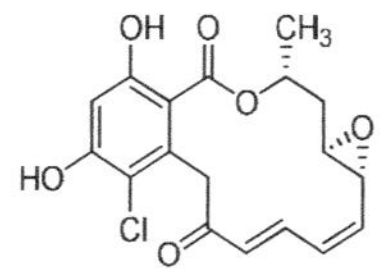	[110]
Phlorotannins and xanthones	pochonin B (**50**)	Tutuila, American Samoa	*H. fuscoatra*	EC_{50}—In Vitro Model of HIV-1 Latency-high-throughput primary cell-based HIV-1 latency assay	39.6 µM	**anti-HIV-1**; reactivation of latent viral loads in CD4+ T-cells	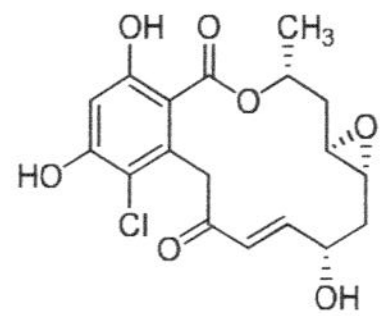	[110]
Auxiliary therapy to HAART therapy—fish oil	pochonin C (**51**)	Tutuila, American Samoa	*H. fuscoatra*	EC_{50}—In Vitro Model of HIV-1 Latency-high-throughput primary cell-based HIV-1 latency assay	6.3 µM	**anti-HIV-1**; reactivation of latent viral loads in CD4+ T-cells	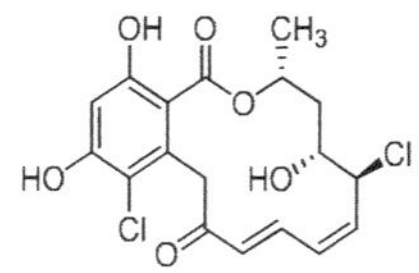	[110]
Others	truncateol O (**52**)	Yongxing Island, Hainan Province of China	sponge-associated fungus *Truncatella angustata*	IC_{50}—Anti-HIV bioassays-VSV-G pseudotyped HIV-1–Luciferase assay system	39 µM	**anti-HIV-1**; inhibition of the HIV replication	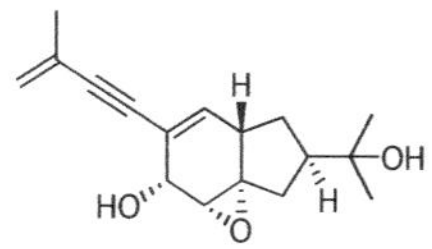	[111]
	truncateol P (**53**)	Yongxing Island, Hainan Province of China	sponge-associated fungus *Truncatella angustata*	IC_{50}—Anti-HIV bioassays-VSV-G pseudotyped HIV-1–Luciferase assay system	16.1 µM	**anti-HIV-1**; inhibition of the HIV replication	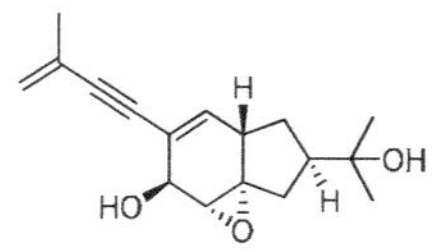	[111]

[a] Tripeptide conjugates of chitosan (a natural marine byproduct), prepared in the laboratory.

Marine sponges are not the sole source of bioactive proteins. For example, Jang et al. reported about a new small hydroxyproline-rich peptide from Alaska Pollack collagen (APHCP, **21**, Figure 8) that exhibits a unique antiviral activity [94]. This peptide is a Gly-Pro-Hyp-Gly-Pro-Hyp-Gly-Pro-Hyp-Gly peptide, and the authors showed that the most important part of a peptide for anti-HIV activity is the hydroxyl group at hydroxyproline, whereas a peptide with only prolines does not exhibit antiviral activity. Its anti-HIV 1 mode of action is manifested through the inhibition of the induced syncytia formation by the interference of an HIV fusion, inhibition of cell lysis, RT activity, and the production of the p24 antigen. It was shown that APHCP can decrease the HIV-1 induced cell lysis at a potency around EC_{50} of 459 μM (EC_{50} against anti-HIV-1 induced cell lysis—MTT assay). Additionally, through the inhibition of the viral RT at EC_{50} at 374 μM, this peptide's crucial role in the inhibition of the conversion of viral RNA to DNA was also confirmed. With EC_{50} of 405 μM, this compound effectively suppressed the p24 production in viral cells, as determined by the Western blot analysis.

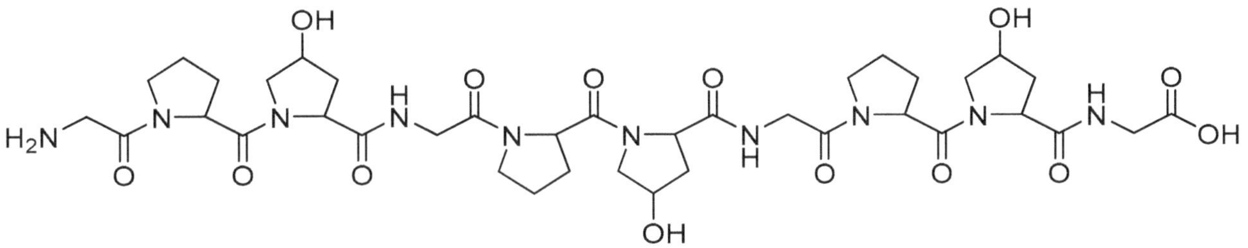

21

Figure 8. Structure of the Alaska Pollack collagen hydroxyl proline (APCHP) peptide (**21**).

Similarly, one new anti-HIV peptide was isolated from *Spirulina maxima* (SM-peptide) [95]–the Leu-Asp-Ala-Val-Asn-Arg peptide, and the authors showed its HIV-1 infection inhibition in a human T cell line MT4. The peptide inhibited cell lysis, p24 antigen production, and HIV-1 RT. Specifically, IC_{50} (obtained by a cell viability assay) against an anti-HIV 1 infection was determined as 0.691 mM, the inhibition of the HIV-1-induced RT activation (RT assay kit) in MT4 cells was at a high 90% at a concentration of 1.093 mM, and the p24 production (p24 antigen production assay) was inhibited at 95% at a concentration of 1.093 mM.

2.5. Alkaloids

Marine organisms are well-established sources of natural alkaloids. Although the term 'alkaloid' seems puzzling and is prone to scientific controversy, alkaloids are generally defined as nitrogen-containing compounds derived from plants and animals. Relatively few alkaloids from marine sources have been found to possess antiretroviral properties and, so far, none have found their clinical use.

Aspernigrin C (**22**, Figure 9) and malformin C (**23,** Figure 9) have been isolated from marine-derived black aspergili, *Aspergillus niger* SCSIO Jcw6F30, and their inhibitory activity against the chemokine receptor subtype 5 (CCR5) tropic HIV-1 SF162 has been evaluated. They show potent inhibition of infection with IC_{50} values 4.7 ± 0.4 μM and 1.4 ± 0.06 μM, which is comparable to the nucleoside reverse transcriptase inhibitor—abacavir (IC_{50} = 0.8 ± 0.1 μM) and the HIV-1 entry inhibitor ADS-J1 (IC_{50} = 0.8 ± 0.1 μM). In comparison to other aspernigrins, it has been suggested that the 2-methylsuccinic moiety is responsible for the potency of aspernigrin C [96].

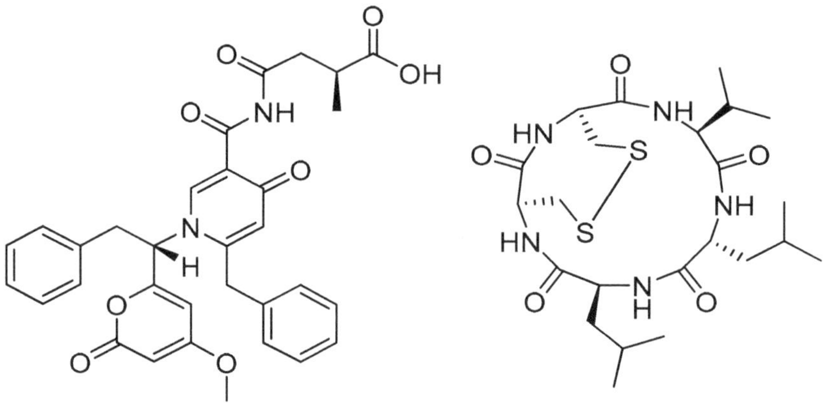

22 23

Figure 9. Structures of aspernigrin C (**22**) and malformin C (**23**).

Thiodiketopiperazine-type alkaloids, eutypellazines A-M, isolated from the EtOAc extract of the fermentation broth of deep-sea sediment fungus *Eutypella sp.* shows potent inhibitory effects against pNL4.3.Env-.Luc co-transfected 293T HIV model cells. Eutypellazine E (**24**, Figure 10) exerts activity in a low micromolar range (IC_{50} = 3.2 ± 0.4 μM), while eutypellazine J (**25**, Figure 10) shows a reactivating effect toward latent HIV-1 in J-Lat A2 cells. This could be used as a promising strategy to expunge the HIV-1 infection by activating latent virus cellular reservoirs in combination with HAART [97].

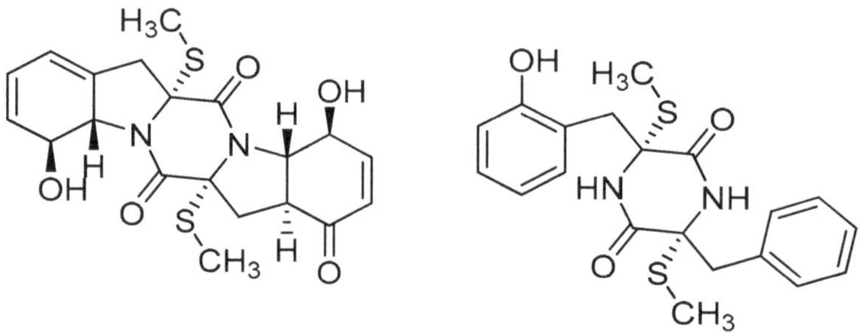

24 25

Figure 10. Structures of eutypellazine E (**24**) and eutypellazine J (**25**).

The *S. carteri* Red Sea sponge extract yields three previously characterized compounds: debromohymenialdisine (DBH) (**26**, Figure 11), hymenialdisine (HD) (**27**, Figure 11), and oroidin (**28**, Figure 11). DBH and HD exhibited a 30–40% inhibition of HIV-1 at 3.1 μM and 13 μM but with associated cytotoxicity. Conversely, oroidin displayed a 50% inhibition of viral replication at 50 μM without observed cytotoxicity. Also, it showed inhibition of HIV-1 reverse transcriptase up to 90% at 25 μMc [98].

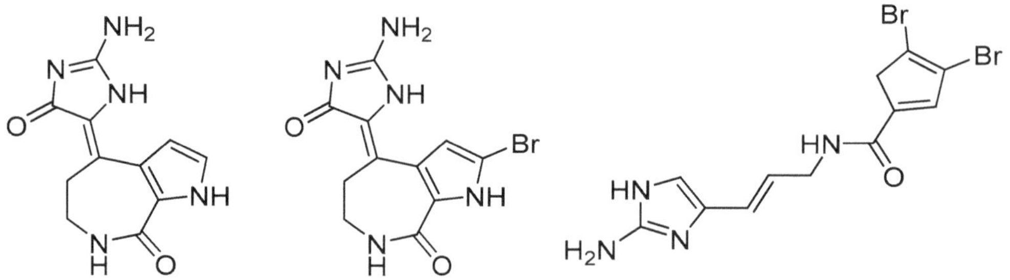

26 27 28

Figure 11. Structures of debromohymenialdisine (**26**), 10Z-hymenialdisine (**27**), and oroidin (**28**).

The two known alkaloids of the aaptamine family containing 1*H*-benz[*de*]-1,6-naphthyridine skeleton, namely 3-(phenetylamino)demethyl(oxy)aaptamine (**29**, Figure 12) and 3-(isopentylamino)demethyl(oxy)aaptamine (**30**, Figure 11), were isolated from the sponge *A. aptos*. They exhibited anti-HIV activity, with inhibitory rates of 88.0% and 72.3%, respectively, at a concentration of 10 μM [99].

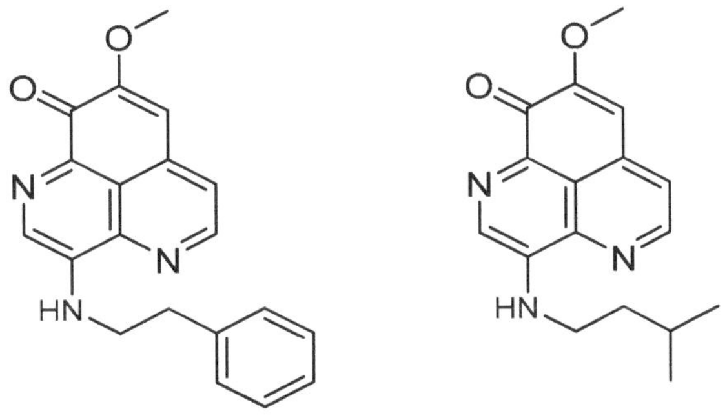

29 **30**

Figure 12. Structures of 3-(phenetylamino)dimethyl(oxo)aaptamine (**29**) and 3-(isopentylamino)dimethyl (oxo)aaptamine (**30**).

Bengamide A (**31**, Figure 13), haliclonycyclamine A+B (**32**, Figure 13) and keramamine C (**33**, Figure 13) inhibit HIV-1 with a 50% effective concentration of 3.8 μM or less. The most potent among them, bengamide A, blocked HIV-1 in a T cell line with an EC_{50} of 0.015 μM (which was comparable to control antiretrovirals indinavir 0.029 μM, efavirenz 0.0024 μM, and raltegravir 0.011 μM) and in peripheral blood mononuclear cells with EC_{50} of 0.032 μM. It was concluded that HIV-1 LTR NF-κB response elements are required for a bengamide A-mediated inhibition of LTR-dependent gene expression [100].

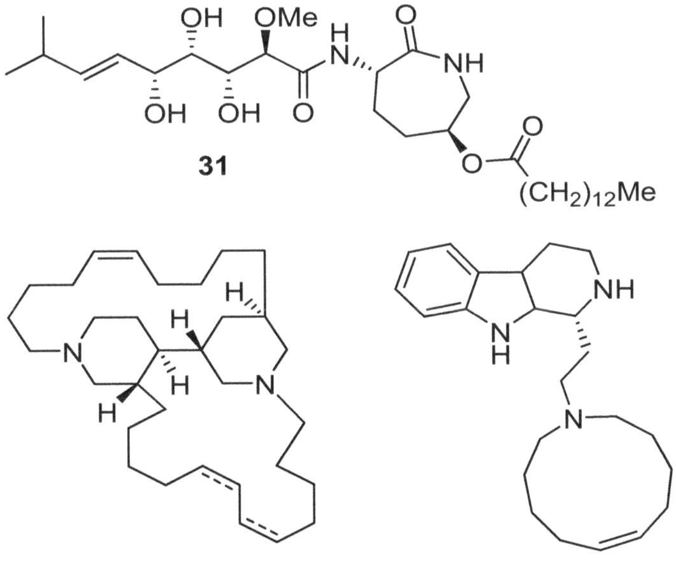

32 **33**

Figure 13. Structures of bengamide A (**31**), haliclonacyclamines A + B (**32**), keramamine C (**33**).

Phenylspirodrimane, stachybotrin D (**34**, Figure 14) isolated from the sponge-derived fungus *Stachybotrys chartarum* MXH-X73, was discovered to be a HIV-1 *RT* inhibitor, which showed inhibitory effects on the wild type (EC_{50} 8.4 μM) and five NNRTI-resistant HIV-1 strains (EC_{50} 7.0; 23.8; 13.3; 14.2; 6.2 μM) [101].

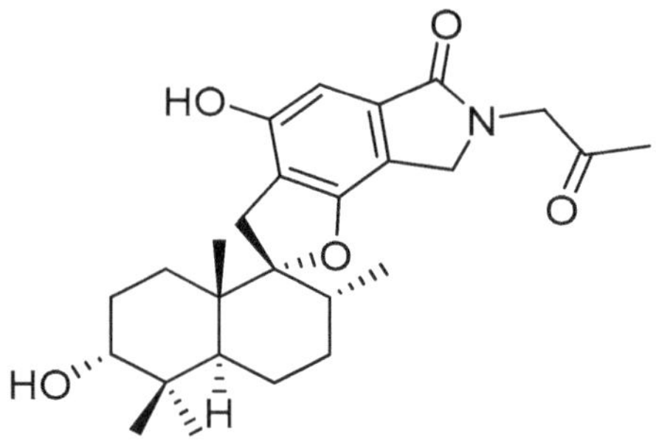

34

Figure 14. Structure of stachybotrin D (**34**).

2.6. Diterpenes

Many terpenes from marine natural products demonstrated anti-HIV properties. Mechanisms of action involve blocking of different steps of the HIV-1 replicative cycle as reverse transcriptase inhibitors, protease inhibitors, or entry inhibitors. Among them, diterpenes from marine algae are nowadays in the spotlight due to their promising anti-HIV activities [102]. Dolabellane diterpenes are compounds from the diterpene group that have recently been extensively studied for their anti-HIV activity. Pardo-Vargas et al. characterized three new dolabellane diterpenes isolated from the marine brown alga *Dictyota pfaffii* from Northeast Brazil: (1R*,2E,4R*,7S,10S*,11S*,12R*)10,18-diacetoxy-7-hydroxy-2,8(17)-dolabelladiene, (1R*,2E,4R*,7R*,10S*,11S*,12R*)10,18-diacetoxy-7-hydroxy-2,8(17)-dolabelladiene, (1R*,2E,4R*,8E,10S*,11S,12R*)10,18-diacetoxy-7-hydroxy-2,8-dolabelladiene, named dolabelladienols A–C (**35–37**, Figure 15), respectively [102]. In particular, the new compounds, dolabelladienols A and B, showed potent anti-HIV-1 activities that can be confirmed with their low IC_{50} values of 2.9 and 4.1 μM and low cytotoxic activity against MT-2 lymphocyte tumor cells. These promising anti-HIV-1 agents were even more active than previously known 2,6-dolabelladienes series.

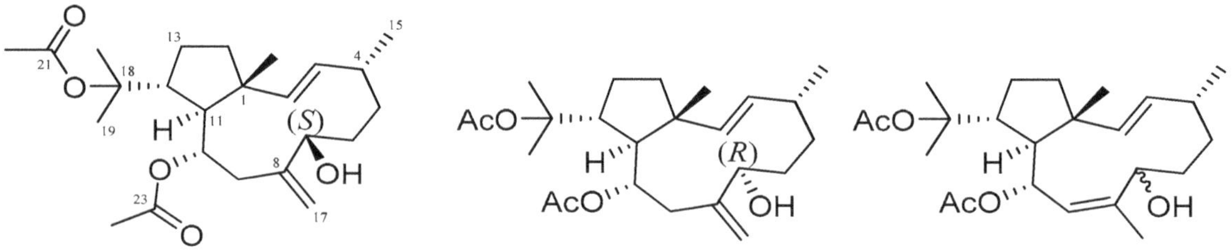

35 **36** **37**

Figure 15. Structures of the new dolabellane diterpenoids dolabelladienols A–C (**35–37**).

De Souza Barros et al. tested marine dolastanes (**38**, **40**, Figure 16) and secodolastane diterpenes (**39**, Figure 16) isolated from the brown alga *Canistrocarpus cervicornis* for anti-HIV-1 activity [103]. They observed that the marine diterpenes **38–40** inhibit the HIV-1 replication in a dose-dependent manner (EC_{50} values of 0.35, 3.67, and 0.794 μM) without a cytotoxic effect (CC_{50} values ranging from 935 to 1910 μM). Additionally, they investigated the virucidal effect of these diterpenes and their potential use as microbicides. Dolastane-diterpenes **38** and **40** showed a potent effect on HIV-1 infectivity, whereas no virucidal effect was observed for secodolastane diterpene **39**, demonstrating another mechanism of antiretroviral activity. Therefore, the authors suggested a potential use of marine dolastanes **38** and **40** as microbicides that could directly inhibit virus infectivity and possibly act before the virus penetrates the target cells [103].

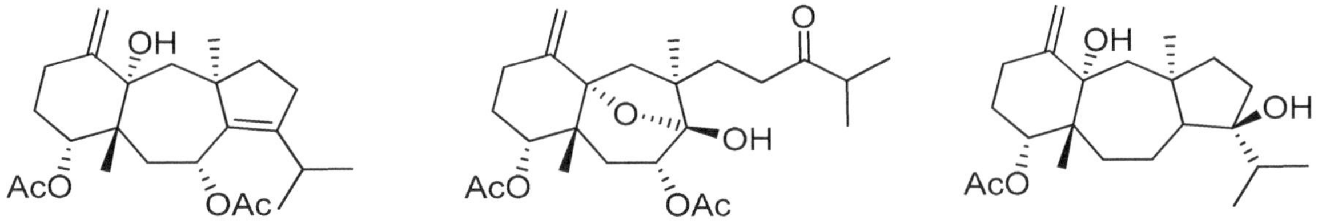

38 39 40

Figure 16. Structures of marine dolastanes (**38** and **40**) and secodolastane diterpene (**39**) derived from *Canistrocarpus cervicornis*.

Dolabelladienetriol from brown alga *Dictyota* spp has also been evaluated as a potential microbicide against HIV-1 in tissue explants. Namely, Stephens et al. examined the 8,10,18-trihydroxy-2,6-dolabelladiene (**41**, Figure 17) in pretreated peripheral blood cells (PBMC) and macrophages along with their protective effect in the ex vivo explant model of the uterine cervix [104]. Pre-treatment of peripheral PBMC and macrophages with dolabelladienotriol showed inhibitory effects on HIV-1 replication. Furthermore, in the explant model dolabelladienetriol inhibited viral replication in a dose-dependent manner from 20 to 99% in concentrations of 0.15 and 14.4 μM without a loss in the viability of the tissue. The authors concluded that this compound has great potential as a possible microbicide. The same compound was also theoretically analyzed as an inhibitor of the wild-type and mutants' HIV-1 reverse transcriptase [105]. Firstly, the structure-activity relationship studies revealed that a low dipole moment and high HOMO (highest occupied molecular orbital)-LUMO (lowest unoccupied molecular orbital) gap values are related to the antiviral activity. Secondly, molecular docking studies with RT wild-type and mutants showed a seahorse-like conformation of 8,10,18-trihydroxy-2,6-dolabelladiene, hydrophobic interactions, and hydrogen bonds with important residues of the binding pocket. Finally, the authors suggested a new derivative of the 8,10,18-trihydroxy-2,6-dolabelladiene with an aromatic moiety in the double bond to improve its biological activity.

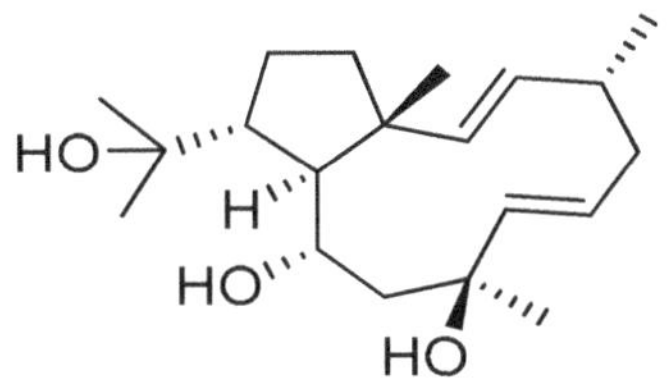

Figure 17. Structure of (1*R*,2*E*,4*R*,6*E*,8*S*,10*S*,11*S*,12*R*)-8,10,18-trihydroxy-2,6-dolabelladiene (**41**).

Although dolabellane diterpenes of brown alga *Dictyota* spp showed a strong anti-HIV-1 activity, this was not confirmed for dolabellane diterpenes isolated from octocorals. Therefore, some chemical transformations have been conducted to improve the anti-HIV-1 potency of the main dolabellane 13-keto-1(*R*),11(*S*)-dolabella-3(*E*),7(*E*),12(18)-triene from Caribbean octocoral *Eunicea laciniata* [106]. Oxygenated dolabellanes derivatives (**42–44**, Figure 18), obtained by epoxidation, epoxide opening, and allylic oxidation of ketodolbellatriene have shown significantly improved antiviral activities and a low cytotoxicity to MT-2 cells, which makes them promising antiviral compounds.

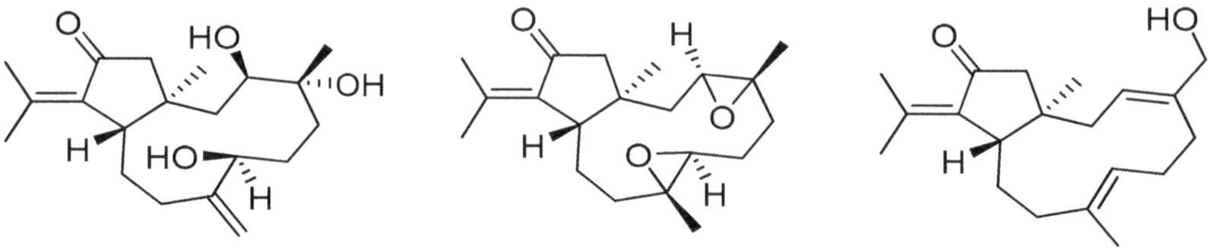

Figure 18. Structures of semi-synthesized oxygenated dolabellanes (**42**–**44**) originally isolated from the Caribbean octocoral *Eunicea laciniata*.

2.7. Phlorotannins and Xanthones

Phlorotannins are tannin derivatives made from several phloroglucinol units linked to each other in different ways. Phlorotannins contain phenyl linkage (fucols), ether linkage (fuhalols and phlorethols), phenyl and ether linkage (fucophloroethols), and dibenzodioxin linkage (eckols) [86,107]. So far, a series of phlorotannins have been identified with potent anti-HIV activity. For example, 8,8′-bieckol and 6,6′-bieckol from marine brown alga *Ecklonia cava* has shown an enhanced HIV-1 inhibitory effect [112,113]. Karadeniz et al. reported that 8,4′′′-dieckol (**45**, Figure 19) is another phlorotannin derivative isolated from the same brown alga that could be used as a drug candidate for the development of new generation anti-HIV therapeutic agents [107]. The compound showed HIV-1 inhibitory activity at noncytotoxic concentrations. More precisely, the results indicated that 8,4′′′-dieckol inhibited the cytopathic effects of HIV-1, including HIV-1 induced syncytia formation, lytic effects, and viral p24 antigen production. Furthermore, 8,4′′′-dieckol inhibited an HIV-1 entry and RT enzyme with the inhibition ratio of 91% at a concentration of 50 μM.

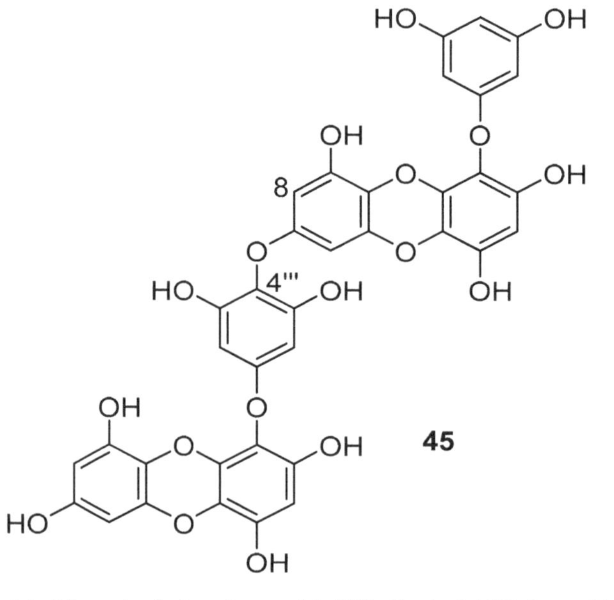

Figure 19. Chemical structure of 8,4′′′-dieckol (**45**) from *E. cava*.

Recently, for the first time, xanthone dimer was identified as a potential anti-HIV-1 agent [108]. Xanthones are secondary metabolites from higher plant families, fungi, and lichen [114,115]. Although structurally related to flavonoids, xanthones are not as frequently encountered in nature [9]. Penicillixanthone A (PXA) (**46**, Figure 20), a natural xanthone dimer, has been isolated from the jellyfish-derived fungus *Aspergillus fumigates* with fourteen other natural products [108]. However, only penicillixanthone A showed inhibitory activities in an HIV infection. Marine-derived PXA displayed potent anti-HIV-1 activity against CCR5-tropic HIV-1 SF162 and CXCR4-tropic HIV-1 NL4-3, with IC_{50} of 0.36 and 0.26 μM, respectively. A molecular docking study confirmed that PXA might bind to either CCR5 or CXCR4 to prevent HIV entry into target cells. Therefore, PXA, as a CCR5/CXCR4 dual-coreceptor antagonist, may be seen as a new potential lead product type for the development of anti-HIV therapeutics.

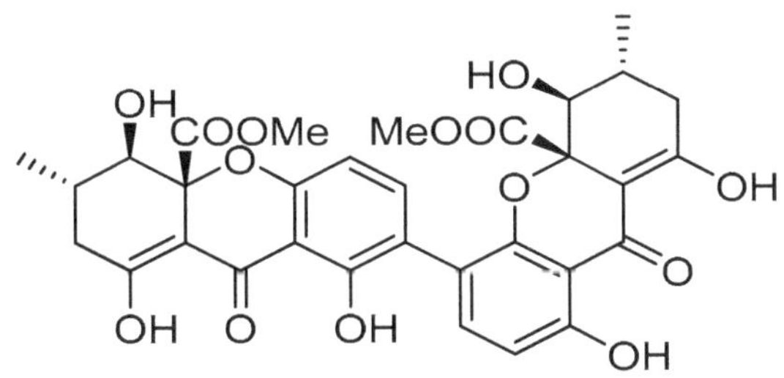

46

Figure 20. Structure of penicillixanthone A (**46**).

2.8. Fish Oil as an Adjuvant to HAART Therapy

HAART therapy can cause severe side effects, e.g., insulin resistance, lipoatrophy, dyslipidemia, and abnormalities of fat distribution. Therefore, finding an adequate diet and supplementation to lower the negative effects of the HAART combination therapy is desirable [116]. Fish oil contains omega-3 polyunsaturated fatty acids (PUFA), eicosapentaenoic (EPA, 20:5n-3) (**47**, Figure 21) and docosahexaenoic (DHA, 22:6n-3) (**48**, Figure 21) acids, which may have beneficial effects for HIV-infected patients. It has been shown that the addition of fish oil to the diet of HIV-infected individuals receiving usual antiretroviral therapy can significantly lower serum triglycerides levels [117], which is highly relevant knowing that HIV dyslipidemia is a serious problem related to an increased frequency of cardiovascular disease.

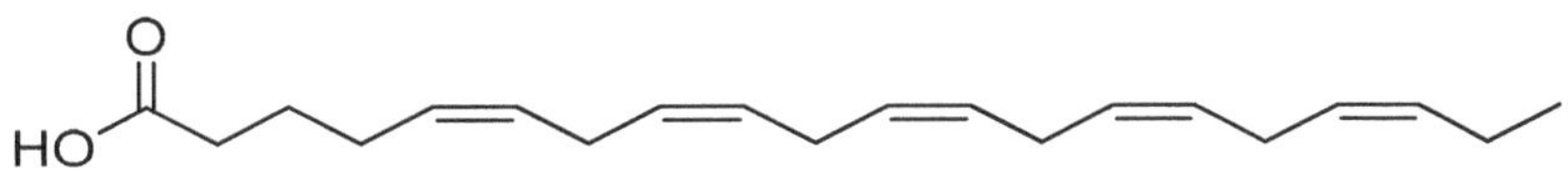

47

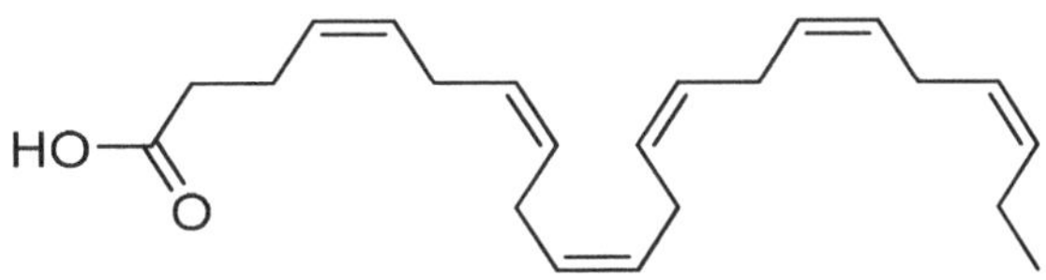

48

Figure 21. Structures of eicosapentanoic (**47**) and docosahexanoic acid (**48**).

Recently, He et al. analyzed the influence of DHA on the locomotor activity in ethanol-treated HIV-1 transgenic rats [109]. The prevalence of alcohol use and alcohol abuse in infected individuals is much higher, and numerous ethanol and HIV-1 viral proteins have synergistic effects on inflammation in the central nervous system [118–120]. HIV remains in the body in its latent form after HAART therapy and, as such, can induce neuroinflammation. DHA depletion has been found to be associated with various neurological abnormalities, and its administration can have a neuroprotective effect. DHA taken daily could reverse the effects of the ethanol negative effect on the locomotor activity in the presence of HIV viral proteins. An in vivo study, using real-time quantitative PCR, showed that the addition of DHA can reduce elevated levels of IL-6, IL-18, and increase the expression of NF-κB in the striatum. This proved the potential of this fish oil constituent as an adjuvant in HIV patients' treatment that can help in lowering the interactive effects of ethanol consumption during HIV infection.

2.9. Others

Resorcyclic acid lactones, namely radicicol (**49**, Figure 22) pochonin B (**50**, Figure 22) and C (**51**, Figure 22) isolated from *H. fuscoatra* exhibited a 92–98% reactivation efficiency of the latent HIV-1 relative to SAHA (subeoylanilide hydroxamic acid, vorinostat, HDAC inhibitor) and EC_{50} of 9.1, 39.6 and 6.3 μM [110]. The reactivation strategy is, indeed, a promising strategy to expunge the HIV-1 infection by reactivating latent viral loads, mainly in CD4 + T-cells, which quickly rebound when antiviral treatment is interrupted. It was noted that all active compounds contain Michael acceptor functionality. The PKC-independent mechanism of reactivation of the latent HIV-1 remains to be elucidated.

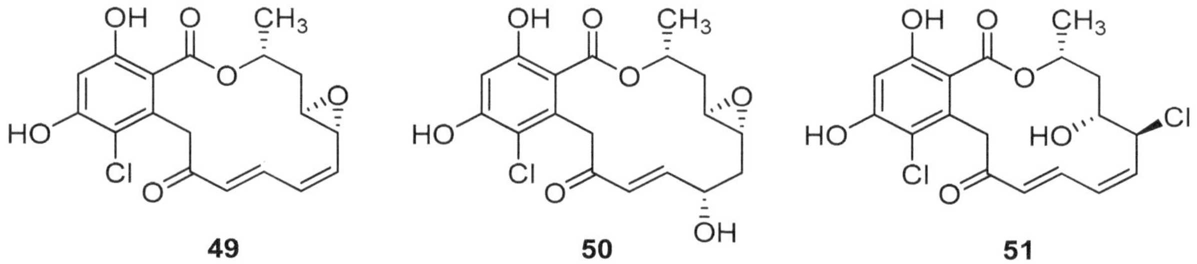

Figure 22. Structures of radicicol (**49**), pochonin B (**50**), pochonin C (**51**).

A team of researchers led by Zhao isolated new isoprenylated cyclohexanols from the sponge-associated fungus *Truncatella angustata* named truncateols O-V [111]. In vitro testing showed that truncateols O and P (**52** and **53**, Figure 23), analogues bearing the alkynyl group in the side chain, exhibit a significant inhibition toward the HIV-1 virus with IC_{50} values of 39.0 μM and 16.1 μM, respectively. These compounds could be considered as new anti-HIV lead compounds due to lower cytotoxicity (CC_{50} > 100 μM) in comparison with the positive control efavirenz (CC_{50} = 40.6 μM).

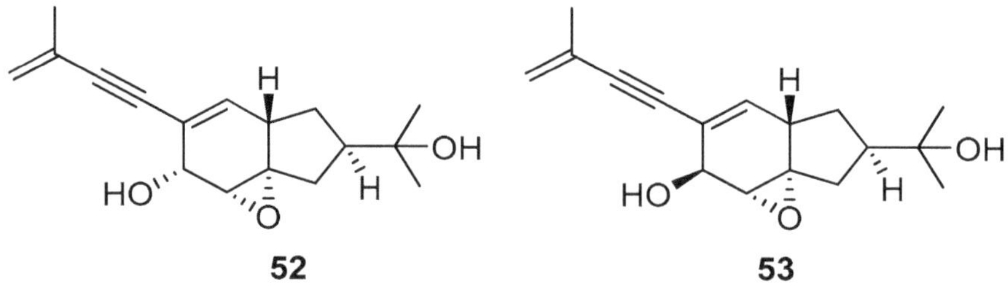

Figure 23. Structures of truncateols O (**52**) and P (**53**).

3. Future Directions in the Anti-HIV Marine Drug Development

Marine organisms have been acknowledged as a precious source of bioactive compounds that may provide novel anti-HIV structures or lead structures for structural optimization. A large amount of evidence from scientific research confirmed a high biological potential of these compounds to treat serious diseases, including infective ones. Some of the marine-derived bioactive compounds discovered much earlier have emerged with novel properties and potential applications after a decade or two. Isolation and structural elucidation of compounds from marine organisms is not an easy task and still carries challenges. Identification of all the compounds is a daunting task, especially with regards to complex structural motifs that may be present in a single marine extract. Taxonomic knowledge is still insufficient to enable unambiguous species classification that can result in the false prediction of chemical constituents and hamper structural analysis. Furthermore, a temporal lag between the discovery, chemical characterization, and associated pharmacological activities is quite common, and the majority of marine metabolites are usually tested for anticancer activity, whereas anti-HIV and other possible biological effects are neglected or mostly not performed due to a lack of funding. Targeted assays and in vivo analyses are similarly performed only for some of the potential candidates, while the translation into clinical trials remains very limited. Thus, the financial gap is certainly a relevant factor contributing to the slow drug development process in this area. In particular, the development of anti-HIV compounds, which act by mechanisms that differ from existing antivirals, requires a well-designed and focused approach to studying the mode of action. Libraries should be created for specifically defined crude extracts, their corresponding simplified fractions as well as for pure compounds for a well-balanced natural product discovery program. Additionally, there exist but few publications in which scientists have tried to modify known compounds of marine origin to improve their bioactivity. We are, however, continuously witnessing advancements in the deep-sea exploration technology, sampling strategies, genome sequencing, genome mining, genetic engineering, chemo-enzymatic synthesis, nanoscale NMR structure determination, and development and optimization of suitable fermentation strategies to ensure a continued supply of unique bioactive compounds from the oceans. Therefore, the grounds have been met for a broad, international effort based on scientific collaboration that would rely on well-equipped infrastructure and human resources as a prerequisite for a full advancement in the field and development of new drug candidates for the pharmaceutical market in the future.

Author Contributions: K.W. devised the main conceptual idea and, together with L.S. and Ž.P., wrote the manuscript parts related to medicinal chemistry. K.W. and Ž.P. performed literature searches and L.S. prepared the table. S.K.P. participated in the manuscript writing and wrote and discussed parts relevant for clinical applications, shaped the paper concept, and performed the final revision.

References

1. AVERT. Symptoms and Stages of HIV Infection. Available online: https://www.avert.org/about-hiv-aids/symptoms-stages (accessed on 12 April 2019).
2. HIV/AIDS. Available online: https://www.who.int/news-room/fact-sheets/detail/hiv-aids (accessed on 12 April 2019).
3. Li, G.; Piampongsant, S.; Faria, N.R.; Voet, A.; Pineda-Peña, A.-C.; Khouri, R.; Lemey, P.; Vandamme, A.-M.; Theys, K. An integrated map of HIV genome-wide variation from a population perspective. *Retrovirology* **2015**, *12*, 18. [CrossRef] [PubMed]
4. Saphire, A.C.S.; Bobardt, M.D.; Zhang, Z.; David, G.; Gallay, P.A. Syndecans Serve as Attachment Receptors for Human Immunodeficiency Virus Type 1 on Macrophages. *J. Virol.* **2001**, *75*, 9187–9200. [CrossRef] [PubMed]
5. Arthos, J.; Cicala, C.; Martinelli, E.; Macleod, K.; Van Ryk, D.; Wei, D.; Xiao, Z.; Veenstra, T.D.; Conrad, T.P.; Lempicki, R.A.; et al. HIV-1 envelope protein binds to and signals through integrin α4β7, the gut mucosal homing receptor for peripheral T cells. *Nat. Immunol.* **2008**, *9*, 301–309. [CrossRef] [PubMed]
6. Cicala, C.; Martinelli, E.; McNally, J.P.; Goode, D.J.; Gopaul, R.; Hiatt, J.; Jelicic, K.; Kottilil, S.; Macleod, K.; O'Shea, A.; et al. The integrin $\alpha_4\beta_7$ forms a complex with cell-surface CD4 and defines a T-cell subset that is highly susceptible to infection by HIV-1. *PNAS* **2009**, *106*, 20877–20882. [CrossRef] [PubMed]
7. Geijtenbeek, T.B.; Kwon, D.S.; Torensma, R.; van Vliet, S.J.; van Duijnhoven, G.C.; Middel, J.; Cornelissen, I.L.; Nottet, H.S.; KewalRamani, V.N.; Littman, D.R.; et al. DC-SIGN, a dendritic cell-specific HIV-1-binding protein that enhances trans-infection of T cells. *Cell* **2000**, *100*, 587–597. [CrossRef]
8. Orloff, G.M.; Orloff, S.L.; Kennedy, M.S.; Maddon, P.J.; McDougal, J.S. Penetration of CD4 T cells by HIV-1. The CD4 receptor does not internalize with HIV, and CD4-related signal transduction events are not required for entry. *J. Immunol.* **1991**, *146*, 2578–2587. [PubMed]
9. Maddon, P.J.; Dalgleish, A.G.; McDougal, J.S.; Clapham, P.R.; Weiss, R.A.; Axel, R. The T4 gene encodes the AIDS virus receptor and is expressed in the immune system and the brain. *Cell* **1986**, *47*, 333–348. [CrossRef]
10. McDougal, J.; Kennedy, M.; Sligh, J.; Cort, S.; Mawle, A.; Nicholson, J. Binding of HTLV-III/LAV to T4+ T cells by a complex of the 110K viral protein and the T4 molecule. *Science* **1986**, *231*, 382–385. [CrossRef]
11. Alkhatib, G. The biology of CCR5 and CXCR4. *Curr. Opin. HIV AIDS* **2009**, *4*, 96–103. [CrossRef]
12. Okoye, A.A.; Picker, L.J. CD4(+) T-cell depletion in HIV infection: Mechanisms of immunological failure. *Immunol. Rev.* **2013**, *254*, 54–64. [CrossRef]

13. Schrager, L.K.; D'Souza, M.P. Cellular and anatomical reservoirs of HIV-1 in patients receiving potent antiretroviral combination therapy. *JAMA* **1998**, *280*, 67–71. [CrossRef] [PubMed]
14. Berkhout, B.; Eggink, D.; Sanders, R.W. Is there a future for antiviral fusion inhibitors? *Curr. Opin. Virol.* **2012**, *2*, 50–59. [CrossRef] [PubMed]
15. Greenberg, M.L.; Cammack, N. Resistance to enfuvirtide, the first HIV fusion inhibitor. *J. Antimicrob. Chemother.* **2004**, *54*, 333–340. [CrossRef] [PubMed]
16. Baldwin, C.E.; Sanders, R.W.; Deng, Y.; Jurriaans, S.; Lange, J.M.; Lu, M.; Berkhout, B. Emergence of a drug-dependent human immunodeficiency virus type 1 variant during therapy with the T20 fusion inhibitor. *J. Virol.* **2004**, *78*, 12428–12437. [CrossRef] [PubMed]
17. Rimsky, L.T.; Shugars, D.C.; Matthews, T.J. Determinants of human immunodeficiency virus type 1 resistance to gp41-derived inhibitory peptides. *J. Virol.* **1998**, *72*, 986–993. [PubMed]
18. Abner, E.; Jordan, A. HIV "shock and kill" therapy: In need of revision. *Antiviral Res.* **2019**, *166*, 19–34. [CrossRef]
19. Hütter, G.; Nowak, D.; Mossner, M.; Ganepola, S.; Müßig, A.; Allers, K.; Schneider, T.; Hofmann, J.; Kücherer, C.; Blau, O.; et al. Long-Term Control of HIV by CCR5 Delta32/Delta32 Stem-Cell Transplantation. *N. Engl. J. Med.* **2009**, *360*, 692–698. [CrossRef] [PubMed]
20. Ananworanich, J.; Robb, M.L. The transient HIV remission in the Mississippi baby: Why is this good news? *J. Int. AIDS Soc.* **2014**, *17*, 19859. [CrossRef]
21. The Lancet HIV. Like London buses, two putative cure cases arrive at once. *Lancet HIV* **2019**, *6*, e205. [CrossRef]
22. Newman, D.J.; Cragg, G.M. Natural Products as Sources of New Drugs from 1981 to 2014. *J. Nat. Prod.* **2016**, *79*, 629–661. [CrossRef]
23. Erakovic Haber, V.; Spaventi, R. Discovery and Development of Novel Drugs. In *Progress in Molecular and Subcellular Biology*; Springer: Cham, Switzerland, 2017; Volume 55, pp. 91–104.
24. Blunt, J.W.; Copp, B.R.; Hu, W.-P.; Munro, M.H.G.; Northcote, P.T.; Prinsep, M.R. Marine natural products. *Nat. Prod. Rep.* **2009**, *26*, 170. [CrossRef] [PubMed]
25. Mori, T.; O'Keefe, B.R.; Sowder, R.C.; Bringans, S.; Gardella, R.; Berg, S.; Cochran, P.; Turpin, J.A.; Buckheit, R.W.; McMahon, J.B.; et al. Isolation and Characterization of Griffithsin, a Novel HIV-inactivating Protein, from the Red Alga *Griffithsia* sp. *J. Biol. Chem.* **2005**, *280*, 9345–9353. [CrossRef] [PubMed]
26. Xue, J.; Gao, Y.; Hoorelbeke, B.; Kagiampakis, I.; Zhao, B.; Demeler, B.; Balzarini, J.; Liwang, P.J. The role of individual carbohydrate-binding sites in the function of the potent anti-HIV lectin griffithsin. *Mol. Pharm.* **2012**, *9*, 2613–2625. [CrossRef] [PubMed]
27. Huang, X.; Jin, W.; Griffin, G.E.; Shattock, R.J.; Hu, Q. Removal of two high-mannose N-linked glycans on gp120 renders human immunodeficiency virus 1 largely resistant to the carbohydrate-binding agent griffithsin. *J. Gen. Virol.* **2011**, *92*, 2367–2373. [CrossRef] [PubMed]
28. Xue, J.; Hoorelbeke, B.; Kagiampakis, I.; Demeler, B.; Balzarini, J.; Liwang, P.J. The griffithsin dimer is required for high-potency inhibition of HIV-1: Evidence for manipulation of the structure of gp120 as part of the griffithsin dimer mechanism. *Antimicrob. Agents Chemother.* **2013**, *57*, 3976–3989. [CrossRef] [PubMed]
29. Gerwick, W.H.; Moore, B.S. Lessons from the Past and Charting the Future of Marine Natural Products Drug Discovery and Chemical Biology. *Chem. Biol.* **2012**, *19*, 85–98. [CrossRef] [PubMed]
30. Martins, A.; Vieira, H.; Gaspar, H.; Santos, S.; Martins, A.; Vieira, H.; Gaspar, H.; Santos, S. Marketed Marine Natural Products in the Pharmaceutical and Cosmeceutical Industries: Tips for Success. *Mar. Drugs* **2014**, *12*, 1066–1101. [CrossRef] [PubMed]
31. Karagozlu, M.Z.; Karadeniz, F.; Kim, S.-K. Anti-HIV activities of novel synthetic peptide conjugated chitosan oligomers. *Int. J. Biol. Macromol.* **2014**, *66*, 260–266. [CrossRef] [PubMed]
32. Ramana, L.N.; Sharma, S.; Sethuraman, S.; Ranga, U.; Krishnan, U.M. Evaluation of chitosan nanoformulations as potent anti-HIV therapeutic systems. *Biochim. Biophys. Acta* **2014**, *1840*, 476–484. [CrossRef]
33. Shohani, S.; Mondanizadeh, M.; Abdoli, A.; Khansarinejad, B.; Salimi-Asl, M.; Ardestani, M.; Ghanbari, M.; Haj, M.; Zabihollahi, R. Trimethyl Chitosan Improves Anti-HIV Effects of Atripla as a New Nanoformulated Drug. *Curr. HIV Res.* **2017**, *15*, 56–65. [CrossRef]
34. Cheung, R.C.F.; Ng, T.B.; Wong, J.H.; Chan, W.Y. Chitosan: An Update on Potential Biomedical and Pharmaceutical Applications. *Mar. Drugs* **2015**, *13*, 5156–5186. [CrossRef] [PubMed]

35. Wijesekara, I.; Pangestuti, R.; Kim, S.-K. Biological activities and potential health benefits of sulfated polysaccharides derived from marine algae. *Carbohydr. Polym.* **2011**, *84*, 14–21. [CrossRef]
36. Jiao, G.; Yu, G.; Zhang, J.; Ewart, H.S. Chemical structures and bioactivities of sulfated polysaccharides from marine algae. *Mar. Drugs* **2011**, *9*, 196–223. [CrossRef] [PubMed]
37. Gupta, S.; Abu-Ghannam, N. Recent developments in the application of seaweeds or seaweed extracts as a means for enhancing the safety and quality attributes of foods. *Innov. Food Sci. Emerg. Technol.* **2011**, *12*, 600–609. [CrossRef]
38. Aquino, R.S.; Grativol, C.; Mourão, P.A.S. Rising from the Sea: Correlations between Sulfated Polysaccharides and Salinity in Plants. *PLoS ONE* **2011**, *6*, e18862. [CrossRef]
39. Torode, T.A.; Marcus, S.E.; Jam, M.; Tonon, T.; Blackburn, R.S.; Hervé, C.; Knox, J.P. Monoclonal Antibodies Directed to Fucoidan Preparations from Brown Algae. *PLoS One* **2015**, *10*, e0118366. [CrossRef] [PubMed]
40. Deniaud-Bouët, E.; Kervarec, N.; Michel, G.; Tonon, T.; Kloareg, B.; Hervé, C. Chemical and enzymatic fractionation of cell walls from Fucales: Insights into the structure of the extracellular matrix of brown algae. *Ann. Bot.* **2014**, *114*, 1203–1216. [CrossRef]
41. Adhikari, U.; Mateu, C.G.; Chattopadhyay, K.; Pujol, C.A.; Damonte, E.B.; Ray, B. Structure and antiviral activity of sulfated fucans from Stoechospermum marginatum. *Phytochemistry* **2006**, *67*, 2474–2482. [CrossRef]
42. Zhang, H.; Wang, J.-Q.; Nie, S.-P.; Wang, Y.-X.; Cui, S.W.; Xie, M.-Y. Sulfated modification, characterization and property of a water-insoluble polysaccharide from Ganoderma atrum. *Int. J. Biol. Macromol.* **2015**, *79*, 248–255. [CrossRef]
43. Witvrouw, M.; De Clercq, E. Sulfated polysaccharides extracted from sea algae as potential antiviral drugs. *Gen. Pharmacol.* **1997**, *29*, 497–511. [CrossRef]
44. Meiyu, G.; Fuchuan, L.; Xianliang, X.; Jing, L.; Zuowei, Y.; Huashi, G. The potential molecular targets of marine sulfated polymannuroguluronate interfering with HIV-1 entry. Interaction between SPMG and HIV-1 rgp120 and CD4 molecule. *Antiviral Res.* **2003**, *59*, 127–135. [CrossRef]
45. Damonte, E.B.; Matulewicz, M.C.; Cerezo, A.S. Sulfated seaweed polysaccharides as antiviral agents. *Curr. Med. Chem.* **2004**, *11*, 2399–2419. [CrossRef] [PubMed]
46. Witvrouw, M.; Schols, D.; Andrei, G.; Snoeck, R.; Ikeda, S.; Pauwels, R.; Van Schepdael, A.; Arnout, J.; Claes, P.; Desmyter, J.; et al. New Polyacetal Polysulphate Active against Human Immunodeficiency Virus and other Enveloped Viruses. *Antivir. Chem. Chemother.* **1992**, *3*, 351–360. [CrossRef]
47. Parish, C.R.; Jakobsen, K.B.; Coombe, D.R.; Bacic, A. Isolation and characterization of cell adhesion molecules from the marine sponge, Ophlitaspongia tenuis. *Biochim. Biophys. Acta* **1991**, *1073*, 56–64. [CrossRef]
48. Lynch, G.; Low, L.; Li, S.; Sloane, A.; Adams, S.; Parish, C.; Kemp, B.; Cunningham, A.L. Sulfated polyanions prevent HIV infection of lymphocytes by disruption of the CD4-gp120 interaction, but do not inhibit monocyte infection. *J. Leukoc. Biol.* **1994**, *56*, 266–272. [CrossRef] [PubMed]
49. Talyshinsky, M.M.; Souprun, Y.Y.; Huleihel, M.M. Anti-viral activity of red microalgal polysaccharides against retroviruses. *Cancer Cell Int.* **2002**, *2*, 8. [CrossRef] [PubMed]
50. Gerenčer, M.; Turecek, P.L.; Kistner, O.; Mitterer, A.; Savidis-Dacho, H.; Barrett, N.P. In vitro and in vivo anti-retroviral activity of the substance purified from the aqueous extract of *Chelidonium majus* L. *Antiviral Res.* **2006**, *72*, 153–156. [CrossRef]
51. Neyts, J.; Snoeck, R.; Schols, D.; Balzarini, J.; Esko, J.D.; Van Schepdael, A.; De Clercq, E. Sulfated polymers inhibit the interaction of human cytomegalovirus with cell surface heparan sulfate. *Virology* **1992**, *189*, 48–58. [CrossRef]
52. Vidhyanandhini, R.; Saravanan, R.; Vairamani, S.; Shanmugam, A. The anticoagulant activity and structural characterization of fractionated and purified glycosaminoglycans from venerid clam Meretrix casta (Chemnitz). *J. Liq. Chromatogr. Relat. Technol.* **2014**, *37*, 917–929. [CrossRef]
53. Li, P.; Sheng, J.; Liu, Y.; Li, J.; Liu, J.; Wang, F. Heparosan-Derived Heparan Sulfate/Heparin-Like Compounds: One Kind of Potential Therapeutic Agents. *Med. Res. Rev.* **2013**, *33*, 665–692. [CrossRef]
54. Ahmadi, A.; Zorofchian Moghadamtousi, S.; Abubakar, S.; Zandi, K. Antiviral Potential of Algae Polysaccharides Isolated from Marine Sources: A Review. *Biomed. Res. Int.* **2015**, *2015*, 1–10. [CrossRef] [PubMed]
55. Rabanal, M.; Ponce, N.M.A.; Navarro, D.A.; Gómez, R.M.; Stortz, C.A. The system of fucoidans from the brown seaweed Dictyota dichotoma: Chemical analysis and antiviral activity. *Carbohydr. Polym.* **2014**, *101*, 804–811. [CrossRef] [PubMed]

56. Thuy, T.T.T.; Ly, B.M.; Van, T.T.T.; Van Quang, N.; Tu, H.C.; Zheng, Y.; Seguin-Devaux, C.; Mi, B.; Ai, U. Anti-HIV activity of fucoidans from three brown seaweed species. *Carbohydr. Polym.* **2015**, *115*, 122–128. [CrossRef] [PubMed]
57. Hoshino, T.; Hayashi, T.; Hayashi, K.; Hamada, J.; Lee, J.B.; Sankawa, U. An antivirally active sulfated polysaccharide from Sargassum horneri (TURNER) C. AGARDH. *Biol. Pharm. Bull.* **1998**, *21*, 730–734. [CrossRef] [PubMed]
58. Schaeffer, D.J.; Krylov, V.S. Anti-HIV Activity of Extracts and Compounds from Algae and Cyanobacteria. *Ecotoxicol. Environ. Saf.* **2000**, *45*, 208–227. [CrossRef] [PubMed]
59. Ueno, M.; Nogawa, M.; Siddiqui, R.; Watashi, K.; Wakita, T.; Kato, N.; Ikeda, M.; Okimura, T.; Isaka, S.; Oda, T.; et al. Acidic polysaccharides isolated from marine algae inhibit the early step of viral infection. *Int. J. Biol. Macromol.* **2019**, *124*, 282–290. [CrossRef]
60. Huang, N.; Wu, M.-Y.; Zheng, C.-B.; Zhu, L.; Zhao, J.-H.; Zheng, Y.-T. The depolymerized fucosylated chondroitin sulfate from sea cucumber potently inhibits HIV replication via interfering with virus entry. *Carbohydr. Res.* **2013**, *380*, 64–69. [CrossRef] [PubMed]
61. Lian, W.; Wu, M.; Huang, N.; Gao, N.; Xiao, C.; Li, Z.; Zhang, Z.; Zheng, Y.; Peng, W.; Zhao, J. Anti-HIV-1 activity and structure–activity-relationship study of a fucosylated glycosaminoglycan from an echinoderm by targeting the conserved CD4 induced epitope. *Biochim. Biophys. Acta* **2013**, *1830*, 4681–4691. [CrossRef]
62. Pirrone, V.; Wigdahl, B.; Krebs, F.C. The rise and fall of polyanionic inhibitors of the human immunodeficiency virus type 1. *Antiviral Res.* **2011**, *90*, 168–182. [CrossRef]
63. Torode, T.A.; Siméon, A.; Marcus, S.E.; Jam, M.; Le Moigne, M.-A.; Duffieux, D.; Knox, J.P.; Hervé, C. Dynamics of cell wall assembly during early embryogenesis in the brown alga Fucus. *J. Exp. Bot.* **2016**, *67*, 6089–6100. [CrossRef]
64. Raimundo, S.C.; Avci, U.; Hopper, C.; Pattathil, S.; Hahn, M.G.; Popper, Z.A. Immunolocalization of cell wall carbohydrate epitopes in seaweeds: Presence of land plant epitopes in Fucus vesiculosus L. (Phaeophyceae). *Planta* **2016**, *243*, 337–354. [CrossRef] [PubMed]
65. Andrade, L.R.; Leal, R.N.; Noseda, M.; Duarte, M.E.R.; Pereira, M.S.; Mourão, P.A.S.; Farina, M.; Amado Filho, G.M. Brown algae overproduce cell wall polysaccharides as a protection mechanism against the heavy metal toxicity. *Mar. Pollut. Bull.* **2010**, *60*, 1482–1488. [CrossRef]
66. Zvyagintseva, T.N.; Shevchenko, N.M.; Chizhov, A.O.; Krupnova, T.N.; Sundukova, E.V.; Isakov, V.V. Water-soluble polysaccharides of some far-eastern brown seaweeds. Distribution, structure, and their dependence on the developmental conditions. *J. Exp. Mar. Bio. Ecol.* **2003**, *294*, 1–13. [CrossRef]
67. Mak, W.; Hamid, N.; Liu, T.; Lu, J.; White, W.L. Fucoidan from New Zealand Undaria pinnatifida: Monthly variations and determination of antioxidant activities. *Carbohydr. Polym.* **2013**, *95*, 606–614. [CrossRef] [PubMed]
68. Fletcher, H.R.; Biller, P.; Ross, A.B.; Adams, J.M.M. The seasonal variation of fucoidan within three species of brown macroalgae. *Algal Res.* **2017**, *22*, 79–86. [CrossRef]
69. Stengel, D.B.; Connan, S.; Popper, Z.A. Algal chemodiversity and bioactivity: Sources of natural variability and implications for commercial application. *Biotechnol. Adv.* **2011**, *29*, 483–501. [CrossRef]
70. Fitton, J.H.; Stringer, D.N.; Karpiniec, S.S. Therapies from Fucoidan: An Update. *Mar. Drugs* **2015**, *13*, 5920–5946. [CrossRef]
71. Astronomo, R.D.; Burton, D.R. Carbohydrate vaccines: Developing sweet solutions to sticky situations? *Nat. Rev. Drug Discov.* **2010**, *9*, 308–324. [CrossRef]
72. Wang, Y.; Ye, X.-S.; Zhang, L.-H. Oligosaccharide assembly by one-pot multi-step strategy. *Org. Biomol. Chem.* **2007**, *5*, 2189. [CrossRef]
73. Astronomo, R.D.; Lee, H.-K.; Scanlan, C.N.; Pantophlet, R.; Huang, C.-Y.; Wilson, I.A.; Blixt, O.; Dwek, R.A.; Wong, C.-H.; Burton, D.R. A Glycoconjugate Antigen Based on the Recognition Motif of a Broadly Neutralizing Human Immunodeficiency Virus Antibody, 2G12, Is Immunogenic but Elicits Antibodies Unable To Bind to the Self Glycans of gp120. *J. Virol.* **2008**, *82*, 6359–6368. [CrossRef]
74. Luallen, R.J.; Lin, J.; Fu, H.; Cai, K.K.; Agrawal, C.; Mboudjeka, I.; Lee, F.-H.; Montefiori, D.; Smith, D.F.; Doms, R.W.; et al. An Engineered Saccharomyces cerevisiae Strain Binds the Broadly Neutralizing Human Immunodeficiency Virus Type 1 Antibody 2G12 and Elicits Mannose-Specific gp120-Binding Antibodies. *J. Virol.* **2008**, *82*, 6447–6457. [CrossRef] [PubMed]

75. Dunlop, D.C.; Ulrich, A.; Appelmelk, B.J.; Burton, D.R.; Dwek, R.A.; Zitzmann, N.; Scanlan, C.N. Antigenic mimicry of the HIV envelope by AIDS-associated pathogens. *AIDS* **2008**, *22*, 2214–2217. [CrossRef] [PubMed]
76. Joyce, J.G.; Krauss, I.J.; Song, H.C.; Opalka, D.W.; Grimm, K.M.; Nahas, D.D.; Esser, M.T.; Hrin, R.; Feng, M.; Dudkin, V.Y.; et al. An oligosaccharide-based HIV-1 2G12 mimotope vaccine induces carbohydrate-specific antibodies that fail to neutralize HIV-1 virions. *PNAS* **2008**, *105*, 15684–15689. [CrossRef] [PubMed]
77. Astronomo, R.D.; Kaltgrad, E.; Udit, A.K.; Wang, S.-K.; Doores, K.J.; Huang, C.-Y.; Pantophlet, R.; Paulson, J.C.; Wong, C.-H.; Finn, M.G.; et al. Defining Criteria for Oligomannose Immunogens for HIV Using Icosahedral Virus Capsid Scaffolds. *Chem. Biol.* **2010**, *17*, 357–370. [CrossRef] [PubMed]
78. Wang, S.-K.; Liang, P.-H.; Astronomo, R.D.; Hsu, T.-L.; Hsieh, S.-L.; Burton, D.R.; Wong, C.-H. Targeting the carbohydrates on HIV-1: Interaction of oligomannose dendrons with human monoclonal antibody 2G12 and DC-SIGN. *PNAS* **2008**, *105*, 3690–3695. [CrossRef] [PubMed]
79. Wang, L.-X. Toward oligosaccharide- and glycopeptide-based HIV vaccines. *Curr. Opin. Drug Discov. Devel.* **2006**, *9*, 194–206. [PubMed]
80. Kumar, K.K.; Reddy, G.S.; Reddy, B.; Shekar, P.C.; Sumanthi, J.; Chandra, K.I.P. Biological role of lectins: A review. *J. Orofac. Sci.* **2012**, *4*, 20. [CrossRef]
81. Balzarini, J. Inhibition of HIV entry by carbohydrate-binding proteins. *Antiviral Res.* **2006**, *71*, 237–247. [CrossRef]
82. Balzarini, J.; Neyts, J.; Schols, D.; Hosoya, M.; Van Damme, E.; Peumans, W.; De Clercq, E. The mannose-specific plant lectins from Cymbidium hybrid and Epipactis helleborine and the (N-acetylglucosamine)n-specific plant lectin from Urtica dioica are potent and selective inhibitors of human immunodeficiency virus and cytomegalovirus replication. *Antiviral Res.* **1992**, *18*, 191–207. [CrossRef]
83. Hansen, J.E.; Nielsen, C.M.; Nielsen, C.; Heegaard, P.; Mathiesen, L.R.; Nielsen, J.O. Correlation between carbohydrate structures on the envelope glycoprotein gp120 of HIV-1 and HIV-2 and syncytium inhibition with lectins. *AIDS* **1989**, *3*, 635–641. [CrossRef]
84. Sato, T.; Hori, K. Cloning, expression, and characterization of a novel anti-HIV lectin from the cultured cyanobacterium, Oscillatoria agardhii. *Fish. Sci.* **2009**, *75*, 743–753. [CrossRef]
85. Akkouh, O.; Ng, T.B.; Singh, S.S.; Yin, C.; Dan, X.; Chan, Y.S.; Pan, W.; Cheung, R.C.F. Lectins with anti-HIV activity: A review. *Molecules* **2015**, *20*, 648–668. [CrossRef] [PubMed]
86. Gogineni, V.; Schinazi, R.F.; Hamann, M.T. Role of Marine Natural Products in the Genesis of Antiviral Agents. *Chem. Rev.* **2015**, *115*, 9655–9706. [CrossRef] [PubMed]
87. Hirayama, M.; Shibata, H.; Imamura, K.; Sakaguchi, T.; Hori, K. High-Mannose Specific Lectin and Its Recombinants from a Carrageenophyta Kappaphycus alvarezii Represent a Potent Anti-HIV Activity Through High-Affinity Binding to the Viral Envelope Glycoprotein gp120. *Mar. Biotechnol.* **2016**, *18*, 144–160. [CrossRef] [PubMed]
88. Vo, T.-S.; Kim, S.-K. Potential Anti-HIV Agents from Marine Resources: An Overview. *Mar. Drugs* **2010**, *8*, 2871–2892. [CrossRef] [PubMed]
89. Cheung, R.C.F.; Ng, T.B.; Wong, J.H. Marine Peptides: Bioactivities and Applications. *Mar. Drugs* **2015**, *13*, 4006–4043. [CrossRef] [PubMed]
90. Qaralleh, H. Chemical and bioactive diversities of marine sponge Neopetrosia. *Bangladesh J. Pharmacol.* **2016**, *11*, 433. [CrossRef]
91. ANEIROS, A.; GARATEIX, A. Bioactive peptides from marine sources: Pharmacological properties and isolation procedures. *J. Chromatogr. B* **2004**, *803*, 41–53. [CrossRef]
92. Shin, H.J.; Rashid, M.A.; Cartner, L.K.; Bokesch, H.R.; Wilson, J.A.; McMahon, J.B.; Gustafson, K.R. Stellettapeptins A and B, HIV-inhibitory cyclic depsipeptides from the marine sponge *Stelletta* sp. *Tetrahedron Lett.* **2015**, *56*, 4215–4219. [CrossRef]
93. Wildeman;Gomez-Archila, L.G.; Galeano, E.; Martínez, A.; Castrillón, F.J.D.; Rugeles, M.T. Bromotyrosine Derivatives from Marine Sponges Inhibit the HIV-1 Replication in Vitro. *Vitae* **2014**, *21*, 114–125.
94. Jang, I.S.; Park, S.J. Hydroxyproline-containing collagen peptide derived from the skin of the Alaska pollack inhibits HIV-1 infection. *Mol. Med. Rep.* **2016**, *14*, 5489–5494. [CrossRef] [PubMed]
95. Jang, I.-S.; Park, S.J. A Spirulina maxima-derived peptide inhibits HIV-1 infection in a human T cell line MT4. *Fish. Aquat. Sci.* **2016**, *19*, 37. [CrossRef]
96. Zhou, X.; Fang, W.; Tan, S.; Lin, X.; Xun, T.; Yang, B.; Liu, S.; Liu, Y. Aspernigrins with anti-HIV-1 activities from the marine-derived fungus Aspergillus niger SCSIO Jcsw6F30. *Bioorg. Med. Chem. Lett.* **2016**, *26*, 361–365. [CrossRef] [PubMed]

97. Niu, S.; Liu, D.; Shao, Z.; Proksch, P.; Lin, W. Eutypellazines A–M, thiodiketopiperazine-type alkaloids from deep sea derived fungus Eutypella sp. MCCC 3A00281. *RSC Adv.* **2017**, *7*, 33580–33590. [CrossRef]
98. O'Rourke, A.; Kremb, S.; Bader, T.; Helfer, M.; Schmitt-Kopplin, P.; Gerwick, W.; Brack-Werner, R.; Voolstra, C. Alkaloids from the Sponge Stylissa carteri Present Prospective Scaffolds for the Inhibition of Human Immunodeficiency Virus 1 (HIV-1). *Mar. Drugs* **2016**, *14*, 28. [CrossRef] [PubMed]
99. Yu, H.-B.; Yang, F.; Sun, F.; Li, J.; Jiao, W.-H.; Gan, J.-H.; Hu, W.-Z.; Lin, H.-W. Aaptamine derivatives with antifungal and anti-HIV-1 activities from the South China Sea sponge Aaptos aaptos. *Mar. Drugs* **2014**, *12*, 6003–6013. [CrossRef] [PubMed]
100. Tietjen, I.; Williams, D.E.; Read, S.; Kuang, X.T.; Mwimanzi, P.; Wilhelm, E.; Markle, T.; Kinloch, N.N.; Naphen, C.N.; Tenney, K.; et al. Inhibition of NF-κB-dependent HIV-1 replication by the marine natural product bengamide A. *Antiviral Res.* **2018**, *152*, 94–103. [CrossRef] [PubMed]
101. Ma, X.; Li, L.; Zhu, T.; Ba, M.; Li, G.; Gu, Q.; Guo, Y.; Li, D. Phenylspirodrimanes with Anti-HIV Activity from the Sponge-Derived Fungus Stachybotrys chartarum MXH-X73. *J. Nat. Prod.* **2013**, *76*, 2298–2306. [CrossRef] [PubMed]
102. Pardo-Vargas, A.; de Barcelos Oliveira, I.; Stephens, P.; Cirne-Santos, C.; de Palmer Paixão, I.; Ramos, F.; Jiménez, C.; Rodríguez, J.; Resende, J.; Teixeira, V.; et al. Dolabelladienols A–C, New Diterpenes Isolated from Brazilian Brown Alga Dictyota pfaffii. *Mar. Drugs* **2014**, *12*, 4247–4259. [CrossRef]
103. de Souza Barros, C.; Cirne-Santos, C.C.; Garrido, V.; Barcelos, I.; Stephens, P.R.S.; Giongo, V.; Teixeira, V.L.; de Palmer Paixão, I.C.N. Anti-HIV-1 activity of compounds derived from marine alga Canistrocarpus cervicornis. *J. Appl. Phycol.* **2016**, *28*, 2523–2527. [CrossRef]
104. Stephens, P.R.S.; Cirne-Santos, C.C.; de Souza Barros, C.; Teixeira, V.L.; Carneiro, L.A.D.; Amorim, L.; dos, S.C.; Ocampo, J.S.P.; Castello-Branco, L.R.R.; de Palmer Paixão, I.C.N. Diterpene from marine brown alga Dictyota friabilis as a potential microbicide against HIV-1 in tissue explants. *J. Appl. Phycol.* **2017**, *29*, 775–780. [CrossRef]
105. Miceli, L.; Teixeira, V.; Castro, H.; Rodrigues, C.; Mello, J.; Albuquerque, M.; Cabral, L.; de Brito, M.; de Souza, A.; Miceli, L.A.; et al. Molecular Docking Studies of Marine Diterpenes as Inhibitors of Wild-Type and Mutants HIV-1 Reverse Transcriptase. *Mar. Drugs* **2013**, *11*, 4127–4143. [CrossRef] [PubMed]
106. Pardo-Vargas, A.; Ramos, F.A.; Cirne-Santos, C.C.; Stephens, P.R.; Paixão, I.C.P.; Teixeira, V.L.; Castellanos, L. Semi-synthesis of oxygenated dolabellane diterpenes with highly in vitro anti-HIV-1 activity. *Bioorg. Med. Chem. Lett.* **2014**, *24*, 4381–4383. [CrossRef] [PubMed]
107. Karadeniz, F.; Kang, K.-H.; Park, J.W.; Park, S.-J.; Kim, S.-K. Anti-HIV-1 activity of phlorotannin derivative 8,4‴-dieckol from Korean brown alga *Ecklonia cava*. *Biosci. Biotechnol. Biochem.* **2014**, *78*, 1151–1158. [CrossRef] [PubMed]
108. Tan, S.; Yang, B.; Liu, J.; Xun, T.; Liu, Y.; Zhou, X. Penicillixanthone A, a marine-derived dual-coreceptor antagonist as anti-HIV-1 agent. *Nat. Prod. Res.* **2017**, 1–5. [CrossRef] [PubMed]
109. He, J.; Huang, W.; Zheng, S.; Vigorito, M.; Chang, S.L. Effects of docosahexaenoic acid on locomotor activity in ethanol-treated HIV-1 transgenic rats. *J. Neurovirol.* **2018**, *24*, 88–97. [CrossRef] [PubMed]
110. Mejia, E.J.; Loveridge, S.T.; Stepan, G.; Tsai, A.; Jones, G.S.; Barnes, T.; White, K.N.; Drašković, M.; Tenney, K.; Tsiang, M.; et al. Study of Marine Natural Products Including Resorcyclic Acid Lactones from Humicola fuscoatra That Reactivate Latent HIV-1 Expression in an in Vitro Model of Central Memory CD4+ T Cells. *J. Nat. Prod.* **2014**, *77*, 618–624. [CrossRef] [PubMed]
111. Zhao, Y.; Liu, D.; Proksch, P.; Zhou, D.; Lin, W. Truncateols O-V, further isoprenylated cyclohexanols from the sponge-associated fungus Truncatella angustata with antiviral activities. *Phytochemistry* **2018**, *155*, 61–68. [CrossRef]
112. Ahn, M.-J.; Yoon, K.-D.; Min, S.-Y.; Lee, J.S.; Kim, J.H.; Kim, T.G.; Kim, S.H.; Kim, N.-G.; Huh, H.; Kim, J. Inhibition of HIV-1 reverse transcriptase and protease by phlorotannins from the brown alga Ecklonia cava. *Biol. Pharm. Bull.* **2004**, *27*, 544–547. [CrossRef]
113. Artan, M.; Li, Y.; Karadeniz, F.; Lee, S.-H.; Kim, M.-M.; Kim, S.-K. Anti-HIV-1 activity of phloroglucinol derivative, 6,6′-bieckol, from Ecklonia cava. *Bioorg. Med. Chem.* **2008**, *16*, 7921–7926. [CrossRef]
114. Cardona, M.L.; Fernández, I.; Pedro, J.R.; Serrano, A. Xanthones from Hypericum reflexum. *Phytochemistry* **1990**, *29*, 3003–3006. [CrossRef]
115. Negi, J.S.; Bisht, V.K.; Singh, P.; Rawat, M.S.M.; Joshi, G.P. Naturally Occurring Xanthones: Chemistry and Biology. *J. Appl. Chem.* **2013**, *2013*, 1–9. [CrossRef]

116. Ahmed, M.; Husain, N.E. Managing dyslipidemia in HIV/AIDS patients: Challenges and solutions. *HIV/AIDS* **2014**, *7*, 1. [CrossRef] [PubMed]
117. Vieira, A.D.S.; Silveira, G.R.M. da Effectiveness of n-3 fatty acids in the treatment of hypertriglyceridemia in HIV/AIDS patients: A meta-analysis. *Cien. Saude Colet.* **2017**, *22*, 2659–2669. [CrossRef] [PubMed]
118. Maria Jose MB, M.N.; MB, M.J.; Agudelo, M.; Yndart, A.; Vargas-Rivera, M.E. Platelets Contribute to BBB Disruption Induced by HIV and Alcohol. *J. Alcohol. Drug Depend.* **2015**, *3*, 1–6. [CrossRef]
119. Flora, G.; Pu, H.; Lee, Y.W.; Ravikumar, R.; Nath, A.; Hennig, B.; Toborek, M. Proinflammatory synergism of ethanol and HIV-1 Tat protein in brain tissue. *Exp. Neurol.* **2005**, *191*, 2–12. [CrossRef] [PubMed]
120. Acheampong, E.; Mukhtar, M.; Parveen, Z.; Ngoubilly, N.; Ahmad, N.; Patel, C.; Pomerantz, R.J. Ethanol strongly potentiates apoptosis induced by HIV-1 proteins in primary human brain microvascular endothelial cells. *Virology* **2002**, *304*, 222–234. [CrossRef]

4

Molecular Mechanisms of the Anti-Cancer Effects of Isothiocyanates from Cruciferous Vegetables in Bladder Cancer

Tomhiro Mastuo, Yasuyoshi Miyata *, Tsutomu Yuno, Yuta Mukae, Asato Otsubo, Kensuke Mitsunari, Kojiro Ohba and Hideki Sakai

Department of Urology, Nagasaki University Graduate School of Biomedical Sciences, Nagasaki 852-8501, Japan; tomozo1228@hotmail.com (T.M.); t.yuno@nagasaki-u.ac.jp (T.Y.); ytmk_n2@yahoo.co.jp (Y.M.); a.06131dpsc@gmail.com (A.O.); ken.mitsunari@gmail.com (K.M.); ohba-k@nagasaki-u.ac.jp (K.O.); hsakai@nagasaki-u.ac.jp (H.S.)

* Correspondence: yasu-myt@nagasaki-u.ac.jp

Abstract: Bladder cancer (BC) is a representative of urological cancer with a high recurrence and metastasis potential. Currently, cisplatin-based chemotherapy and immune checkpoint inhibitors are used as standard therapy in patients with advanced/metastatic BC. However, these therapies often show severe adverse events, and prolongation of survival is unsatisfactory. Therefore, a treatment strategy using natural compounds is of great interest. In this review, we focused on the anti-cancer effects of isothiocyanates (ITCs) derived from cruciferous vegetables, which are widely cultivated and consumed in many regions worldwide. Specifically, we discuss the anti-cancer effects of four ITC compounds—allyl isothiocyanate, benzyl isothiocyanate, sulforaphane, and phenethyl isothiocyanate—in BC; the molecular mechanisms underlying their anti-cancer effects; current trends and future direction of ITC-based treatment strategies; and the carcinogenic potential of ITCs. We also discuss the advantages and limitations of each ITC in BC treatment, furthering the consideration of ITCs in treatment strategies and for improving the prognosis of patients with BC.

Keywords: allyl isothiocyanate; benzyl isothiocyanate; sulforaphane; phenethyl isothiocyanate; bladder cancer

---

1. Introduction

Bladder cancer (BC) is recognized as a representative of urological cancer (UC), but it has specific pathological characteristics and treatment strategies. BC shows a high recurrence and metastasis potential, even if radical operation is performed [1,2]. Regarding treatment strategies, only two regimens have been approved as effective methods: platinum-based chemotherapy, including gemcitabine and cisplatin combination therapy and MVAC therapy, and immune checkpoint inhibitors, such as pembrolizumab [3–5]. Unfortunately, these regimens have shown relatively severe adverse events, including renal dysfunction, neutropenia, and immunogenic abnormalities, and it is currently difficult to predict therapeutic effects [3,4,6]. Although there is an improved prognosis of BC patients undergoing these therapies, prolongation of survival is far from satisfactory, especially in patients with advanced/metastatic disease. Currently, new anti-cancer drugs for UC are under development, some of which are expected to be approved for the treatment of advanced/metastatic BC in the near feature [7,8]. However, there is little information on the safety and adverse events of these new drugs.

Based on these facts, as well as the artificially produced anti-cancer drugs, treatment strategies employing natural compounds have garnered special interest for various types of malignancies. There is a general consensus that considering treatment strategies using natural product(s) is important for improving the quality of life and prognosis of cancer patients. In fact, there is a report that curcumin, a natural occurring polyphenol derived from turmeric (*Curcuma longa*), had anti-cancer effects via suppression of cancer cell proliferation, invasion, and metastasis in lung cancer cells [9]. The authors also showed that regulation of microRNA expression plays important roles in the curcumin-induced anti-cancer effects [9]. Furthermore, Yiqi Huayu Jiedu decoction, which comprises various Chinese herbs and natural compounds, was reported to increase the anti-cancer effects of standard chemotherapy in patients with stage III gastric cancer after radical gastrectomy and improve the quality of life of patients [10]. In addition to these reports, several reviews and *in vivo* and *in vitro* studies have demonstrated that a variety of natural products possess anti-cancer potential and can avoid the undesirable effects of standard therapies of malignancies [11–14].

Regarding BC, multiple studies showed that a variety of natural products have anti-cancer effects and maintain quality of life, including *Evodia rutaecarpa* or curcumin [15,16]. Several reports also demonstrated the relationship between natural products and prevention of carcinogenesis, clinicopathological features, and anti-cancer effects in BC [17,18]. In previous studies, we showed the anti-cancer effects, clinical usefulness, and pathological mechanisms of green tea polyphenol or royal jelly in urological cancers, including BC [19–25]. Although green tea and royal jelly are eaten in some parts of Asia and Western countries, this is not the case globally. In contrast, cruciferous vegetables, such as broccoli, kale, cauliflower, bock choy, and horseradish, are widely cultivated in many regions and are commonly eaten worldwide. Isothiocyanates (ITCs) are naturally occurring products of cruciferous vegetables, and researchers have investigated their health benefits and efficacy in the treatment of various diseases, including malignancies. Although some reviews mentioned the anti-cancer effects of ITCs in BC, there is relatively little comprehensive information on the molecular mechanisms of the ITC anti-cancer effects in BC cells [26–28]. In addition, comprehensive information on each ITC member, including allyl isothiocyanate (AITC), benzyl isothiocyanate (BITC), sulforaphane (SFN), and phenethyl isothiocyanate (PEITC), is limited. Therefore, in this review, we discuss the anti-cancer effects and efficacy of ITCs in BC cells obtained by *in vivo* and *in vitro* studies. In particular, we focus on the changes in malignant behaviors and cancer-related molecules by ITC members in BC cells. Furthermore, we provide future direction of ITC-based therapy for patients with BC.

2. Isothiocyanates in Cruciferous Vegetables

Cruciferous vegetables are classified in the family Brassicaceae/Cruciferae. Several *in vivo*, *in vitro*, and epidemiological studies have shown that cruciferous vegetables inhibit carcinogenesis of BC [27,29,30]. However, in contrast to these reports, a study suggested that cruciferous vegetable intake is not significantly associated with reduced BC risk [31]. Thus, there are controversial results regarding the relationship between cruciferous vegetables and cancer risk in UC. Additionally, there is limited knowledge on the molecular mechanisms of the anti-cancer effects of cruciferous vegetables.

ITCs are naturally present in cruciferous vegetables and are produced by the hydrolysis of glucosinolates [32]. There is a general agreement that ITCs are beneficial for human health via various mechanisms, such as their anti-microbial activity, prevention of cardiovascular disease, and improvement of fasting glucose levels [33,34]. ITCs are also reported to exhibit anti-carcinogenic activities in various cancer types, including BC [27,33,35,36]. ITCs include the compounds AITC, BITC, SFN, and PEITC (Figure 1), each of which has multiple activities, including anti-cancer effects [37]. In the following sections, we will present the changes in malignant aggressiveness and molecular expression/activity in BC by each ITC member.

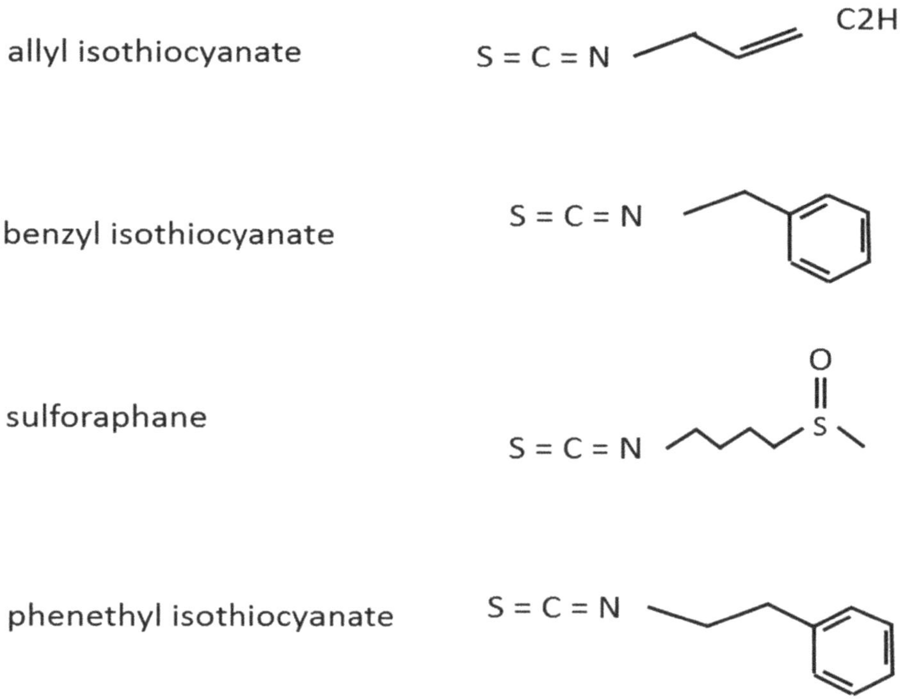

Figure 1. Structures of the isothiocyanate members.

2.1. Allyl Isothiocyanate

AITC is a volatile and water-insoluble compound derived from various cruciferous vegetables that exhibits multiple functions, such as anti-inflammation, neuroprotection, and anti-bacterial activity [38,39]. In addition, AITC is reported to have anti-cancer effects in various types of malignancies [40–42]. However, a study showed that AITC had no significant inhibitory effects on cell proliferation or stimulation of apoptosis in the human breast cancer cell line MDA-MB-231 [43]. Nevertheless, other studies have highlighted the potential advantages of AITC in BC treatment, as the major route of excretion of orally administered AITC is through urine, demonstrating relatively high bioavailability in urine and bladder tissue compared with other organs [44,45]. In this section, we will introduce the anti-cancer effects of AITC in BC and provide future direction for novel treatment strategies using AITC.

2.1.1. In Vitro Studies

The anti-cancer effects of AITC and its molecular mechanisms have been investigated in various BC cell lines; for instance, AITC was found to lead to morphological changes and inhibit the cell proliferation of the human BC cell lines RT4 and T24 [46]. AITC was also reported to affect cell cycle arrest and apoptosis of RT4 and T24 cells [44]. Moreover, the cytotoxic effects of AITC were confirmed in another BC cell line (UM-UC-3 cells) [47], and the percentages of apoptotic cells increased in an AITC dose-dependent manner in three different BC cell lines (UM-UC-3, UM-UC-6, and T24) [48]. This same study demonstrated that AITC-induced apoptosis is mediated by a mitochondrion-mediated system, including activation of caspase-9, caspase-3, lamin B1, and poly ADP-ribose polymerase (PARP) as well as Bcl-2 phosphorylation at Ser-70 by c-Jun N-terminal kinase (JNK) [48].

These anti-cancer effects, such as anti-proliferation and pro-apoptosis, of AITC are speculated to be independent from TP53—an important regulator of cell death—because RT4 cells possess wild-type TP53, while T24 and UM-UC-3 cells possess mutated TP53 [49]. Moreover, the anti-cancer effects of AITC involved different molecular mechanisms between RT4 and T24 cells. In RT4 cells, AITC treatment increased S100P and Bax levels and decreased Bcl-2 levels; meanwhile, Bax, Bcl-2, and anillin levels increased while S100P levels decreased in T24 cells [46]. The Bax/Bcl-2 pathway is speculated to be a key modulator of AITC in RT4 cells, with anillin and S100P mainly functioning in this system [46].

Thus, these *in vitro* studies demonstrated that the anti-cancer effects of AITC in BC cells are dependent on the pathological and molecular characteristics of cancer cells.

Molecular mechanisms of the AITC-induced anti-cancer effect in BC cells are shown in Table 1. To our knowledge, there are only two *in vitro* studies on this topic, warranting further research to discuss treatment strategies using ITCs.

Table 1. *In vitro* molecular mechanism of the anti-cancer effects of allyl isothiocyanate.

Anti-Cancer Effect	Underlying Molecular Mechanisms	Reference
Cell growth ↓	Increased S100P and Bax expression and decreased Bcl-2 expression in RT4 cells	Sávio et al., 2015 [46]
Cell growth ↓	Increased Bcl-2, Bax, and anillin expression and decreased S100P expression in T24 cells	Sávio et al., 2015 [46]
Apoptosis ↑	Regulation of mitochondrion-mediated mechanisms and Bcl-2 phosphorylation	Geng et al., 2011 [48]

Bcl, B-cell lymphoma-2; Bax, Bcl-2-associated X protein.

2.1.2. *N*-acetylcysteine Conjugate Allyl Isothiocyanate

AITC is mainly excreted in urine as *N*-acetylcysteine conjugate (NAC-AITC). In human and rat BC cells (UM-UC-3 and AY-27 cells, respectively), NAC-AITC inhibits cell proliferation and regulates cell cycle arrest and apoptosis [50]. The anti-cancer effects of NAC-AITC were found associated with downregulation of α-tubulin, β-tubulin/ and vascular endothelial growth factor and activation of caspase-3. Moreover, the authors conclude that the anti-cancer effects of NAC-AITC, including prevention and treatment of cancer are superior to AITC in terms of pharmacokinetic and physical properties. Similar anti-tumor growth activity was found in an orthotopic rat BC model, wherein bladder tumor weight in the NAC-AITC group is significantly lower than that in control ($p = 0.0213$) [50]. In addition, NAC-AITC suppressed muscle invasion of BC cells (NAC-AITC group = 30%; control = 79%). Similar to the BC cell lines, α- and β-tubulin, vascular endothelial growth factor, and cleaved caspase-3 were found associated with the *in vivo* anti-cancer effects [50].

2.1.3. In Vivo Studies

Dietary administration of a freeze-dried, aqueous extract of broccoli sprouts that included AITC was found to reduce the incidence, multiplicity, and size of BC in an *N*-butyl-*N*-(4-hydroxybutyl) nitrosamine (BBN)-induced rat BC model [51]. However, the detailed molecular mechanisms of this anti-cancer effect were not clearly defined. Another study showed that oral intake of AITC-rich mustard seed powder inhibits tumor growth and muscle invasion in an orthotopic rat BC model via regulation of apoptosis, cell cycle, and angiogenic potential [52]; downregulation of vascular endothelial growth factor and cyclin B1 and upregulation of caspase-3 and cleavage of PARP were found associated with these anti-cancer effects [52].

When AITC is stably stored as its glucosinolate precursor (sinigrin) in mustard seed powder (MSP-1), a study revealed that sinigrin itself is not bioactive, whereas hydrated MSP-1 leads to apoptosis and G2/M phase arrest in bladder cancer cell lines *in vitro*. In an orthotopic rat bladder cancer model, oral MSP-1 inhibited bladder cancer growth by 34.5% ($P < 0.05$) and blocked muscle invasion by 100%. The anti-cancer activity of AITC delivered as MSP-1 appears to be more robust than that of pure AITC. Therefore, MSP-1 may be an attractive delivery vehicle for AITC, as it strongly inhibits bladder cancer development and progression [52].

2.1.4. Combination Therapy of Allyl Isothiocyanate and Conventional Anti-cancer Agents

The cyclooxygenase (COX)-2-plastaglandin (PG) E2-system is an important pathological mechanism of carcinogenesis, tumor growth, and progression in UC [53–55]. Therefore, COX-2 inhibitors have been suggested as chemoprotective and therapeutic agents in a variety of cancers [56–58]. The synergistic effects of a combination of COX-2 inhibitors and other standard therapy have also been reported [59,60]. Celecoxib, a selective COX-2 inhibitor, is used for various pathological conditions worldwide. Thus, to clarify the anti-cancer effects of a combination of celecoxib and AITC, *in vitro* studies employing AY-27 bladder cancer cells and *in vivo* studies with the F344/AY-27 rat bladder urothelial cell carcinoma model were performed [61]. *In vitro*, AITC first showed no significant impact on COX-2 expression, and PGE2 production was confirmed. However, when the growth inhibitory effects of AITC and celecoxib were analyzed, growth inhibition of AY-27 cells by AITC was not altered by celecoxib addition. The authors thus speculated that the COX-2-mediated anti-tumor growth effects of celecoxib did not reach detectable levels due to excessive dilution of PGE2 in the culture medium. On the other hand, *in vivo* studies employing an animal model with orthotopic BC showed that combination therapy of AITC (1 mg/Kg) and celecoxib (10 mg/Kg) suppresses tumor growth and muscle invasion and that these anti-cancer effects are stronger compared with those of AITC or celecoxib alone. Inhibition of tumor-related angiogenesis regulated by vascular endothelial growth was found to play a crucial role in these anti-cancer effects.

Another combination therapy employed AITC and cisplatin, a standard anti-cancer drug for patients with BC [62]. *In vitro* studies with lung cancer cells (HOP62) and ovarian cancer cells (2008) showed that the variabilities of both cancer cell lines are significantly inhibited by a combination of AITC and cisplatin, whose inhibitory effects are stronger compared with those of AITC or cisplatin alone. The anti-proliferative effects were confirmed by colony formation assays, and when relationships between cell death and the combination therapy were examined, levels of pro-apoptotic molecules (caspase-3) were found increased and anti-apoptotic molecules (Bcl-2 and survivin) decreased; thus, this combination can suppress tumor growth *in vitro*. Mechanistically, regulation of cell cycle, β-tubulin depletion, and microtubule dysfunction are associated with the anti-cancer effects of AITC and cisplatin. Finally, the combination index of ATIC and cisplatin in lung cancer cells indicates a synergistic interaction. Indeed, *in vivo* studies with A549-derived lung cancer xenograft tumor models showed decreases in tumor volumes after combination therapy (AITC = 50 mg/Kg and cisplatin = 6 mg/kg), whereas tumor volumes increased after AITC (50 mg/Kg) or cisplatin (6 mg/kg) monotherapy. Overall, the anti-cancer effect parameters (i.e., maximum tumor growth inhibition, tumor doubling time, and frequency of partial response and complete response) are remarkably better after combination therapy than after either monotherapy. Furthermore, AITC + cisplatin therapy exhibits no toxicity, including maximum weight loss of pretreatment bodyweight.

2.1.5. Clinical Trials and Future Direction of Allyl Isothiocyanate-Based Therapy

Recently, an *in vitro* study employing the macrophage cell line RAW 264.7 and human BC cell line HT1376 was conducted to clarify the anti-inflammatory activity and anti-cancer effect of AITC nanoparticles [63]. The results showed that AITC nanoparticles inhibit cancer cell proliferation and migration; however, these anti-cancer effects are dependent on AITC concentration; inhibition of cancer cell proliferation and migration is achieved at 70 mg L^{-1} and 8.75 mg L^{-1} of AITC nanoparticles, respectively. AITC nanoparticles were also found to suppress production of lipopolysaccharide-induced tumor necrosis factor (TNF)-α, interleukin (IL)-6, nitric oxide (NO), and inducible NO synthase in macrophage cells, and their anti-inflammatory effects are stronger than those of AITC or nanoparticles alone. The authors thus suggested that AITC nanoparticles can be a valuable treatment strategy for BC via their regulation of inflammation, immunity, and oxidative stress.

Other novel strategies employing AITC are currently under development. For example, the anti-cancer effects of AITC-conjugated silicon quantum dots were examined in human umbilical vein endothelial cells (HUVECs) and human hepatocellular carcinoma cells (HepG2) [64]. Interestingly, high doses of AITC (40–320 μM) were found to significantly inhibit HepG2 cell viability, whereas low doses (5 μM) significantly stimulated cancer cell viability. Similar trends were confirmed for cancer cell migration (inhibition at 20 μM AITC and stimulation at 2.5 μM) and angiogenesis (HUVEC tube formation ability is suppressed at > 5 μM but stimulated at even lower doses of 1.25 and 2.5 μM AITC). Thus, there is a possibility that the anti-cancer effects of AITC are dependent on its concentration and that low concentrations of AITC may have detrimental effects via increased cancer cell proliferation, migration, and angiogenesis in hepatocellular carcinoma. The authors further showed that AITC-conjugated silicon quantum dots overcame the limitation of AITC in the same analysis. Therefore, AITC-conjugated silicon quantum dots are suggested as a useful drug delivery system for AITC in cancer patients. Although there are no data in BC, AITC is also predicted to have biphasic effects of anti-cancer effects and angiogenesis. Therefore, we suggest additional *in vivo* and *in vitro* studies of the silicon quantum dot system in BC to elucidate new treatment strategies for patients.

2.2. *Benzyl Isothiocyanate*

Similar to other ITC members, BITC has immunomodulatory, anti-microbial, and anti-oxidative activities under various pathological conditions [34,65,66] Several studies have also shown that BITC possesses anti-cancer and chemopreventive effects in various types of malignancies [67–69]. However, there is limited information on its anti-cancer effects and molecular mechanisms in UC.

2.2.1. In Vitro Studies

Similar to AITC, BITC has shown anti-proliferative and pro-apoptotic activity in BC cells [70,71]; however, the pro-apoptotic activity of BITC is stronger compared with that of other ITC members, including AITC and SFN. Moreover, caspase-9 is the main regulator of BITC-induced apoptosis in UM-UC-3 cells, although all ITC members exhibit pro-apoptotic activities via activation of caspase-3, 8, and 9 [70,72]. Additionally, mitochondrial activities are targets of BITC, and BITC-induced changes are regulated by various members of the Bcl-2 family, including Bcl-2, Bax, Bak, and Bcl-xl [70].

As previously mentioned, ITCs are primarily disposed and concentrated in the urine as NAC conjugates. UC originates from urothelial cells and is constantly exposed to urine in the urinary tract. Therefore, studies have focused on the anti-cancer effects of NAC-conjugated BITC in BC cells [71] and found that it suppresses BC cell growth through anti-proliferative and pro-apoptotic activities. Activation of caspase-3, 8, and 9; cell cycle arrest in phases S and G2/M; and regulation of Cdc25C were associated with the anti-proliferative function of NAC-conjugated BITC. The authors confirmed, however, that longer treatment durations or higher doses of NAC-conjugated BITC are necessary to exert similar effects as those of BITC.

miRNAs are major modulators of carcinogenesis, malignant aggressiveness, and outcome in UC [73,74] and several miRNAs are closely associated with cisplatin sensitivity of BC cells [75]. miR-99a-5p, a tumor suppressor, exhibits anti-proliferative and pro-apoptotic activities in UC [76–78]. One study demonstrated that BITC treatment upregulates miR-99a-5p expression in the BC cell lines 5637 and T24 [76], which leads to decreased mRNA and protein levels of IGF-1R, FGF-R3, and mTOR in both BC cell lines. The authors also demonstrated a molecular mechanism associated with regulation of BC cell survival and apoptosis by BITC. Taken together, these findings indicate that BITC exhibits anti-cancer effects via regulation of cell survival in UC. Another study elucidated the anti-cancer effects of BITC-induced miR-99a expression in BC cells [79] and reported that BITC enhances miR-99a expression in 5637 and T24 BC cells, which is associated with ERK activation and nuclear transcriptional activation of c-Jun/(activator protein) AP-1. Thus, the authors suggested that BITC stimulates miR-99a expression via regulation of the ERK/AP-1 pathway in BC and demonstrated the anti-cancer effects of miR-99a in UC. Nevertheless, there is a general consensus that the anti-carcinogenic and anti-cancer effects of miR-99a represent a complex mechanism in BC cells [80–82]. Therefore, this information is useful for understanding the biological function of BITC in BC. The molecular mechanisms of the anti-cancer effects of BITC are shown in Table 2.

Table 2. *In vitro* molecular mechanisms of the anti-cancer effects of benzyl isothiocyanate.

Anti-Cancer Effect	Underlying Molecular Mechanisms	Reference
Cell growth ↓	Suppression of IGF1R, FGFR3, and mTOR activation by miR-99a-5p upregulation	Liu et al., 2019 [76]
Apoptosis ↑	Via caspase-9, a major regulator, and Bcl-2, Bax, Bak, and Bcl-xl	Tang & Zhang, 2005 [70]
Apoptosis ↑	Stimulation of caspase-3, 8, and 9 and cell cycle arrest in the same phases by Cdc25C	Tang et al., 2006 [71]

IGF1R, insulin-like growth factor 1 receptor; FGFR, fibroblast growth factor receptor; mTOR, mechanistic target of rapamycin; Bcl, B-cell lymphoma-2; Bax, Bcl-2-associated X protein; Bak, BCL2-antagonist/killer.

2.2.2. In Vivo Studies

In a rat model of BBN-induced BC, oral intake of BITC suppressed the incidence of neoplastic pathological changes, such as dysplasia, papilloma, and carcinoma, and multiplicities in a dose-dependent manner (10, 100, or 1,000 ppm BITC) [83]. Notably, epithelial hyperplasia of the bladder was found in rats treated with 100 or 1,000 ppm BITC without BBN [83]. The same researchers also demonstrated the carcinogenic potential of BITC in this BC animal model [84]. Therefore, the toxicity and risk of BITC in BC treatment should be considered; this is further detailed later in the text (see Section 2.1).

2.2.3. Combination Therapy of Benzyl Isothiocyanate and Cisplatin

As mentioned in Section 2.4, combination therapy of ITCs and cisplatin is expected to have better anti-cancer effects than those of ITCs or cisplatin alone. Indeed, several reports showed that BITC enhances the anti-cancer effects of cisplatin in lung cancer cells (NCI-H596), head and neck squamous cell carcinoma cells (HN12, HN8, and HN30), and leukemia cells (HL-60) [85–87]; there are no similar studies in BC cells, however.

2.3. *Sulforaphane*

SFN can be found in cruciferous vegetables, such as broccoli, cauliflower, brussel sprouts, cabbage, kale, and kohlrabi [88]. SFN is reported to regulate cancer cell survival via inhibition of cell proliferation and stimulation of apoptosis in a variety of cancers [89,90]. Among the ITC members, SFN has been the most widely investigated regarding its pathological roles and molecular mechanisms both *in vivo* and *in vitro*.

2.3.1. In Vitro Studies: Cell Cycle-, Caspase- and Bcl-2-Related Molecules

Regarding the relationships between SFN and cell survival, including cell proliferation, cell cycle, and death, various mechanisms have been suggested. For example, SFN was reported to induce growth arrest and apoptosis in a BC cell line (5637 cells) [91]. Moreover, induction and stimulation of cyclin B1 and Cdk1 were found associated with the anti-proliferative effects of SFN, whereas activation of caspase-3, 8, and 9 and PARP corresponded to its pro-apoptotic effects; these SFN-induced anti-cancer effects are speculated to be regulated via reactive oxygen species (ROS)-dependent mechanisms [91]. Another study showed that SFN treatment suppresses cell viability in a dose-dependent manner and induces apoptosis in T24 human BC cells via regulation of caspase-3, caspase-9, and PARP [92]. Moreover, the SFN-induced apoptosis of BC cells is mediated by dysregulation of mitochondria function, cytochrome *c* release, and Bcl-2-related pathways [92].

Other studies focused on the relationships between cell cycle-related molecules and SFN. For instance, after 10–40 μM SFN treatment for 24 or 48 h, T24 cell viability is significantly suppressed with IC50 values of 26.9 ± 1.12 μM (24 h) or 15.9 ± 0.76 μM (48 h) [93]. Conversely, 20 μM SFN treatment for 24 or 48 h resulted in apoptotic features, such as cell shrinkage, condensed chromatin, and apoptotic bodies, in the same BC cells; increased numbers of apoptotic cells were confirmed by flow cytometry [93]. SFN is also associated with blocking cell cycle progression at G0/G1 phase. In addition to its pro-apoptotic activities, upregulation of the cyclin-dependent kinase inhibitor p27 plays crucial roles in the 20 μM SFN-induced anti-cancer effects in BC cells, whereas p16 or cyclin D1 expression does not [93]. Thus, regulation of cell cycle-related molecules and mitochondrial function, caspases, and the Bcl-2 protein family represent the molecular mechanisms of SFN-induced anti-proliferative and pro-apoptotic activities in BC cells.

2.3.2. In Vitro Studies: Oxidative Stress, Endoplasmic Reticulum Stress, and Growth Factors

As mentioned above, many investigators believe that the anti-cancer effects of SFN in BC are mainly associated with caspase- and mitochondria-related pathways. Nevertheless, there are other cancer-related factors involved. For instance, SFN can inhibit DNA damage induced by chemical carcinogens in BC T24 cells [94]. Moreover, SFN-induced oxidative stress through ROS has been suggested as a key modulator [91,92]. Nuclear factor erythroid 2-related factor-2 (Nrf2) regulation and endoplasmic reticulum (ER) stress are also associated with SFN and carcinogenesis, pathological behavior, and cell survival in UC [28,92]. Notably, these Nrf2 and ER signaling pathways are important factors in the response to oxidative stress and anti-oxidative activities [28,92,95]. A study showed that enhanced insulin-like growth-factor-binding protein-3 (IGFBP-3) and suppressed nuclear factor-kappa B (NF-κB) expression by SFN are associated with the anti-proliferative effect of SFN in the BC cell line BIU87. Interestingly, the authors also found that SFN stimulates apoptosis and cell cycle arrest at the G2/M phase, resulting from IGFBP-3 and NF-κB regulation [96]. As IGFBP-3 and NF-κB are known to possess pro-apoptotic and anti-apoptotic functions, respectively, in various malignancies [97,98], this stimulation of apoptosis by SPN via increased IGFBP-3 and decreased NF-κB levels are in agreement with established findings. Another report on the relationship between SFN-induced anti-cancer effects and growth factors demonstrated that 20 μM SFN leads to a 2.6-, 3.0-, or 3.1-fold increase in the G_2/M phase compared with that of controls in three BC cell lines (RT4, J82, and UM-UC-3, respectively) [99]. In addition, SFN induces apoptosis in RT4 and UM-UC-3 cells. Thus, these findings indicate that upregulation of caspase-3/7 and PARP activity and downregulation of survivin, EGFR, and HER2/neu are the underlying molecular mechanisms.

TNF-related apoptosis-inducing ligand (TRAIL) is recognized as an initiator of apoptosis. Its dysregulation has been identified in various malignant cells, including BC [100,101]. As a result, resistance to TRAIL is associated with high malignant potential and worse prognosis for patients with BC [102]. SFN treatment however, has been reported to reverse the pro-apoptotic activity of TRAIL in TRAIL-resistant BC cells [103]; the SFN-induced mechanisms were found associated with apoptosis-related molecules (e.g., caspases, mitochondrial membrane potential, Bid, and death receptor 5) and oxidative stress-related factors (e.g., ROS and Nrf2).

The anti-cancer effects of SFN under hypoxic conditions in BC cell lines have also been reported [88]; in RT112 cells, 20 μM SFN inhibited cancer cell proliferation by 26.1 ± 4.1% and 39.7 ± 5.2% under normoxia and hypoxia, respectively ($P < 0.05$), with similar results observed for RT4 cells (normoxia, 29.7 ± 4.6%; hypoxia, 48.3 ± 5.2%). Tumor tissues, especially those within the center, are generally under hypoxic conditions due to the oxygen consumption of the tumor to support its growth. Thus, these findings indicate that SFN can suppress cell proliferation under hypoxic conditions in BC with rapid tumor growth compared with that under normoxia and relatively slow growth. Interestingly, the same study also showed that SFN suppresses glycolytic metabolism under hypoxia by decreasing the nuclear translocation of hypoxia-inducible factor-1α, thereby reducing its protein levels [88]. Suppression of glycolytic metabolism in cancer cells is important for inhibiting tumor growth and progression as high glycolytic metabolism leads to increased cancer cell proliferation. Overall, the findings demonstrate that SFN plays several roles in suppressing malignant aggressiveness, such as by decreasing cancer cell proliferation, in BC cells.

2.3.3. In Vitro Studies: Inflammation, Epithelial-to-Mesenchymal Transition, Epigenesis, and Others

In addition to reducing BC cell survival, SFN inhibits malignant aggressiveness by suppressing inflammation, cancer cell invasion, and metastasis. Several studies have shown that SFN downregulates

COX-2 expression in BC cells via regulation of p38 mitogen-activated protein kinase (MAPK) and NF-κB [104–106]. Moreover, p38 MARK is positively associated with glutathione transferase and thioredoxin reductase-1—both antioxidant enzymes—following SFN treatment [105]. Furthermore, SFN can inhibit epithelial-to-mesenchymal transition (EMT)—an important mediator of cancer cell invasion and metastasis—via regulation of COX-2/matrix metalloproteinase (MMP)-2, -9/ZEB1, Snail, and miR-200c/ZEB1 in BC cells [106].

SFN was found to inhibit histone status in BC cells, which is associated with reduced levels of histone H1 phosphorylation via modification of histone acetyltransferase and histone deacetylase activity [26]. Changes in histone H1 status were previously reported to be associated with carcinogenesis and prognosis of BC [107]. Based on these findings, SFN is speculated to inhibit carcinogenesis and progression of BC via epigenetic modification [26].

Recently, the physiological and pathological roles of gut microbiota have garnered great interest. Research has shown how they affect systematic metabolism, inflammation, and the immune system, contributing to carcinogenesis, malignant potential, and cancer progression, of which similar findings have been reported in UC [108–110]. Interestingly, SFN was found to normalize gut microbiota dysbiosis by increasing the abundance of *Bacteroides fragilis* and *Clostridium* cluster I in a BBN-induced BC animal model [111], suppressing BBN-induced histological changes, including sub-mucosal capillary growth. While the detailed mechanisms of the anti-carcinogenic function of SFN in this model is not fully clear, normalization of intestinal flora has been shown to repair intestinal barrier dysfunction and injured mucosal epithelium via regulation of tight junction proteins, including ZO-1, claudin-1, occludin, and mucin-2 [111]. Moreover, SFN plays crucial roles in the inflammatory status of this model, as it decreases pro-inflammatory factors such as IL-6 and secretory immunoglobin A, which are increased by carcinogenesis [111]. The authors conclude that these gut microbiota-related beneficial effects of SFN led to its anti-carcinogenic effects in BC via complex mechanisms that involve inflammation and the immune system [111]. A summary of the molecular mechanisms of the anti-cancer effects of SFN is shown in Table 3.

Table 3. *In vitro* molecular mechanisms of the anti-cancer effects of sulforaphane.

Anti-Cancer Effect	Underlying Molecular Mechanisms	Reference
Cell growth ↓	Increased IGFBP-3 expression and decreased NF-κB expression	Dang et al., 2014 [96]
Cell growth ↓	Increased cyclin B1 and Cdk1 phosphorylation and their complex effects	Park et al., 2014 [91]
Cell growth ↓	Suppression of HIF-1α-mediated glycolytic metabolism under hypoxic conditions	Xia et al., 2019 [88]
Apoptosis ↑	Increased expression of the cyclin-dependent kinase inhibitor p27	Shan et al., 2006 [93]
Apoptosis ↑	Increased caspase-3/7 and PARP expression and decreased survivin, EGFR, and HER2/neu expression	Abboui et al., 2012 [99]
Apoptosis ↑	Increased IGFBP-3 expression and decreased NF-κB expression	Dang et al., 2014 [96]
Apoptosis ↑	Activation of ROS-mediated caspase-3/9 and PARP, ER stress, and Nrf2	Jo et al., 2014 [92]
Apoptosis ↑	Activation of caspase-3, 8, and 9 and PARP via ROS-dependent pathways	Park et al., 2014 [91]
Apoptosis ↑	Reversal of TRAIL activity via regulation of caspases, MMP, DR5, ROS, and Nrf2	Jin et al., 2018 [103]
Invasion ↓	Regulation of EMT and COX-2/MMP2,9/ZEB1, Snail, and miR-200c/ZEB1 pathways	Shan et al., 2013 [93]
Migration ↓	Regulation of autophagy activation	Bao et al., 2014 [112]

IGFBP, insulin-like growth-factor-binding protein; NF-κB, nuclear factor-kappa B; HIF, hypoxia-inducible factor; PARP, poly ADP-ribose polymerase; EGFR, epidermal growth factor receptor; HER, human EGFR-related; ROS, reactive oxygen species; ER, endoplasmic reticulum; Nrf2, nuclear factor erythroid 2-related factor; MMP, matrix metalloproteinase; DR5, death receptor 5; EMT, epithelial-to-mesenchymal transition; COX, cyclooxygenase.

2.3.4. In Vivo Studies

In vivo studies with the chemical-induced BC animal model have shown that SFN inhibits carcinogenesis, tumor growth, and progression via a complex mechanism that includes prevention of DNA damage [94]. In a murine UM-UC-3 xenograft model, tumor growth rates and tumor weights in the SFN group were found lower than in the control group (not significant and $p < 0.05$, respectively) [51]. Furthermore, this model showed decreases in tumor volumes in SFN-treated mice (12 mg/kg bodyweight for 5 weeks) with an inhibitory rate of 63% via increased caspase-3 and cytochrome *c* expression and decreased survivin expression [113]. In addition to the apoptosis-related pathways, several other molecules have been suggested to be associated with the anti-cancer effects of SFN, based on *in vivo* studies. Thus, further *in vivo* studies are essential for understanding the efficacy and limitations of an SFN-based treatment strategy against BC.

2.3.5. Combination Therapy of Sulforaphane and Other Therapeutic Agents

Although several clinical trials on the anti-cancer effects of SFN and broccoli sprout extracts have been performed, the results were unsatisfactory [114,115]; for example, no or minimum effects are detected on serum and tissue biomarkers of patients with prostate and breast cancer. Although a similar clinical trial has not been performed for patients with BC, the clinical effects of SFN monotherapy are also predicted to be unsatisfactory. Therefore, the efficacy of a combination therapy of SFN and other therapeutic agents was investigated in BC cells.

A combination therapy of acetazolamide (AZ; a carbonic anhydrase inhibitor) and SFN showed suppressed proliferative and clonogenic effects and stimulated apoptotic activity via caspase-3 and PARP activation [116]. In addition, the PI3K/Akt signaling pathway was found to play an important role in the anti-cancer effects of this combination therapy. The authors thus conclude that AZ + SFN is a potential therapeutic strategy for BC. Another study examined the effects of two ITCs (AITC + SFN) on the lung cancer cell line A549 [117]; their anti-carcinogenic effects showed higher inhibitory effects on tumor growth and cancer cell migration and greater stimulation of apoptosis compared with that of ATIC or SFN alone. Moreover, oxidative stress, including ROS, is associated with these activities. Although this study was not performed on BC cells, we believe that a combination of different ITCs may be effective for the prevention and treatment of BC. Indeed, in the BC cell line UM-UC-3, pro-apoptotic activity of BITC or PEITC alone is stronger than that of AITC or SFN alone [72]. Moreover, ≥20 μM SFN significantly suppresses cell proliferation in the BC cell line BIU87, whereas 10 μM SFN had no significant effect [96,112]. Therefore, more detailed studies on the combination of various ITC types, dosages, and durations are necessary to identify the most efficacious combination therapy of the ITC members.

Nevertheless, there are potential limitations of SFN-based therapies. Novel immunotherapy strategies, such as immune checkpoint inhibitors, have been recently established as standard therapy for patients with advanced/metastatic BC [118,119]. While we speculate that a combination of immunotherapy and SFN may be useful for the prevention and treatment of BC, a combination of SFN with T cell-mediated cancer immunotherapies is not recommended because SFN can function both as an anti- and pro-carcinogenic factor due to its effects on tumor and immune cells [120].

2.4. Phenethyl Isothiocyanate

Similar to other ITC members, PEITC can suppress carcinogenesis and malignant aggressiveness in various types of malignancies [121]. Suppression of various cancer-promoting characteristics, such as cancer cell proliferation, invasion, and angiogenesis, via regulation of the Bcl-2 protein family, caspases, and matrix metalloproteinases are reported as the potential molecular mechanisms underlying the tumor-suppressive activities of PEITC [121–123].

2.4.1. In Vitro Studies

PEITC was shown to have anti-cancer regulatory effects on cancer cell survival and apoptosis in BC cells [124]; PEITC inhibits cell viability in a dose-dependent manner and enhances apoptotic potential, as measured by caspases activities in T24 cells [124]. However, as shown in Table 4, the detailed molecular mechanisms underlying these anti-cancer effects in BC cells are not fully understood. It was reported that PEITC inhibits cell proliferation and stimulates apoptosis in the human adriamycin (ADM)-resistant bladder carcinoma cell line T24/ADM [123]. Interestingly, this study showed that PEITC increases intracellular drug accumulation potential and DNA topoisomerase II expression, and decreases multidrug resistance-related factors, such as multidrug resistance gene (MDR1), multidrug resistance-associated protein (MRP1), and glutathione S-transferase π [123]. In general, such changes by PEITC lead to increased chemosensitivity. Additionally, the authors clarified the detailed molecular mechanism underlying multidrug resistance reversal potential, which includes downregulation of NF-κB, survivin, Twist, and Akt and upregulation of PTEN and JNK by PEITC. As chemotherapeutic regimens including ADM are the standard therapy for patients with advanced UC [125,126], these findings highlight PEITC as a potential therapeutic agent for BC treatment, especially in patients with drug-resistant BC [123]. While we agree with their conclusion, clinical trials testing this hypothesis have yet to be performed.

Table 4. *In vitro* molecular mechanism of the anti-cancer effects of phenethyl isothiocyanate.

Anti-Cancer Effect	Underlying Molecular Mechanisms	Reference
Apoptosis ↑	Via caspase-9, a major regulator, and Bcl-2, Bax, Bak, and Bcl-xl	Tang & Zhang, 2005 [70]
Apoptosis ↑	Decreased NF-κB, survivin, Twist, and Akt expression and increased PTEN and JNK expression	Tang et al., 2013 [123]

Bcl, B-cell lymphoma-2; Bax, Bcl-2-associated X protein; Bak, BCL2-antagonist/killer; NF-κB, nuclear factor-kappa B; JNK, c-Jun N-terminal kinase.

Although BITC has been suggested to suppress cell growth by upregulating miR-99a expression via regulation of the c-Jun/AP-1 pathway in BC [79,80], this pathway plays no significant role in the anti-proliferative effects of PEITC in BC cells [127]. *In vitro* molecular mechanisms of the anti-cancer effects of PEITC are shown in Table 4.

2.4.2. In Vivo Studies

PEITC is suggested to play crucial roles in preventing the initiation step of carcinogenesis and inhibiting tumor progression in a variety of malignancies [121]. However, in a chemically BBN-induced BC animal model using male human c-Ha-ras proto-oncogene transgenic rats, microscopic BC is observed in the BBN alone (16 weeks) and BBN (8 weeks) → PEITC (8 weeks) groups; but not in the PEITC (8 weeks) → BBN (8 weeks) group [128]. This finding indicates that PEITC can inhibit the carcinogenic process after initiation. However, a conclusion cannot be drawn due to the limited information on *in vivo* SFN activities in BC.

2.4.3. Combination Therapy of Phenethyl Isothiocyanate and Other Therapeutic Agents

We previously introduced a novel treatment strategy that combines AITC and cisplatin for lung cancer cells (Section 2.1.4). Similarly, the efficacy of a combination therapy of PEITC and cisplatin was demonstrated in several studies. For instance, cervical cancer cells (HeLa) treated for 24 h with 5 μM PEITC and 10 μM cisplatin show typical features of apoptosis, such as cell shrinkage, membrane blebbing, and cell detachment, with a 4-fold increase in caspase-3 activity; these significant changes are not observed for either treatment alone [122]. The same study also showed that PEITC increases the pro-apoptotic activity of cisplatin in C33A cervical cancer and MCF-7 breast cancer cells; interestingly, this pro-apoptotic activity is not detected in normal human mammary epithelial MCF-10A cells [122]. Another study on non-small cell lung cancer cells (A549) showed that the percentage cell survival after treatment with AITC (15 μM) or cisplatin (5 μM) alone is 79.2 ± 3.8% and 55.9 ± 3.4%, respectively, whereas cell survival in the combination group is 46.2 ± 2.7% [129]. Notably, when PITC and cisplatin are co-encapsulated in liposomal nanoparticles, A549 cell survival further decreased to 33.3 ± 2.9% [129]. Similar results were obtained in another non-small cell lung cancer cells (H596), where the percentage cell survival after treatment with liposomal-PEITC-cisplatin or free PITC + cisplatin is 55.0 ± 9.5% and 28.6 ± 6.3%, respectively ($p < 0.001$) [129]. Moreover, the liposomal nanoparticles containing both PEITC and cisplatin have the advantage of increased circulation time in the bloodstream and accumulation in tumors [130]. Therefore, co-encapsulated PITC and cisplatin in liposomal nanoparticles may be a potential therapeutic strategy for advanced/metastatic UC.

3. Carcinogenic Potential of Isothiocyanates

There is general consensus that all ITC members possess anti-cancer effects in BC cells. However, several studies have also suggested the carcinogenic potential of ITCs in BC. In this section, we will discuss the relationships between BITC, SFN, and PEITC and carcinogenic changes in BC. To our knowledge, AITC has not been shown to promote tumorigenesis and carcinoma in BC; nevertheless, we cannot conclude that AITC has no carcinogenic potential as there is limited information on the biological and pathological effects of AITC in BC.

3.1. Carcinogenic Potential of Benzyl Isothiocyanate

In a two-stage carcinogenesis model, rats treated with BITC and with BBN initiation show neoplastic lesions, including papillary or nodular-hyperplasia (100%), papilloma (38%), and carcinoma (100%); these frequencies are higher than in rats under a basal diet (57%, 5%, and 24%, respectively) [131]. The frequencies of papilloma and carcinoma are also lower than those in rats with initiation + BITC (papilloma = 17% and carcinoma = 0%) and rats without initiation. Therefore, BITC may enhance the carcinogenic process in rats with initiation alone. However, in a BBN-induced BC rat model, oral administration of 10, 100, or 1,000 ppm BBN suppresses carcinogenic pathological changes [83]; moreover, epithelial hyperplasia of the urinary bladder is detected in rats treated with 100 or 1,000 ppm BITC, even without BBN [83]. Furthermore, the same research group showed that these neoplastic changes increase in rats with initiation treatment of 500 ppm BBN and subsequent low dose (25 ppm) BBN exposure, and their frequencies are further increased by additional treatment with 100 and 1000 ppm BITC in a dose-dependent manner [84]. In a similar experiment without initiation treatment, dysplasia, papilloma, and carcinoma were rare, although almost all rats had hyperplasia, except for the control and 100 ppm BITC groups [84]. Thus, BITC may stimulate carcinogenesis in a high-risk population of BBN-induced BC cases [83,84,132].

3.2. Carcinogenic Potential of Sulforaphane

As shown in a previous study, ≥20 μM SFN decreases cell viability and migration of T24 BC cells [112]. However, the study also showed that a low concentration of SFN promotes BC cell proliferation and migration [112], where 1–5 μM SFN or 2.5 and 3.75 SFN increase cell growth to approximately 120–130% and cell migration to 128 and 133% compared with those of control [112]. Thus, a biphasic effect of SFN on cell growth and migration of BC cells was suggested. Mechanistically, activation of autophagy by SFN is speculated to be associated with upregulated cell migration in an *in vivo* study using the autophagy inhibitor 3-methyladenine in T24 cells. The authors also found an enhanced protective effect in conjunction with selenium against free radical-induced cell death. Although this mechanism was confirmed in human hepatocyte cells (HHL-5) and breast cancer cells (MCF-7) rather than in BC cells, the benefits, and risks of SFN have been shown to be dependent on its doses and interactions with the microenvironment, including autophagy and selenium.

3.3. Carcinogenic Potential of Phenethyl Isothiocyanate

In an animal model of dimethylbenzanthracene-induced mammary carcinogenesis, continuous oral administration of 1200 ppm PEITC induces hyperplasia in the urinary bladder [133]. However, another study showed a high frequency of carcinoma (11 of 12 rats; 91.7%) with oral administration of 0.1% PEITC in rats for 48 weeks [134]; the authors thus conclude that PEITC has carcinogenic activities in the rat urinary bladder. By contrast, in a two-stage carcinogenesis model, rats treated with PEITC with BBN initiation exhibit papillary or nodular-hyperplasia (100%), papilloma (24%), and carcinoma (100%). Meanwhile, frequencies of papilloma (17%) and carcinoma (33%) are lower in rats without initiation than in those with initiation [131]. In studies showing the carcinogenic potential of PEITC according to initiation, specifically in a rat medium-term multi-organ carcinogenesis model, oral treatment with 0.1% PEITC after the initiation period leads to incidences of papillary or nodular-hyperplasia and tumors [135]. However, the authors showed that PEITC provided during the initiation period is not associated with carcinogenic activity [135]. These findings suggest that PEITC may stimulate carcinogenesis of UC during the post-initiation period. Another study, however, demonstrated that PEITC increases the incidences of papillary or nodular hyperplasia, dysplasia, and carcinoma in a dose-dependent manner; thus, > 0.01% PEITC enhances rat urinary bladder carcinogenesis and > 0.05% PEITC has tumorigenic potential. [136]. Collectively, these findings indicate that carcinogenic potential of PEITC administration may be modulated by complex mechanisms that involve timing and dosage.

When 0.1% BITC or 0.1% PEITC is administered in the diet to 6-week-old F344 rats for 1, 2, 3, and 7 days, a significant reduction of urinary pH levels compared to the normal control is detected, starting at day 1 [132]. Similarly, a reduction is detected in the urinary concentration of Na and Cl, whereas K is reduced. The same study also showed that thickness of the urinary bladder urothelium is significantly increased by administration of both BITC and PEITC and that inflammation, vacuolation, erosion, and apoptosis/single cell necrosis occur in the urinary bladder lesion; these morphological changes are not observed in normal control rats [132]. Furthermore, the cell proliferation potential, evaluated by the BrdU labeling index in male rats treated with BITC and female rats with BITC + PEITC, is significantly higher than that of control rats [132]. By contrast, when 0.1% BITC or 0.1% PEITC is administered for 14 days, histopathological simple hyperplasia and papillary/nodular hyperplasia are detected in 100% and 86% and 100% and 60% of the cases, respectively [132]. The authors thus suggest that continuous proliferation of bladder epithelial cells by BITC and PEITC plays important roles in pathological changes, including inflammation and the early stage of carcinogenesis [132]. Taken together, these findings are extremely important for the consideration of ITC treatment strategies, especially BITC and PEITC, for UC. However, we should note the difference in administered levels of ITCs in these studies. Although the mean daily consumption of BITC and PEITC in rats was approximately 80 mg/kg/day [132], these levels do not reflect human physiological conditions, i.e., 30 g of fresh watercress = 7.6 mg of PEITC per person and 0.8 mg from fresh (0.5 mg) and cooked (0.3 mg) Swede-turnips = 0.28 mg/person/day of PEITC [137,138].

4. Further Considerations

As previously mentioned, ITCs exhibit their anti- and pro-carcinogenic activities via complex mechanisms. In this review, we mainly introduced the findings of pre-clinical *in vivo* and *in vitro* studies for easier understanding across the field. However, we would be remiss if we do not mention that other cancer-related factors and signaling molecules affect the biological activities and anti-cancer effects of ITCs in malignancies. These include direct/indirect interactions with Nrf2 and NF-κB, the Nrf2-Kelch-like ECH-associated protein (Keap) 1-antioxidant response element (ARE) signaling pathway, and antioxidant enzymes, such as NAD(P)H quinone reductase (NQO1) and glutathione S transferases (GSTs), through the Nrf2-Keap1-ARE signaling pathway are closely associated with ITC-induced bioactivity [139–141]. We would like to emphasize that further basic research is essential for uncovering the utility and limitations of ITCs in cancer treatment, including BC.

Another important issue to consider is the carcinogenic risk factors of BC, which are affected by a variety of harmful chemical compounds (e.g., cigarette smoke) or physiologically active substances (e.g., sex hormones) [142–144]. With regards to cigarette smoke, cytochrome P450 and phase II detoxification enzymes, such as DOQ1, GSTs, and glucuronosyltransferase inhibit the formation of carcinogenic compounds from tobacco-specific carcinogens, and PEITC modulates such cancer preventive activities [145]. This finding supports the hypothesis that PEITC may suppress the tobacco-related cancer risk in smokers. Indeed, a clinical trial showed that metabolic activation of a tobacco-specific lung carcinogen is significantly suppressed by PEIT treatment [146]. We believe that the cancer risk of BC in smokers may be suppressed by ITCs though similar anti-carcinogenic mechanisms, and thus there is value in performing such clinical trials for BC. Furthermore, the frequency of BC is known to be remarkably higher in men than in women, which is perhaps due to the testosterone-androgen receptor pathways [147]. Interestingly, PEITC was reported to suppress testosterone-induced cancer cell proliferation by downregulating the testosterone-androgen receptor pathway in prostate cancer [148]. Meanwhile, other research has shown that estrogen-mediated pathways are associated with malignant potential and tumor growth of BC [143,144]. In addition, SFN was found to regulate tumor growth of breast cancer cells by modulating estrogen activities [149]. Unfortunately, there is little information on the influence of ITC-mediated sex hormone activity on the malignant potential of BC. Nevertheless, there is a possibility that ITCs affect carcinogenesis and malignant aggressiveness by regulating sex hormones in BC. This highlights the need for designing studies to identify the biological roles of ITCs according to patient background and environment, including occupation, diet, and health habits.

5. Conclusions

In this review, we discussed the anti-cancer effects of ITCs in BC. The research suggests that all ITC members can suppress carcinogenesis, tumor development, and progression *in vivo* and *in vitro*. Furthermore, regulation of cell proliferation, cell cycle, and apoptosis play crucial roles in the ITC-induced anti-cancer effects, and such phenomena are mainly regulated by complex mechanisms involving caspases, Bcl-2 family proteins, and mitochondrial activities. While changes in cancer-related molecules by ITCs may correspond to anti-cancer mechanisms in BC cells, some ITCs may have neoplastic and carcinogenic potential in BC. To clarify this issue, more detailed studies at the molecular level are essential. While there is a possibility that ITC-based treatment strategies can improve prognosis in patients with BC, further clinical trials with well-designed protocols are required to establish the optimal doses and types of ITCs for application in BC treatment [112]. In addition, it would be fruitful to investigate the anti-cancer effects and clinical utility of combination therapies of ITCs and new therapeutic strategies, including immunotherapy and gene therapy, for patients with BC.

Author Contributions: Conceptualization, Y.M.; supervision, H.S.; writing—original draft preparation, T.M., Y.M., T.Y., Y.M., A.O., K.M. and K.O. All authors have read and agreed to the published version of the manuscript. The authors declare that the content of this paper has not been published or submitted for publication elsewhere.

References

1. Metts, M.C.; Metts, J.C.; Milito, S.J.; Thomas, C.R., Jr. Bladder cancer: A review of diagnosis and management. *J. Natl. Med. Assoc.* **2000**, *92*, 285–294. [PubMed]
2. Siegel, R.L.; Miller, K.D.; Jemal, A. Cancer statistics, 2019. *CA Cancer J. Clin.* **2019**, *69*, 7–34. [CrossRef] [PubMed]
3. Von der Maase, H.; Hansen, S.W.; Roberts, J.T.; Dogliotti, L.; Oliver, T.; Moore, M.J.; Bodrogi, I.; Albers, P.; Knuth, A. Gemcitabine and cisplatin versus methotrexate, vinblastine, doxorubicin, and cisplatin in advanced or metastatic bladder cancer: Results of a large, randomized, multinational, multicenter, phase III study. *J. Clin. Oncol.* **2000**, *18*, 3068–3077. [CrossRef] [PubMed]
4. Tripathi, A.; Plimack, E.R. Immunotherapy for Urothelial Carcinoma: Current Evidence and Future Directions. *Curr. Urol Rep.* **2018**, *19*, 109. [CrossRef]
5. Wang, H.; Liu, J.; Fang, K.; Ke, C.; Jiang, Y.; Wang, G.; Yang, T.; Chen, T.; Shi, X. Second-line treatment strategy for urothelial cancer patients who progress or are unfit for cisplatin therapy: A network meta-analysis. *BMC Urol.* **2019**, *19*, 125. [CrossRef]
6. Tan, W.P.; Tan, W.S.; Inman, B.A. PD-L1/PD-1 Biomarker for Metastatic Urothelial Cancer that Progress Post-platinum Therapy: A Systematic Review and Meta-analysis. *Bladder. Cancer* **2019**, *5*, 211–223. [CrossRef]
7. Hanna, K.S. Clinical Overview of Enfortumab Vedotin in the Management of Locally Advanced or Metastatic Urothelial Carcinoma. *Drugs* **2019**, in press. [CrossRef]
8. Sharma, P.; Sohn, J.; Shin, S.J.; Oh, D.Y.; Keam, B.; Lee, H.J.; Gizzi, M.; Kalinka, E.; de Vos, F.Y.F.L. Efficacy and Tolerability of Tremelimumab in Locally Advanced or Metastatic Urothelial Carcinoma Patients Who Have Failed First-Line Platinum-Based Chemotherapy. *Clin. Cancer Res* **2019**, in press.

9. Wan Mohd Tajuddin, W.N.B.; Lajis, N.H.; Abas, F.; Othman, I.; Naidu, R. Mechanistic Understanding of Curcumin's Therapeutic Effects in Lung Cancer. *Nutrients* **2019**, *11*, 989. [CrossRef]
10. Shu, P.; Tang, H.; Zhou, B.; Wang, R.; Xu, Y.; Shao, J.; Qi, M.; Xia, Y.; Huang, W.; Liu, S. Effect of Yiqi Huayu Jiedu decoction on stages II and III gastric cancer: A multicenter, prospective, cohort study. *Medicine* **2019**, *98*, e17875. [CrossRef]
11. Cullen, J.K.; Simmons, J.L.; Parsons, P.G.; Boyle, G.M. Topical treatments for skin cancer. Oral Intake of Royal Jelly Has Protective Effects Against Tyrosine Kinase Inhibitor-Induced Toxicity in Patients with Renal Cell Carcinoma: A Randomized, Double-Blinded, Placebo-Controlled Trial. *Adv. Drug Deliv. Rev.* **2019**, in press.
12. Emsen, B.; Ozdemir, O.; Engin, T.; Togar, B.; Cavusoglu, S.; Turkez, H. Inhibition of growth of U87MG human glioblastoma cells by Usnea longissima Ach. *An. Acad. Bras. Cienc.* **2019**, *91*, e20180994. [CrossRef] [PubMed]
13. Huang, Z.; Wei, P. Compound Kushen Injection for gastric cancer: A protocol of systematic review and meta-analysis. *Med. Baltimore* **2019**, *98*, e17927. [CrossRef] [PubMed]
14. Kim, K.I.; Kong, M.; Lee, S.H.; Lee, B.J. The efficacy and safety of Kyung-Ok-Ko on cancer-related fatigue in lung cancer patients: Study protocol for a randomized, patients-assessor blind, placebo-controlled, parallel-group, single-center trial. *Medicine* **2019**, *98*, e17717. [CrossRef]
15. Shi, C.S.; Li, J.M.; Chin, C.C.; Kuo, Y.H.; Lee, Y.R.; Huang, Y.C. Evodiamine Induces Cell Growth Arrest, Apoptosis and Suppresses Tumorigenesis in Human Urothelial Cell Carcinoma Cells. *Anticancer Res.* **2017**, *37*, 1149–1159.
16. Falke, J.; Parkkinen, J.; Vaahtera, L.; Hulsbergen-van de Kaa, C.A.; Oosterwijk, E.; Witjes, J.A. Curcumin as Treatment for Bladder Cancer: A Preclinical Study of Cyclodextrin-Curcumin Complex and BCG as Intravesical Treatment in an Orthotopic Bladder Cancer Rat Model. *Biomed. Res. Int.* **2018**, *2018*, 9634902. [CrossRef]
17. Yang, H.Y.; Chen, P.C.; Wang, J.D. Chinese herbs containing aristolochic acid associated with renal failure and urothelial carcinoma: A review from epidemiologic observations to causal inference. *Biomed. Res. Int.* **2014**, *2014*, 569325. [CrossRef]
18. Křížová, L.; Dadáková, K.; Kašparovská, J.; Kašparovský, T. Isoflavones. *Molecules* **2019**, *24*, 1076. [CrossRef]
19. Sagara, Y.; Miyata, Y.; Nomata, K.; Hayashi, T.; Kanetake, H. Green tea polyphenol suppresses tumor invasion and angiogenesis in N-butyl-(-4-hydroxybutyl) nitrosamine-induced bladder cancer. *Cancer Epidemiol.* **2010**, *34*, 350–354. [CrossRef]
20. Matsuo, T.; Miyata, Y.; Asai, A.; Sagara, Y.; Furusato, B.; Fukuoka, J.; Sakai, H. Green Tea Polyphenol Induces Changes in Cancer-Related Factors in an Animal Model of Bladder Cancer. *PLoS ONE* **2017**, *12*, e0171091. [CrossRef]
21. Araki, K.; Miyata, Y.; Ohba, K.; Nakamura, Y.; Matsuo, T.; Mochizuki, Y.; Sakai, H. *Medicines* **2018**, *6*, 2. [CrossRef] [PubMed]
22. Miyata, Y.; Matsuo, T.; Araki, K.; Nakamura, Y.; Sagara, Y.; Ohba, K.; Sakai, H. Anticancer Effects of Green Tea and the Underlying Molecular Mechanisms in Bladder Cancer. *Medicines* **2018**, *5*, 87. [CrossRef] [PubMed]
23. Miyata, Y.; Sakai, H. Anti-Cancer and Protective Effects of Royal Jelly for Therapy-Induced Toxicities in Malignancies. *Int. J. Mol. Sci.* **2018**, *19*, 3270. [CrossRef] [PubMed]
24. Yasuda, T.; Miyata, Y.; Nakamura, Y.; Sagara, Y.; Matsuo, T.; Ohba, K.; Sakai, H. High Consumption of Green Tea Suppresses Urinary Tract Recurrence of Urothelial Cancer *via* Down-regulation of Human Antigen-R Expression in Never Smokers. *In Vivo* **2018**, *32*, 721–729. [CrossRef] [PubMed]
25. Miyata, Y.; Shida, Y.; Hakariya, T.; Sakai, H. Anti-Cancer Effects of Green Tea Polyphenols Against Prostate Cancer. *Molecules* **2019**, *24*, 193. [CrossRef] [PubMed]
26. Abbaoui, B.; Telu, K.H.; Lucas, C.R.; Thomas-Ahner, J.M.; Schwartz, S.J.; Clinton, S.K.; Freitas, M.A.; Mortazavi, A. The impact of cruciferous vegetable isothiocyanates on histone acetylation and histone phosphorylation in bladder cancer. *J. Proteomics* **2017**, *156*, 94–103. [CrossRef] [PubMed]
27. Abbaoui, B.; Lucas, C.R.; Riedl, K.M.; Clinton, S.K.; Mortazavi, A. Cruciferous Vegetables, Isothiocyanates, and Bladder Cancer Prevention. *Mol. Nutr. Food Res.* **2018**, *62*, e1800079. [CrossRef]
28. Leone, A.; Diorio, G.; Sexton, W.; Schell, M.; Alexandrow, M.; Fahey, J.W.; Kumar, N.B. Sulforaphane for the chemoprevention of bladder cancer: Molecular mechanism targeted approach. *Oncotarget* **2017**, *8*, 35412–35424. [CrossRef]

29. Tang, L.; Zirpoli, G.R.; Guru, K.; Moysich, K.B.; Zhang, Y.; Ambrosone, C.B.; McCann, S.E. Consumption of raw cruciferous vegetables is inversely associated with bladder cancer risk. *Cancer Epidemiol. Biomarkers Prev.* **2008**, *17*, 938–944. [CrossRef]
30. Vieira, A.R.; Vingeliene, S.; Chan, D.S.; Aune, D.; Abar, L.; Navarro Rosenblatt, D.; Greenwood, D.C.; Norat, T. Fruits, vegetables, and bladder cancer risk: A systematic review and meta-analysis. *Cancer Med.* **2015**, *4*, 136–146. [CrossRef]
31. Xu, C.; Zeng, X.T.; Liu, T.Z.; Zhang, C.; Yang, Z.H.; Li, S.; Chen, X.Y. Fruits and vegetables intake and risk of bladder cancer: A PRISMA-compliant systematic review and dose-response meta-analysis of prospective cohort studies. *Med. Baltimore* **2015**, *94*, e759. [CrossRef] [PubMed]
32. Shapiro, T.A.; Fahey, J.W.; Wade, K.L.; Stephenson, K.K.; Talalay, P. Chemoprotective glucosinolates and isothiocyanates of broccoli sprouts: Metabolism and excretion in humans. *Cancer Epidemiol. Biomarkers Prev.* **2001**, *10*, 501–508. [PubMed]
33. Palliyaguru, D.L.; Yuan, J.M.; Kensler, T.W.; Fahey, J.W. Isothiocyanates: Translating the Power of Plants to People. *Mol. Nutr. Food Res.* **2018**, *62*, e1700965. [CrossRef] [PubMed]
34. Romeo, L.; Iori, R.; Rollin, P.; Bramanti, P.; Mazzon, E. Isothiocyanates: An Overview of Their Antimicrobial Activity against Human Infections. *Molecules* **2018**, *23*, 624. [CrossRef]
35. Novío, S.; Cartea, M.E.; Soengas, P.; Freire-Garabal, M.; Núñez-Iglesias, M.J. Effects of Brassicaceae Isothiocyanates on Prostate Cancer. *Molecules* **2016**, *21*, 626. [CrossRef]
36. Martin, S.L.; Royston, K.J.; Tollefsbol, T.O. The Role of Non-Coding RNAs and Isothiocyanates in Cancer. *Mol. Nutr. Food Res.* **2018**, *62*, e1700913. [CrossRef]
37. Mitsiogianni, M.; Koutsidis, G.; Mavroudis, N.; Trafalis, D.T.; Botaitis, S.; Franco, R.; Zoumpourlis, V.; Amery, T.; Galanis, A. The Role of Isothiocyanates as Cancer Chemo-Preventive, Chemo-Therapeutic and Anti-Melanoma Agents. *Antioxidants* **2019**, *8*, E106. [CrossRef]
38. Aytac, Z.; Dogan, S.Y.; Tekinay, T.; Uyar, T. Release and antibacterial activity of allyl isothiocyanate/β-cyclodextrin complex encapsulated in electrospun nanofibers. *Colloids Surf. B Biointerfaces* **2014**, *120*, 125–131. [CrossRef]
39. Subedi, L.; Venkatesan, R.; Kim, S.Y. Neuroprotective and Anti-Inflammatory Activities of Allyl Isothiocyanate through Attenuation of JNK/NF-κB/TNF-α Signaling. *Int. J. Mol. Sci.* **2017**, *18*, 1423. [CrossRef]
40. Chen, N.G.; Chen, K.T.; Lu, C.C.; Lan, Y.H.; Lai, C.H.; Chung, Y.T.; Yang, J.S.; Lin, Y.C. Allyl isothiocyanate triggers G2/M phase arrest and apoptosis in human brain malignant glioma GBM 8401 cells through a mitochondria-dependent pathway. *Oncol. Rep.* **2010**, *24*, 449–455.
41. Qin, G.; Li, P.; Xue, Z. Effect of allyl isothiocyanate on the viability and apoptosis of the human cervical cancer HeLa cell line *in vitro*. *Oncol. Lett.* **2018**, *15*, 8756–8760. [CrossRef] [PubMed]
42. Rajakumar, T.; Pugalendhi, P.; Thilagavathi, S.; Ananthakrishnan, D.; Gunasekaran, K. Allyl isothiocyanate, a potent chemopreventive agent targets AhR/Nrf2 signaling pathway in chemically induced mammary carcinogenesis. *Mol. Cell Biochem.* **2018**, *437*, 1–12. [CrossRef]
43. Sayeed, M.A.; Bracci, M.; Ciarapica, V.; Malavolta, M.; Provinciali, M.; Pieragostini, E.; Gaetani, S.; Monaco, F.; Lucarini, G. Allyl Isothiocyanate Exhibits No Anticancer Activity in MDA-MB-231 Breast Cancer Cells. *Int. J. Mol. Sci.* **2018**, *19*, 145. [CrossRef] [PubMed]
44. Savio, A.L.; da Silva, G.N.; de Camargo, E.A.; Salvadori, D.M. Cell cycle kinetics, apoptosis rates, DNA damage and TP53 gene expression in bladder cancer cells treated with allyl isothiocyanate (mustard essential oil). *Mutat. Res.* **2014**, *762*, 40–46. [CrossRef] [PubMed]
45. Kim, Y.J.; Lee, D.H.; Ahn, J.; Chung, W.J.; Jang, Y.J.; Seong, K.S.; Moon, J.H.; Ha, T.Y.; Jung, C.H. Pharmacokinetics, Tissue Distribution, and Anti-Lipogenic/Adipogenic Effects of Allyl-Isothiocyanate Metabolites. *PLoS ONE* **2015**, *10*, e0132151.
46. Sávio, A.L.; da Silva, G.N.; Salvadori, D.M. Inhibition of bladder cancer cell proliferation by allyl isothiocyanate (mustard essential oil). *Mutat. Res.* **2015**, *771*, 29–35. [CrossRef]
47. Blažević, I.; Đulović, A.; Maravić, A.; Čikeš Čulić, V.; Montaut, S.; Rollin, P. Antimicrobial and Cytotoxic Activities of Lepidium latifolium L.; Hydrodistillate, Extract and Its Major Sulfur Volatile Allyl Isothiocyanate. *Chem. Biodivers.* **2019**, *16*, e1800661. [CrossRef]
48. Geng, F.; Tang, L.; Li, Y.; Yang, L.; Choi, K.S.; Kazim, A.L.; Zhang, Y. Allyl isothiocyanate arrests cancer cells in mitosis, and mitotic arrest in turn leads to apoptosis via Bcl-2 protein phosphorylation. *J. Biol. Chem.* **2011**, *286*, 32259–32267. [CrossRef]

49. Hinata, N.; Shirakawa, T.; Zhang, Z.; Matsumoto, A.; Fujisawa, M.; Okada, H.; Kamidono, S.; Gotoh, A. Radiation induces p53-dependent cell apoptosis in bladder cancer cells with wild-type- p53 but not in p53-mutated bladder cancer cells. *Urol. Res.* **2003**, *31*, 387–396. [CrossRef]
50. Bhattacharya, A.; Li, Y.; Geng, F.; Munday, R.; Zhang, Y. The principal urinary metabolite of allyl isothiocyanate, N-acetyl-S-(N-allylthiocarbamoyl)cysteine, inhibits the growth and muscle invasion of bladder cancer. *Carcinogenesis* **2012**, *33*, 394–398. [CrossRef]
51. Munday, R.; Mhawech-Fauceglia, P.; Munday, C.M.; Paonessa, J.D.; Tang, L.; Munday, J.S.; Lister, C.; Wilson, P.; Fahey, J.W. Inhibition of urinary bladder carcinogenesis by broccoli sprouts. *Cancer Res.* **2008**, *68*, 1593–1600. [CrossRef] [PubMed]
52. Bhattacharya, A.; Li, Y.; Wade, K.L.; Paonessa, J.D.; Fahey, J.W.; Zhang, Y. Allyl isothiocyanate-rich mustard seed powder inhibits bladder cancer growth and muscle invasion. *Carcinogenesis* **2010**, *31*, 2105–2110. [CrossRef] [PubMed]
53. Miyata, Y.; Kanda, S.; Nomata, K.; Eguchi, J.; Kanetake, H. Expression of cyclooxygenase-2 and EP4 receptor in transitional cell carcinoma of the upper urinary tract. *J. Urol.* **2005**, *173*, 56–60. [CrossRef] [PubMed]
54. Miyata, Y.; Ohba, K.; Kanda, S.; Nomata, K.; Eguchi, J.; Hayashi, T.; Kanetake, H. Pathological function of prostaglandin E2 receptors in transitional cell carcinoma of the upper urinary tract. *Virchows Arch.* **2006**, *448*, 822–829. [CrossRef] [PubMed]
55. Van Kessel, K.E.; Zuiverloon, T.C.; Alberts, A.R.; Boormans, J.L.; Zwarthoff, E.C. Targeted therapies in bladder cancer: An overview of in vivo research. *Nat. Rev. Urol.* **2015**, *12*, 681–694. [CrossRef] [PubMed]
56. Benelli, R.; Venè, R.; Ferrari, N. Prostaglandin-endoperoxide synthase 2 (cyclooxygenase-2), a complex target for colorectal cancer prevention and therapy. *Transl. Res.* **2018**, *196*, 42–61. [CrossRef] [PubMed]
57. Ferreira, T.; Campos, S.; Silva, M.G.; Ribeiro, R.; Santos, S.; Almeida, J.; Pires, M.J.; Gil da Costa, R.M.; Córdova, C. The Cyclooxigenase-2 Inhibitor Parecoxib Prevents Epidermal Dysplasia in HPV16-Transgenic Mice: Efficacy and Safety Observations. *Int. J. Mol. Sci.* **2019**, *20*, 3902. [CrossRef]
58. Umezawa, S.; Higurashi, T.; Komiya, Y.; Arimoto, J.; Horita, N.; Kaneko, T.; Iwasaki, M.; Nakagama, H.; Nakajima, A. Chemoprevention of colorectal cancer: Past, present, and future. *Cancer Sci.* **2019**, *110*, 3018–3026. [CrossRef]
59. Mascan, B.; Marignol, L. Aspirin in the Management of Patients with Prostate Cancer Undergoing Radiotherapy: Friend or Foe? *Anticancer Res.* **2018**, *38*, 1897–1902.
60. Guo, Q.; Li, Q.; Wang, J.; Liu, M.; Wang, Y.; Chen, Z.; Ye, Y.; Guan, Q.; Zhou, Y. A comprehensive evaluation of clinical efficacy and safety of celecoxib in combination with chemotherapy in metastatic or postoperative recurrent gastric cancer patients: A preliminary, three-center, clinical trial study. *Medicine (Baltimore)* **2019**, *98*, e16234. [CrossRef]
61. Bhattacharya, A.; Li, Y.; Shi, Y.; Zhang, Y. Enhanced inhibition of urinary bladder cancer growth and muscle invasion by allyl isothiocyanate and celecoxib in combination. *Carcinogenesis* **2013**, *34*, 2593–2599. [CrossRef] [PubMed]
62. Ling, X.; Westover, D.; Cao, F.; Cao, S.; He, X.; Kim, H.R.; Zhang, Y.; Chan, D.C.; Li, F. Synergistic effect of allyl isothiocyanate (AITC) on cisplatin efficacy in vitro and in vivo. *Am. J. Cancer Res.* **2015**, *5*, 2516–2530. [PubMed]
63. Chang, W.J.; Chen, B.H.; Inbaraj, B.S.; Chien, J.T. Preparation of allyl isothiocyanate nanoparticles, their anti-inflammatory activity towards RAW 264.7 macrophage cells and anti-proliferative effect on HT1376 bladder cancer cells. *J. Sci Food Agric.* **2019**, *99*, 3106–3116. [CrossRef] [PubMed]
64. Liu, P.; Behray, M.; Wang, Q.; Wang, W.; Zhou, Z.; Chao, Y.; Bao, Y. Anti-cancer a ctivities of allyl isothiocyanate and its conjugated silicon quantum dots. *Sci. Rep.* **2018**, *18*, 1084. [CrossRef]
65. Ibrahim, A.; Al-Hizab, F.A.; Abushouk, A.I.; Abdel-Daim, M.M. Nephroprotective Effects of Benzyl Isothiocyanate and Resveratrol Against Cisplatin-Induced Oxidative Stress and Inflammation. *Front. Pharmacol.* **2018**, *9*, 1268. [CrossRef]
66. Tang, Y.; Naito, S.; Abe-Kanoh, N.; Ogawa, S.; Yamaguchi, S.; Zhu, B.; Murata, Y.; Nakamura, Y. Benzyl isothiocyanate attenuates the hydrogen peroxide-induced interleukin-13 expression through glutathione S-transferase P induction in T lymphocytic leukemia cells. *J. Biochem. Mol. Toxicol.* **2018**, *32*, e22054. [CrossRef]

67. Huang, Y.P.; Jiang, Y.W.; Chen, H.Y.; Hsiao, Y.T.; Peng, S.F.; Chou, Y.C.; Yang, J.L.; Hsia, T.C.; Chung, J.G. Benzyl Isothiocyanate Induces Apoptotic Cell Death Through Mitochondria-dependent Pathway in Gefitinib-resistant NCI-H460 Human Lung Cancer Cells *In Vitro*. *Anticancer Res.* **2018**, *38*, 5165–5176. [CrossRef]
68. Ma, L.; Chen, Y.; Han, R.; Wang, S. Benzyl isothiocyanate inhibits invasion and induces apoptosis via reducing S100A4 expression and increases PUMA expression in oral squamous cell carcinoma cells. *Braz. J. Med. Biol. Res.* **2019**, *52*, e8409. [CrossRef]
69. Xie, B.; Zhao, L.; Guo, L.; Liu, H.; Fu, S.; Fan, W.; Lin, L.; Chen, J.; Wang, B.; Fan, L.; et al. Benzyl isothiocyanate suppresses development and metastasis of murine mammary carcinoma by regulating the Wnt/β-catenin pathway. *Mol. Med. Rep.* **2019**, *20*, 1808–1818. [CrossRef]
70. Tang, L.; Zhang, Y. Mitochondria are the primary target in isothiocyanate-induced apoptosis in human bladder cancer cells. *Mol. Cancer Ther.* **2005**, *4*, 1250–1259. [CrossRef]
71. Tang, L.; Li, G.; Song, L.; Zhang, Y. The principal urinary metabolites of dietary isothiocyanates, N-acetylcysteine conjugates, elicit the same anti-proliferative response as their parent compounds in human bladder cancer cells. *Anticancer Drugs* **2006**, *17*, 297–305. [CrossRef] [PubMed]
72. Tang, L.; Zhang, Y. Dietary isothiocyanates inhibit the growth of human bladder carcinoma cells. *J. Nutr.* **2004**, *134*, 2004–2010. [CrossRef] [PubMed]
73. Izquierdo, L.; Ingelmo-Torres, M.; Mallofré, C.; Lozano, J.J.; Verhasselt-Crinquette, M.; Leroy, X.; Colin, P.; Comperat, E.; Roupret, M.; Alcaraz, A.; et al. Prognostic value of microRNA expression pattern in upper tract urothelial carcinoma. *BJU Int.* **2014**, *113*, 813–821. [CrossRef]
74. Braicu, C.; Cojocneanu-Petric, R.; Chira, S.; Truta, A.; Floares, A.; Petrut, B.; Achimas-Cadariu, P.; Berindan-Neagoe, I. Clinical and pathological implications of miRNA in bladder cancer. *Int. J. Nanomed.* **2015**, *10*, 791–800. [CrossRef] [PubMed]
75. Nordentoft, I.; Birkenkamp-Demtroder, K.; Agerbæk, M.; Theodorescu, D.; Ostenfeld, M.S.; Hartmann, A.; Borre, M.; Ørntoft, T.F.; Dyrskjøt, L. miRNAs associated with chemo-sensitivity in cell lines and in advanced bladder cancer. *BMC Med. Genomics* **2012**, *5*, 40. [CrossRef] [PubMed]
76. Liu, Y.; Li, B.; Yang, X.; Zhang, C. MiR-99a-5p inhibits bladder cancer cell proliferation by directly targeting mammalian target of rapamycin and predicts patient survival. *J. Cell Biochem.* **2019**, *120*, 19330–19337. [CrossRef] [PubMed]
77. Inamoto, T.; Uehara, H.; Akao, Y.; Ibuki, N.; Komura, K.; Takahara, K.; Takai, T.; Uchimoto, T.; Saito, K. A Panel of MicroRNA Signature as a Tool for Predicting Survival of Patients with Urothelial Carcinoma of the Bladder. *Dis. Markers* **2018**, *2018*, 5468672. [CrossRef]
78. Tsai, T.F.; Lin, J.F.; Chou, K.Y.; Lin, Y.C.; Chen, H.E.; Hwang, T.I. miR-99a-5p acts as tumor suppressor via targeting to mTOR and enhances RAD001-induced apoptosis in human urinary bladder urothelial carcinoma cells. *Onco Targets Ther.* **2018**, *11*, 239–252. [CrossRef]
79. Tsai, T.F.; Chen, P.C.; Lin, Y.C.; Chou, K.Y.; Chen, H.E.; Ho, C.Y.; Lin, J.F.; Hwang, T.I. Benzyl isothiocyanate promotes miR-99a expression through ERK/AP-1-dependent pathway in bladder cancer cells. *Environ. Toxicol.* **2020**, *35*, 47–54. [CrossRef]
80. Feng, Y.; Kang, Y.; He, Y.; Liu, J.; Liang, B.; Yang, P.; Yu, Z. microRNA-99a acts as a tumor suppressor and is down-regulated in bladder cancer. *BMC Urol.* **2014**, *14*, 50. [CrossRef]
81. Tsai, T.F.; Lin, Y.C.; Chen, H.E.; Chou, K.Y.; Lin, J.F.; Hwang, T.I.S. Involvement of the insulin-like growth factor I receptor and its downstream antiapoptotic signaling pathway is revealed by dysregulated micro-RNA in bladder carcinoma. *Urol Sci.* **2014**, *25*, 58–64. [CrossRef]
82. Ganji, S.M.; Saidijam, M.; Amini, R.; Mousavi-Bahar, S.H.; Shabab, N.; Seyedabadi, S.; Mahdavinezhad, A. Evaluation of MicroRNA-99a and MicroRNA-205 Expression Levels in Bladder Cancer. *Int J. Mol. Cell Med.* **2017**, *6*, 87–95. [PubMed]
83. Okazaki, K.; Yamagishi, M.; Son, H.Y.; Imazawa, T.; Furukawa, F.; Nakamura, H.; Nishikawa, A.; Masegi, T.; Hirose, M. Simultaneous treatment with benzyl isothiocyanate, a strong bladder promoter, inhibits rat urinary bladder carcinogenesis by N-butyl-N-(4-hydroxybutyl)nitrosamine. *Nutr. Cancer* **2002**, *42*, 211–216. [CrossRef] [PubMed]

84. Okazaki, K.; Umemura, T.; Imazawa, T.; Nishikawa, A.; Masegi, T.; Hirose, M. Enhancement of urinary bladder carcinogenesis by combined treatment with benzyl isothiocyanate and N-butyl-N-(4-hydroxybutyl)nitrosamine in rats after initiation. *Cancer Sci.* **2003**, *94*, 948–952. [CrossRef]
85. Di Pasqua, A.J.; Hong, C.; Wu, M.Y.; McCracken, E.; Wang, X.; Mi, L.; Chung, F.L. Sensitization of non-small cell lung cancer cells to cisplatin by naturally occurring isothiocyanates. *Chem. Res. Toxicol.* **2010**, *23*, 1307–1309. [CrossRef]
86. Lee, Y.; Kim, Y.J.; Choi, Y.J.; Lee, J.W.; Lee, S.; Chung, H.W. Enhancement of cisplatin cytotoxicity by benzyl isothiocyanate in HL-60 cells. *Food Chem. Toxicol.* **2012**, *50*, 2397–2406. [CrossRef]
87. Wolf, M.A.; Claudio, P.P. Benzyl isothiocyanate inhibits HNSCC cell migration and invasion, and sensitizes HNSCC cells to cisplatin. *Nutr. Cancer* **2014**, *66*, 285–294. [CrossRef]
88. Xia, Y.; Kang, T.W.; Jung, Y.D.; Zhang, C.; Lian, S. Sulforaphane Inhibits Nonmuscle Invasive Bladder Cancer Cells Proliferation through Suppression of HIF-1α-Mediated Glycolysis in Hypoxia. *J. Agric. Food Chem.* **2019**, *67*, 7844–7854. [CrossRef]
89. Bernkopf, D.B.; Daum, G.; Brückner, M.; Behrens, J. Sulforaphane inhibits growth and blocks Wnt/β-catenin signaling of colorectal cancer cells. *Oncotarget* **2018**, *9*, 33982–33994. [CrossRef]
90. Kan, S.F.; Wang, J.; Sun, G.X. Sulforaphane regulates apoptosis- and proliferation-related signaling pathways and synergizes with cisplatin to suppress human ovarian cancer. *Int. J. Mol. Med.* **2018**, *42*, 2447–2458. [CrossRef]
91. Park, H.S.; Han, M.H.; Kim, G.Y.; Moon, S.K.; Kim, W.J.; Hwang, H.J.; Park, K.Y.; Choi, Y.H. Sulforaphane induces reactive oxygen species-mediated mitotic arrest and subsequent apoptosis in human bladder cancer 5637 cells. *Food Chem. Toxicol.* **2014**, *64*, 157–165. [CrossRef] [PubMed]
92. Jo, G.H.; Kim, G.Y.; Kim, W.J.; Park, K.Y.; Choi, Y.H. Sulforaphane induces apoptosis in T24 human urinary bladder cancer cells through a reactive oxygen species-mediated mitochondrial pathway: The involvement of endoplasmic reticulum stress and the Nrf2 signaling pathway. *Int. J. Oncol.* **2014**, *45*, 1497–1506. [CrossRef] [PubMed]
93. Shan, Y.; Sun, C.; Zhao, X.; Wu, K.; Cassidy, A.; Bao, Y. Effect of sulforaphane on cell growth, G(0)/G(1) phase cell progression and apoptosis in human bladder cancer T24 cells. *Int. J. Oncol.* **2006**, *29*, 883–888. [CrossRef] [PubMed]
94. Ding, Y.; Paonessa, J.D.; Randall, K.L.; Argoti, D.; Chen, L.; Vouros, P.; Zhang, Y. Sulforaphane inhibits 4-aminobiphenyl-induced DNA damage in bladder cells and tissues. *Carcinogenesis* **2010**, *31*, 1999–2003. [CrossRef] [PubMed]
95. Cullinan, S.B.; Diehl, J.A. Coordination of ER and oxidative stress signaling: The PERK/Nrf2 signaling pathway. *Int. J. Biochem. Cell Biol.* **2006**, *38*, 317–332. [CrossRef] [PubMed]
96. Dang, Y.M.; Huang, G.; Chen, Y.R.; Dang, Z.F.; Chen, C.; Liu, F.L.; Guo, Y.F.; Xie, X.D. Sulforaphane inhibits the proliferation of the BIU87 bladder cancer cell line via IGFBP-3 elevation. *Asian Pac. J. Cancer Prev.* **2014**, *15*, 1517–1520. [CrossRef] [PubMed]
97. Baxter, R.C. IGF binding proteins in cancer: Mechanistic and clinical insights. *Nat. Rev. Cancer.* **2014**, *14*, 329–341. [CrossRef]
98. Patel, M.; Horgan, P.G.; McMillan, D.C.; Edwards, J. NF-κB pathways in the development and progression of colorectal cancer. *Transl. Res.* **2018**, *197*, 43–56. [CrossRef]
99. Abbaoui, B.; Riedl, K.M.; Ralston, R.A.; Thomas-Ahner, J.M.; Schwartz, S.J.; Clinton, S.K.; Mortazavi, A. Inhibition of bladder cancer by broccoli isothiocyanates sulforaphane and erucin: Characterization, metabolism, and interconversion. *Mol. Nutr. Food Res.* **2012**, *56*, 1675–1687. [CrossRef]
100. Hao, L.; Zhao, Y.; Li, Z.G.; He, H.G.; Liang, Q.; Zhang, Z.G.; Shi, Z.D.; Zhang, P.Y.; Han, C.H. Tumor necrosis factor-related apoptosis-inducing ligand inhibits proliferation and induces apoptosis of prostate and bladder cancer cells. *Oncol. Lett.* **2017**, *13*, 3638–3640. [CrossRef]
101. Yuan, S.Y.; Shiau, M.Y.; Ou, Y.C.; Huang, Y.C.; Chen, C.C.; Cheng, C.L.; Chiu, K.Y.; Wang, S.S.; Tsai, K.J. Miconazole induces apoptosis via the death receptor 5-dependent and mitochondrial-mediated pathways in human bladder cancer cells. *Oncol. Rep.* **2017**, *37*, 3606–3616. [CrossRef] [PubMed]
102. Levidou, G.; Thymara, I.; Saetta, A.A.; Papanastasiou, P.; Pavlopoulos, P.; Sakellariou, S.; Fragkou, P.; Patsouris, E.; Korkolopoulou, P. TRAIL and osteoprotegerin (OPG) expression in bladder urothelial carcinoma: Correlation with clinicopathological parameters and prognosis. *Pathology* **2013**, *45*, 138–144. [CrossRef] [PubMed]

103. Jin, C.Y.; Molagoda, I.M.N.; Karunarathne, W.A.H.M.; Kang, S.H.; Park, C.; Kim, G.Y.; Choi, Y.H. TRAIL attenuates sulforaphane-mediated Nrf2 and sustains ROS generation, leading to apoptosis of TRAIL-resistant human bladder cancer cells. *Toxicol. Appl. Pharmacol.* **2018**, *352*, 132–141. [CrossRef] [PubMed]
104. Shan, Y.; Wu, K.; Wang, W.; Wang, S.; Lin, N.; Zhao, R.; Cassidy, A.; Bao, Y. Sulforaphane down-regulates COX-2 expression by activating p38 and inhibiting NF-kappaB-DNA-binding activity in human bladder T24 cells. *Int. J. Oncol.* **2009**, *34*, 1129–1134. [PubMed]
105. Shan, Y.; Wang, X.; Wang, W.; He, C.; Bao, Y. p38 MAPK plays a distinct role in sulforaphane-induced up-regulation of ARE-dependent enzymes and down-regulation of COX-2 in human bladder cancer cells. *Oncol. Rep.* **2010**, *23*, 1133–1138.
106. Shan, Y.; Zhang, L.; Bao, Y.; Li, B.; He, C.; Gao, M.; Feng, X.; Xu, W.; Zhang, X.; Wang, S. Epithelial-mesenchymal transition, a novel target of sulforaphane via COX-2/MMP2, 9/Snail, ZEB1 and miR-200c/ZEB1 pathways in human bladder cancer cells. *J. Nutr. Biochem.* **2013**, *24*, 1062–1069. [CrossRef]
107. Telu, K.H.; Abbaoui, B.; Thomas-Ahner, J.M.; Zynger, D.L.; Clinton, S.K.; Freitas, M.A.; Mortazavi, A. Alterations of histone H1 phosphorylation during bladder carcinogenesis. *J. Proteome Res.* **2013**, *12*, 3317–3326. [CrossRef]
108. Schwabe, R.F.; Jobin, C. The microbiome and cancer. *Nat. Rev. Cancer.* **2013**, *13*, 800–812. [CrossRef]
109. Markowski, M.C.; Boorjian, S.A.; Burton, J.P.; Hahn, N.M.; Ingersoll, M.A.; Maleki Vareki, S.; Pal, S.K.; Sfanos, K.S. The Microbiome and Genitourinary Cancer: A Collaborative Review. *Eur. Urol.* **2019**, *75*, 637–646. [CrossRef]
110. Nagano, T.; Otoshi, T.; Hazama, D.; Kiriu, T.; Umezawa, K.; Katsurada, N.; Nishimura, Y. Novel cancer therapy targeting microbiome. *Onco. Targets Ther.* **2019**, *12*, 3619–3624. [CrossRef]
111. He, C.; Huang, L.; Lei, P.; Liu, X.; Li, B.; Shan, Y. Sulforaphane Normalizes Intestinal Flora and Enhances Gut Barrier in Mice with BBN-Induced Bladder Cancer. *Mol. Nutr. Food Res.* **2018**, *62*, e1800427. [CrossRef] [PubMed]
112. Bao, Y.; Wang, W.; Zhou, Z.; Sun, C. Benefits and risks of the hormetic effects of dietary isothiocyanates on cancer prevention. *PLoS ONE* **2014**, *9*, e114764. [CrossRef]
113. Wang, F.; Shan, Y. Sulforaphane retards the growth of UM-UC-3 xenographs, induces apoptosis, and reduces survivin in athymic mice. *Nutr. Res.* **2012**, *32*, 374–380. [CrossRef]
114. Alumkal, J.J.; Slottke, R.; Schwartzman, J.; Cherala, G.; Munar, M.; Graff, J.N.; Beer, T.M.; Ryan, C.W.; Koop, D.R. A phase II study of sulforaphane-rich broccoli sprout extracts in men with recurrent prostate cancer. *Invest. N. Drugs* **2015**, *33*, 480–489. [CrossRef]
115. Atwell, L.L.; Hsu, A.; Wong, C.P.; Stevens, J.F.; Bella, D.; Yu, T.W.; Pereira, C.B.; Lohr, C.V.; Christensen, J.M.; Dashwood, R.H.; et al. Absorption and chemopreventive targets of sulforaphane in humans following consumption of broccoli sprouts or a myrosinase-treated broccoli sprout extract. *Mol. Nutr. Food Res.* **2015**, *59*, 424–433. [CrossRef]
116. Islam, S.S.; Mokhtari, R.B.; Akbari, P.; Hatina, J.; Yeger, H.; Farhat, W.A. Simultaneous Targeting of Bladder Tumor Growth, Survival, and Epithelial-to-Mesenchymal Transition with a Novel Therapeutic Combination of Acetazolamide (AZ) and Sulforaphane (SFN). *Target Oncol.* **2016**, *11*, 209–227. [CrossRef]
117. Rakariyatham, K.; Yang, X.; Gao, Z.; Song, M.; Han, Y.; Chen, X.; Xiao, H. Synergistic chemopreventive effect of allyl isothiocyanate and sulforaphane on non-small cell lung carcinoma cells. *Food Funct.* **2019**, *10*, 893–902. [CrossRef]
118. Jiang, D.M.; Sridhar, S.S. Prime time for immunotherapy in advanced urothelial cancer. *Asia Pac. J. Clin. Oncol.* **2018**, *14* (Suppl. S5), 24–32. [CrossRef]
119. Fan, Z.; Liang, Y.; Yang, X.; Li, B.; Cui, L.; Luo, L.; Jia, Y.; Wang, Y.; Niu, H. A meta-analysis of the efficacy and safety of PD-1/PD-L1 immune checkpoint inhibitors as treatments for metastatic bladder cancer. *Onco Targets Ther.* **2019**, *12*, 1791–1801. [CrossRef]
120. Liang, J.; Hänsch, G.M.; Hübner, K.; Samstag, Y. Sulforaphane as anticancer agent: A double-edged sword? Tricky balance between effects on tumor cells and immune cells. *Adv. Biol. Regul.* **2019**, *71*, 79–87. [CrossRef]
121. Gupta, P.; Wright, S.E.; Kim, S.H.; Srivastava, S.K. Phenethyl isothiocyanate: A comprehensive review of anti-cancer mechanisms. *Biochim. Biophys. Acta.* **2014**, *1846*, 405–424. [PubMed]

122. Wang, X.; Govind, S.; Sajankila, S.P.; Mi, L.; Roy, R.; Chung, F.L. Phenethyl isothiocyanate sensitizes human cervical cancer cells to apoptosis induced by cisplatin. *Mol. Nutr. Food Res.* **2011**, *55*, 1572–1581. [CrossRef] [PubMed]
123. Tang, K.; Lin, Y.; Li, L.M. The role of phenethyl isothiocyanate on bladder cancer ADM resistance reversal and its molecular mechanism. *Anat. Rec. Hoboken* **2013**, *296*, 899–906. [CrossRef] [PubMed]
124. Pullar, J.M.; Thomson, S.J.; King, M.J.; Turnbull, C.I.; Midwinter, R.G.; Hampton, M.B. The chemopreventive agent phenethyl isothiocyanate sensitizes cells to Fas-mediated apoptosis. *Carcinogenesis* **2004**, *25*, 765–772. [CrossRef]
125. Teply, B.A.; Kim, J.J. Systemic therapy for bladder cancer—A medical oncologist's perspective. *J. Solid Tumors* **2014**, *4*, 25–35. [CrossRef]
126. Zargar, H.; Shah, J.B.; van Rhijn, B.W.; Daneshmand, S.; Bivalacqua, T.J.; Spiess, P.E.; Black, P.C.; Kassouf, W.; Collaborators. Neoadjuvant Dose Dense MVAC versus Gemcitabine and Cisplatin in Patients with cT3-4aN0M0 Bladder Cancer Treated with Radical Cystectomy. *J. Urol.* **2018**, *199*, 1452–1458. [CrossRef]
127. Yao, S.; Zhang, Y.; Li, J. c-jun/AP-1 activation does not affect the antiproliferative activity of phenethyl isothiocyanate, a cruciferous vegetable-derived cancer chemopreventive agent. *Mol. Carcinog.* **2006**, *45*, 605–612. [CrossRef]
128. Tachibana, H.; Gi, M.; Kato, M.; Yamano, S.; Fujioka, M.; Kakehashi, A.; Hirayama, Y.; Koyama, Y.; Tamada, S.; Nakatani, T.; et al. Carbonic anhydrase 2 is a novel invasion-associated factor in urinary bladder cancers. *Cancer Sci.* **2017**, *108*, 331–337. [CrossRef]
129. Sun, M.; Shi, Y.; Dang, U.J.; Di Pasqua, A.J. Phenethyl Isothiocyanate and Cisplatin Co-Encapsulated in a Liposomal Nanoparticle for Treatment of Non-Small Cell Lung Cancer. *Molecules* **2019**, *24*, 801. [CrossRef]
130. Yang, Y.-T.; Shi, Y.; Jay, M.; Di Pasqua, A.J. Enhanced toxicity of cisplatin with chemosensitizer phenethyl isothiocyanate toward non-small cell lung cancer cells when delivered in liposomal nanoparticles. *Chem. Res. Toxicol.* **2014**, *27*, 946–948. [CrossRef]
131. Hirose, M.; Yamaguchi, T.; Kimoto, N.; Ogawa, K.; Futakuchi, M.; Sano, M.; Shirai, T. Strong promoting activity of phenylethyl isothiocyanate and benzyl isothiocyanate on urinary bladder carcinogenesis in F344 male rats. *Int. J. Cancer* **1998**, *77*, 773–777. [CrossRef]
132. Akagi, K.; Sano, M.; Ogawa, K.; Hirose, M.; Goshima, H.; Shirai, T. Involvement of toxicity as an early event in urinary bladder carcinogenesis induced by phenethyl isothiocyanate, benzyl isothiocyanate, and analogues in F344 rats. *Toxicol. Pathol.* **2003**, *31*, 388–396. [CrossRef] [PubMed]
133. Lubet, R.A.; Steele, V.E.; Eto, I.; Juliana, M.M.; Kelloff, G.J.; Grubbs, C.J. Chemopreventive efficacy of anethole trithione, N-acetyl-L-cysteine, miconazole and phenethylisothiocyanate in the DMBA-induced rat mammary cancer model. *Int. J. Cancer.* **1997**, *72*, 95–101. [CrossRef]
134. Sugiura, S.; Ogawa, K.; Hirose, M.; Takeshita, F.; Asamoto, M.; Shirai, T. Reversibility of proliferative lesions and induction of non-papillary tumors in rat urinary bladder treated with phenylethyl isothiocyanate. *Carcinogenesis* **2003**, *24*, 547–553. [CrossRef]
135. Ogawa, K.; Futakuchi, M.; Hirose, M.; Boonyaphiphat, P.; Mizoguchi, Y.; Miki, T.; Shirai, T. Stage and organ dependent effects of 1-*O*-hexyl-2,3,5-trimethylhydroquinone, ascorbic acid derivatives, n-heptadecane-8,10-dione and phenylethyl isothiocyanate in a rat multiorgan carcinogenesis model. *Int. J. Cancer* **1998**, *76*, 851–856. [CrossRef]
136. Ogawa, K.; Hirose, M.; Sugiura, S.; Cui, L.; Imaida, K.; Ogiso, T.; Shirai, T. Dose dependent promotion by phenylethyl isothiocyanate, a known chemopreventer, of two-stage rat urinary bladder and liver carcinogenesis. *Nutr. Cancer* **2001**, *40*, 134–139. [CrossRef]
137. Sones, K.; Heaney, R.K.; Fenwick, G.R. An estimate of the mean daily Intake of glucosinolates from cruciferous vegetables in the UK. *J. Sci. Food Agric.* **1984**, *35*, 712–720. [CrossRef]
138. Chung, F.L.; Morse, M.A.; Eklind, K.I.; Lewis, J. Quatitation of human uptake of the anticarcinogen phenethyl isothiocyanate after a watercress meal. *Cancer Epidemiol. Biomark. Prev.* **1992**, *1*, 383–388.
139. Krajka-Kuźniak, V.; Paluszczak, J.; Szaefer, H.; Baer-Dubowska, W. The activation of the Nrf2/ARE pathway in HepG2 hepatoma cells by phytochemicals and subsequent modulation of phase II and antioxidant enzyme expression. *J. Physiol. Biochem.* **2015**, *71*, 227–738. [CrossRef]
140. Becker, T.M.; Juvik, J.A. The Role of Glucosinolate Hydrolysis Products from Brassica Vegetable Consumption in Inducing Antioxidant Activity and Reducing Cancer Incidence. *Diseases* **2016**, *4*, 22. [CrossRef]

141. Soundararajan, P.; Kim, J.S. Anti-Carcinogenic Glucosinolates in Cruciferous Vegetables and Their Antagonistic Effects on Prevention of Cancers. *Molecules* **2018**, *23*, 2983. [CrossRef] [PubMed]
142. Cumberbatch, M.G.K.; Jubber, I.; Black, P.C.; Esperto, F.; Figueroa, J.D.; Kamat, A.M.; Kiemeney, L.; Lotan, Y.; Pang, K.; Silverman, D.T. Epidemiology of Bladder Cancer: A Systematic Review and Contemporary Update of Risk Factors in 2018. *Eur. Urol.* **2018**, *74*, 784–795. [CrossRef] [PubMed]
143. Ou, Z.; Wang, Y.; Chen, J.; Tao, L.; Zuo, L.; Sahasrabudhe, D.; Joseph, J.; Wang, L.; Yeh, S. Estrogen receptor β promotes bladder cancer growth and invasion via alteration of miR-92a/DAB2IP signals. *Exp. Mol. Med.* **2018**, *50*, 152. [CrossRef] [PubMed]
144. Ye, X.; Guo, J.; Zhang, H.; Meng, Q.; Ma, Y.; Lin, R.; Yi, X.; Lu, H.; Bai, X.; Cheng, J. The enhanced expression of estrogen-related receptor α in human bladder cancer tissues and the effects of estrogen-related receptor α knockdown on bladder cancer cells. *J. Cell Biochem.* **2019**, *120*, 13841–13852. [CrossRef]
145. Ioannides, C.; Konsue, N. A principal mechanism for the cancer chemopreventive activity of phenethyl isothiocyanate is modulation of carcinogen metabolism. *Drug Metab. Rev.* **2015**, *47*, 356–373. [CrossRef]
146. Yuan, J.M.; Stepanov, I.; Murphy, S.E.; Wang, R.; Allen, S.; Jensen, J.; Strayer, L.; Adams-Haduch, J.; Upadhyaya, P.; Le, C. Clinical Trial of 2-Phenethyl Isothiocyanate as an Inhibitor of Metabolic Activation of a Tobacco-Specific Lung Carcinogen in Cigarette Smokers. *Cancer Prev. Res.* **2016**, *9*, 396–405. [CrossRef]
147. Sanguedolce, F.; Cormio, L.; Carrieri, G.; Calò, B.; Russo, D.; Menin, A.; Pastore, A.L.; Greco, F.; Bozzini, G.; Galfano, A. Role of androgen receptor expression in non-muscle-invasive bladder cancer: A systematic review and meta-analysis. *Histol. Histopathol.* **2019**, in press.
148. Beklemisheva, A.A.; Feng, J.; Yeh, Y.A.; Wang, L.G.; Chiao, J.W. Modulating testosterone stimulated prostate growth by phenethyl isothiocyanate via Sp1 and androgen receptor down-regulation. *Prostate* **2007**, *67*, 863–870. [CrossRef]
149. Gianfredi, V.; Vannini, S.; Moretti, M.; Villarini, M.; Bragazzi, N.L.; Izzotti, A.; Nucci, D. Sulforaphane and Epigallocatechin Gallate Restore Estrogen Receptor Expression by Modulating Epigenetic Events in the Breast Cancer Cell Line MDA-MB-231: A Systematic Review and Meta-Analysis. *J. Nutrigenet. Nutrigenomics* **2017**, *10*, 126–135. [CrossRef]

5

Evaluating the Anti-cancer Efficacy of a Synthetic Curcumin Analog on Human Melanoma Cells and Its Interaction with Standard Chemotherapeutics

Krishan Parashar [1], Siddhartha Sood [1], Ali Mehaidli [1], Colin Curran [1], Caleb Vegh [1], Christopher Nguyen [1], Christopher Pignanelli [1], Jianzhang Wu [2], Guang Liang [2], Yi Wang [2] and Siyaram Pandey [1,*]

1 Department of Chemistry and Biochemistry, University of Windsor, 401 Sunset Avenue, Windsor, ON N9B 3P4, Canada
2 Chemical Biology Research Center, School of Pharmaceutical Sciences, Whenzhou Medical University, University Town, Chashan, Wenzhou 325035, China
* Correspondence: spandey@uwindsor.ca

Academic Editor: Kyoko Nakagawa-Goto

Abstract: Melanoma is the leading cause of skin-cancer related deaths in North America. Metastatic melanoma is difficult to treat and chemotherapies have limited success. Furthermore, chemotherapies lead to toxic side effects due to nonselective targeting of normal cells. Curcumin is a natural product of *Curcuma longa* (turmeric) and has been shown to possess anti-cancer activity. However, due to its poor bioavailability and stability, natural curcumin is not an effective cancer treatment. We tested synthetic analogs of curcumin that are more stable. One of these derivatives, Compound A, has shown significant anti-cancer efficacy in colon, leukemia, and triple-negative inflammatory breast cancer cells. However, the effects of Compound A against melanoma cells have not been studied before. In this study, for the first time, we demonstrated the efficacy of Compound A for the selective induction of apoptosis in melanoma cells and its interaction with tamoxifen, taxol, and cisplatin. We found that Compound A induced apoptosis selectively in human melanoma cells by increasing oxidative stress. The anti-cancer activity of Compound A was enhanced when combined with tamoxifen and the combination treatment did not result in significant toxicity to noncancerous cells. Additionally, Compound A did not interact negatively with the anti-cancer activity of taxol and cisplatin. These results indicate that Compound A could be developed as a selective and effective melanoma treatment either alone or in combination with other non-toxic agents like tamoxifen.

Keywords: melanoma; curcumin analog; apoptosis; oxidative stress; drug–drug interaction; tamoxifen; taxol; cisplatin

1. Introduction

Melanoma is an aggressive malignancy that emerges from the uncontrolled division of melanocytes and contributes to the larger part of skin cancer deaths [1]. Global incidence of melanoma has increased significantly, with rates rising in Europe and North America [2–4]. Fortunately, melanoma is easily treatable by surgical removal if detected early [5]. Deep melanoma tumors, however, tend to metastasize to lymph nodes and spread to other parts of the body [5,6]. Hence, at advanced stages surgery is not adequate and treatment becomes more difficult. Further treatment options include chemotherapy, radiation, and immunotherapy [7]. Melanoma is known to be highly resistant, thus limiting the effectiveness of these therapies [7,8]. Most chemotherapies are genotoxic or target cytoskeleton structures in cancer cells to induce cell death. However, this targeting is nonselective as it kills normal cells, which leads to severe toxicity.

Recent research has focused on targeting mitochondria, oxidative stress, and metabolic vulnerabilities to induce cancer cell death selectively [9]. Cancer cells shift their metabolism from oxidative phosphorylation to glycolysis, which reduces mitochondrial permeabilization and promotes mitochondrial stability [10–13]. The shift to glycolysis and the up-regulation of anti-apoptotic proteins, enables cancer cells to resist apoptosis [11–13]. Induction of cancer cell death selectively can occur through targeting the unique characteristics of cancerous cells. For example, analogs of the natural compound pancratistatin (PST) were able to induce apoptosis selectively in cancer cells through disrupting the mitochondrial membrane potential and the release of apoptogenic factors [14,15]. Cancer cells also display higher basal levels of reactive oxygen species (ROS), which promotes tumor proliferation and progression [16,17]. However, excessive ROS levels lead to damage of important biomolecules including DNA and protein, thus resulting in cell death [18]. Cancer cells depend on up-regulated expression of antioxidant enzymes to survive. Therefore, external sources of ROS or agents that stimulate oxidative stress may target cancer cells selectively [16]. For example, the natural compound piperlongumine induces cell death selectively through targeting the oxidative pathway [14]. An enhanced cytotoxic effect was observed when piperlongumine was combined with a pancratistatin analog, an activator of the intrinsic pathway of apoptosis through mitochondrial targeting [15].

Curcumin is a natural compound isolated from the *Curcuma longa* plant and has been shown to inhibit cancer growth and induce apoptosis in cancer cells [19,20]. Curcumin is pleiotropic and affects the activity of signaling molecules in a variety of pathways including inflammation [21]. Interestingly, curcumin has been shown to induce cell death through increasing ROS [20,22,23]. Due to poor bioavailability and stability, curcumin is not effective in vivo models and therefore could not advance to clinical success [24]. However, synthetic analogs of natural curcumin could have increased chemical stability and bioavailability. Therefore, these molecules should have the potential to be developed as cancer-selective drugs. Furthermore, a more potent analog could be synthesized that may have very high anti-cancer activity at low concentrations.

We synthesized several novel analogs of curcumin and screened them on various cancer cell lines [24]. Previously, we have demonstrated that two analogs, Compounds A and I, were the most effective in inducing apoptosis selectively in different cancer cell lines including triple-negative breast and p53-negative colorectal cancer cells [24]. Furthermore, these analogs induced cell death at lower doses compared to natural curcumin and the induction of apoptosis was driven by oxidative stress selectively in cancer cells. Compound A was also found to be effective in inhibiting human tumor growth xenografted in nude mice when administered intraperitoneally. This suggested that Compound A is biostable as well as bioavailable. Additionally, Compound A was shown to be well tolerated in mice. However, the anti-cancer activity of Compound A and other analogs of curcumin had yet to be studied in human melanoma cells. The interactions of these compounds with standard chemotherapies have also not been investigated.

Tamoxifen (TAM) is a non-genotoxic drug used to treat and prevent estrogen receptor (ER) positive breast cancer [25]. Though tamoxifen functions as an ER antagonist, it has also been shown to target and disrupt the mitochondria [25,26]. Previous work demonstrated that tamoxifen sensitized cancer cell mitochondria, thereby enhancing the anti-cancer efficacy of PST in ER negative breast cancer, and melanoma cells [27,28]. In a previous study, natural curcumin was combined with tamoxifen, which resulted in a synergistic induction of cell death selective to melanoma cells [29]. Conversely, this combination treatment did not result in significant cell death in noncancerous cells. Cell death was attributed to apoptosis as well as autophagy, a pro-survival or pro-death process, which occurs in response to stress [30,31]. Given that Compound A is more effective than natural curcumin, it is imperative to also investigate the interaction of Compound A with tamoxifen on human melanoma cells.

The objective of this study was to investigate the efficacy of novel synthetic curcumin analogs against human melanoma cells and demonstrate the possible mechanism of induction of apoptosis. We determined the effect of combining Compound A with tamoxifen in melanoma cells. We also investigated the drug–drug interactions of Compound A in combination with the standard chemotherapeutics taxol and cisplatin. Through screening the analogs on melanoma cells, Compound A was determined to be the most effective and selective in reducing cell viability. We have observed the selective induction of apoptosis by Compound A in two different melanoma cell lines. Furthermore, the effective doses of Compound A were well tolerated in normal human fibroblasts. Investigation into the mechanism revealed that cell death was triggered through induction of oxidative stress. The combination treatment of low doses of Compound A and tamoxifen resulted in an enhancement of apoptosis in human melanoma cells. Lastly, Compound A did not interfere with the anti-cancer activity of taxol and cisplatin. In conclusion, in this paper we demonstrate for the first time the anti-cancer activity of Compound A against human melanoma cells. These results may lead to the development of a non-toxic treatment that induces apoptosis selectively in melanoma cells through targeting oxidative vulnerabilities. Additionally, we demonstrate that Compound A has the potential to be developed as an adjuvant with tamoxifen and as a safer and effective melanoma treatment.

2. Results

2.1. Compounds A and I Induce Cell Death Effectively and Selectively in Human Melanoma Cells

The WST-1 colorimetric assay was utilized 48 h post treatment to determine the anti-cancer efficacy of curcumin (Figure 1) and synthetic analogs of curcumin (A-J), on A375 melanoma cells (Figure 2). Overall these analogs were more effective in reducing cell viability in A375 cells than natural curcumin. Natural curcumin was almost ineffective in reducing the viability of A375 cells even up to 20 μM (Figure 3C). However, various synthetic analogs were effective in reducing the viability of these cells at lower doses. The viability data for Compound A, I, and curcumin (for structures see Figure 1) were re-plotted as bar graphs for better comparison (Figure 3A–C). Compounds A and I were the most effective in reducing cell viability as demonstrated by lower IC_{50} values (approximately 1 and 2 μM, respectively; Figure 3A,B). The effective doses of Compounds A and I were tested on noncancerous normal human fibroblasts (NHF) and were well tolerated (Figure 3D,E). Similarly, natural curcumin did not reduce cell viability in NHF cells at different doses as indicated in Figure 3F. These results indicate selective toxicity of Compounds A and I to melanoma cells. It is important to note that Compound H was very effective in killing cancer cells at lower doses but was not taken for further study due to similar toxicity to normal cells, as determined previously [24]. Thus, Compounds A and I were chosen for further investigation with regards to the mode of cell death and mechanism.

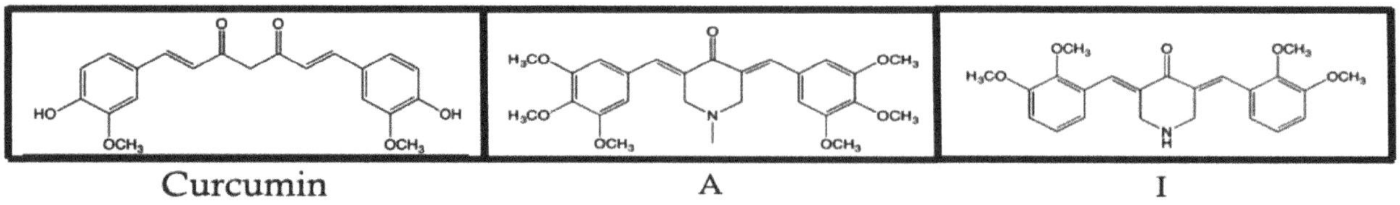

Figure 1. Structures of curcumin and analogs A and I. Previously published in Pignanelli et al. [24].

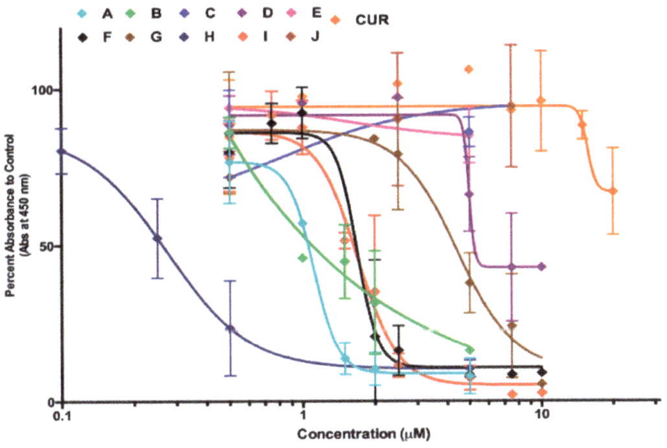

Figure 2. Effect of various curcumin analogs on cell viability of A375 melanoma cells. A375 melanoma cells were treated with natural curcumin (CUR) and curcumin analogs (A-J) for 48 h. The WST-1 assay was performed as described in the materials and methods section. Values are expressed as a mean ± SD from at least three independent experiments. The x-axis represents concentration (μM) and the y-axis represents absorbance (% of control). Graph obtained using the log (inhibitor) vs. response—variable slope (four parameters) curve on GraphPrism6.

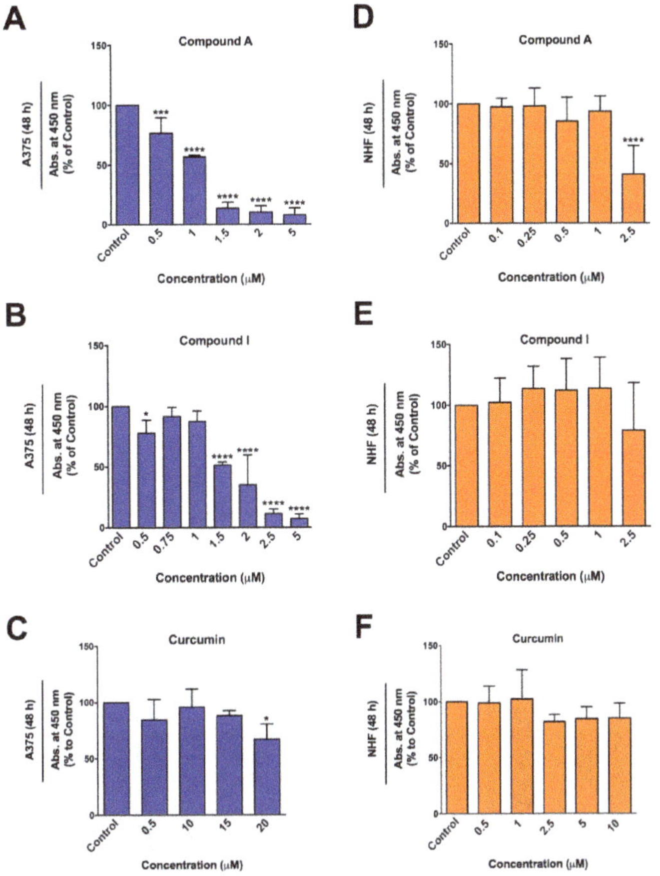

Figure 3. Compounds A and I selectively reduce cell viability in human melanoma cells. (**A–C**) A375 melanoma cells and (**D–F**) noncancerous normal human fibroblasts (NHF) were treated with Compound A, Compound I, and curcumin for 48 h. The WST-1 assay was performed as described in the materials and methods section. A375 cell viability data from Figure 1 were re-plotted as bar graphs to produce Figure 3 (A–C). Values are expressed as a mean ± SD from at least three independent experiments. The x-axis represents concentration (μM) and the y-axis represents absorbance (% of control).

2.2. Compounds A and I Induce Apoptosis Selectively in Human Melanoma Cells

The Annexin V binding assay and propidium iodide (PI) staining was utilized to distinguish early and late stage apoptosis, respectively. A375 (Figure 4A) and NHF (Figure 4B) cells were treated for 48 h with Compound A, Compound I, and curcumin. Compounds A and I induced apoptosis effectively in A375 melanoma cells at significantly lower doses compared to natural curcumin (Figure 4A). As shown in Figure 4A, Compound A induced significant apoptosis at 0.25 µM and 0.5 µM doses whereas limited induction of apoptosis was observed by natural curcumin only at 10 µM dose. Interestingly, the doses of Compound A that were greatly toxic to melanoma cells did not induce apoptosis significantly in noncancerous normal human fibroblasts 48 h following treatment (Figure 4B). However, significant apoptotic induction was observed at higher doses of Compound I (2 µM) and curcumin (10 µM). These results were supported by cellular and nuclear morphology following staining of A375 cells with Hoechst and propidium iodide (Figure 4E). The images revealed morphological changes indicative of apoptosis such as cell shrinkage, nuclear condensation, and PI positive signals (indicating permeability) in cancer cells.

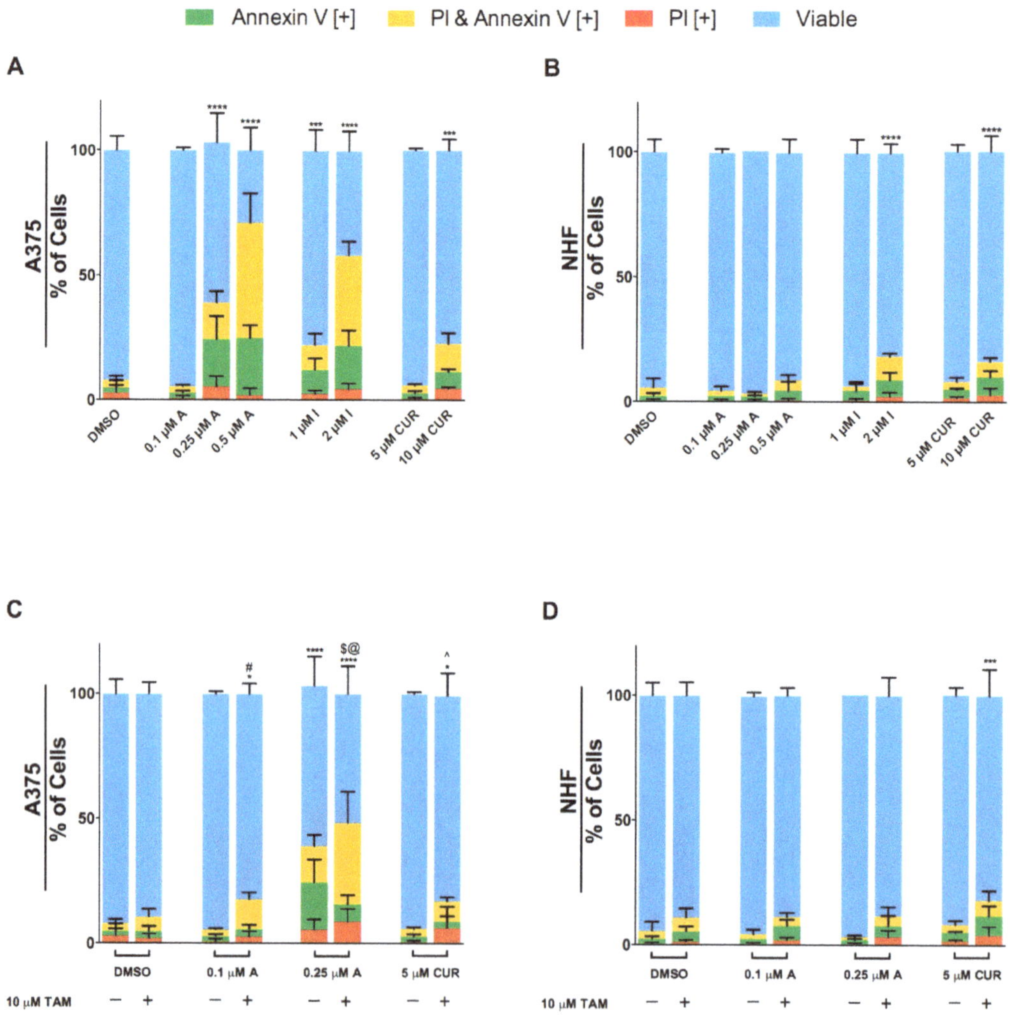

Figure 4. *Cont.*

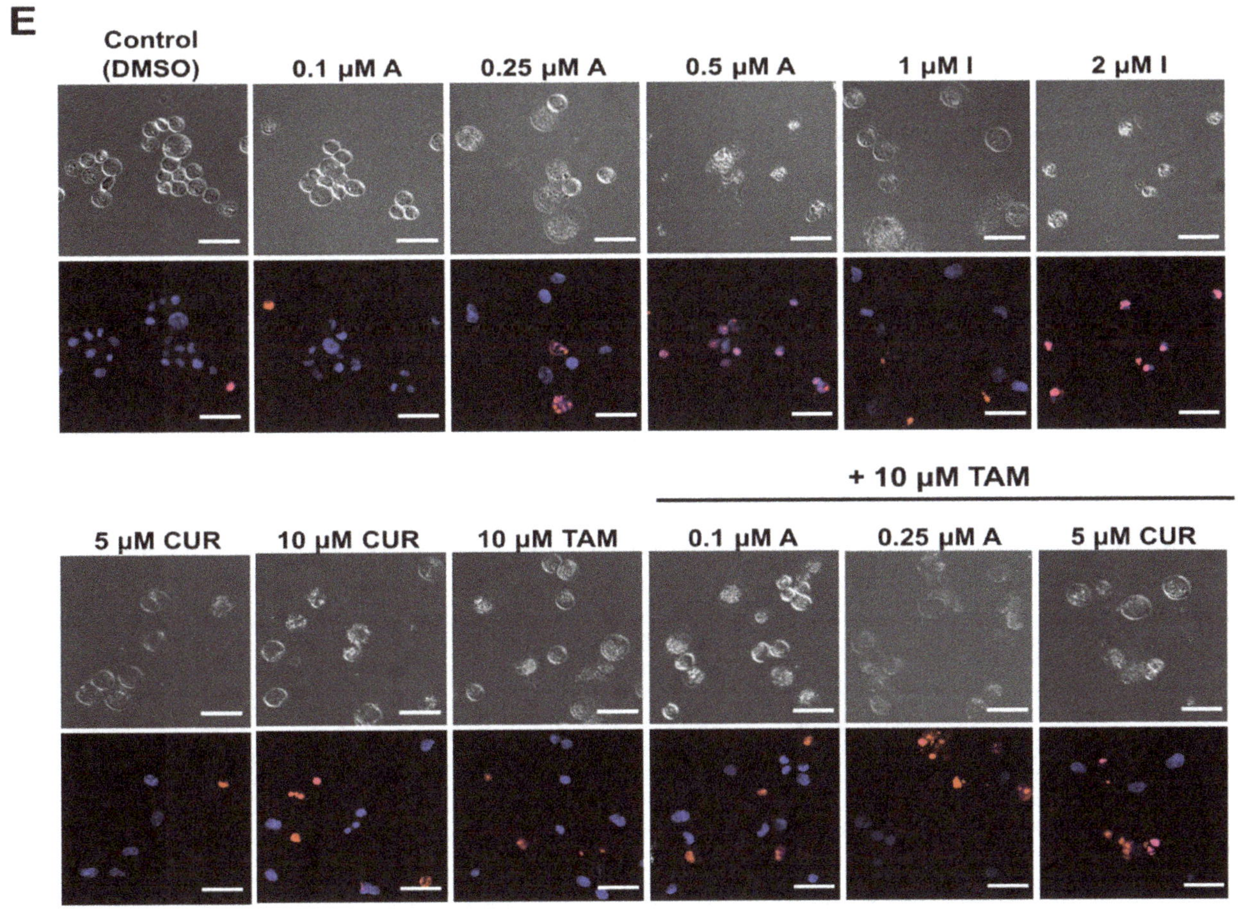

Figure 4. Compounds A and I induce apoptosis selectively and Compound A interacts positively with tamoxifen. (**A**) A375 melanoma cells and (**B**) noncancerous normal human fibroblasts (NHF) were treated with the indicated compounds for 48 h then stained with Annexin V and PI to quantify apoptosis, as described in the materials and methods section. Image based cytometry was utilized to assess apoptosis. The *y*-axis represents the percent of cells positive for Annexin V (green), PI (red), Annexin V and PI (orange), or cells negative for Annexin V and PI (blue). Values are expressed as mean ± SD from three independent experiments. (**C**) A375 melanoma cells and (**D**) NHF cells were treated with Compound A and curcumin alone and in combination with tamoxifen for 48 h. Please note, the data of Compound A and curcumin alone shown in Figure 4A,B were used again in Figure 4C,D, respectively along with the combination treatments for direct comparison. **p* < 0.05 vs. DMSO control (comparison of viable cells only); ***p* < 0.01 vs. DMSO control (comparison of viable cells only); ****p* < 0.001 vs. DMSO control (comparison of viable cells only); *****p* < 0.0001 vs. DMSO control (comparison of viable cells only); #*p* < 0.05 vs. 0.1 μM Compound A alone (comparison of viable cells only); $*p* < 0.05 vs. 0.25 μM Compound A alone (comparison of viable cells only); ^*p* < 0.05 vs. 5 μM CUR alone (comparison of viable cells only); @p < 0.05 vs. tamoxifen treatment alone (comparison of viable cells only). (**E**) A375 micrographs at 48 h. Top: Bright field images at 400× magnification. Bottom: Fluorescent images stained with PI (red) and Hoechst (blue). Scale bar = 100 μm. Micrographs are representative of three independent experiments. A = Compound A, I = Compound I, CUR = Curcumin, TAM = Tamoxifen.

2.3. Enhancement of the Anti-cancer Activity of Compound A in Combination with Tamoxifen

Tamoxifen as such does not have strong anti-cancer activity against melanoma cells. Previously it has been reported that tamoxifen in combination with curcumin demostrated sufficient cytotoxicity against melanoma cells [29]. We investigated whether the synthetic curcumin derivative, Compound A would show a similar enhancement wth tamoxifen. A375 cells were treated with Compound A and tamoxifen alone or in combination for 48 h and apoptosis was monitored using Annexin V binding assay and propidium iodide staining. As shown in Figure 4C, there was a clear enhancement of cell death inducing activity of Compound A by tamoxifen particularly at low doses of Compound A (0.1 µM and 0.25 µM). These results were supported by fluorescent micrographs of A375 cells treated with the indicated compounds for 48 h followed by staining with Hoechst and propidium iodide (Figure 4E). On the other hand, the same combination did not show significant toxicity to normal human fibroblasts (Figure 4D).

2.4. Interaction of Compound A with Taxol and Cisplatin in Two Melanoma Cell Lines

We investigated the effect of Compound A on the cell-death-inducing activity of taxol and cisplatin on human melanoma cells. A375 (Figure 5A) and G361 (Figure 5B) cells were treated with a range of taxol and cisplatin doses in the presence or absence of 0.1 µM Compound A. The Annexin V and propidium iodide staining revealed that there was no enhancement of cell death by the combination treatments in A375 cells. In G361 cells, an enhancement was observed when 0.01 µM of taxol was combined with 0.1 µM Compound A, relative to taxol alone. However, there seems to be no enhancement at higher doses of taxol in G361 cells. We did not observe any enhancement of cisplatin when combined with Compound A in G361 cells.

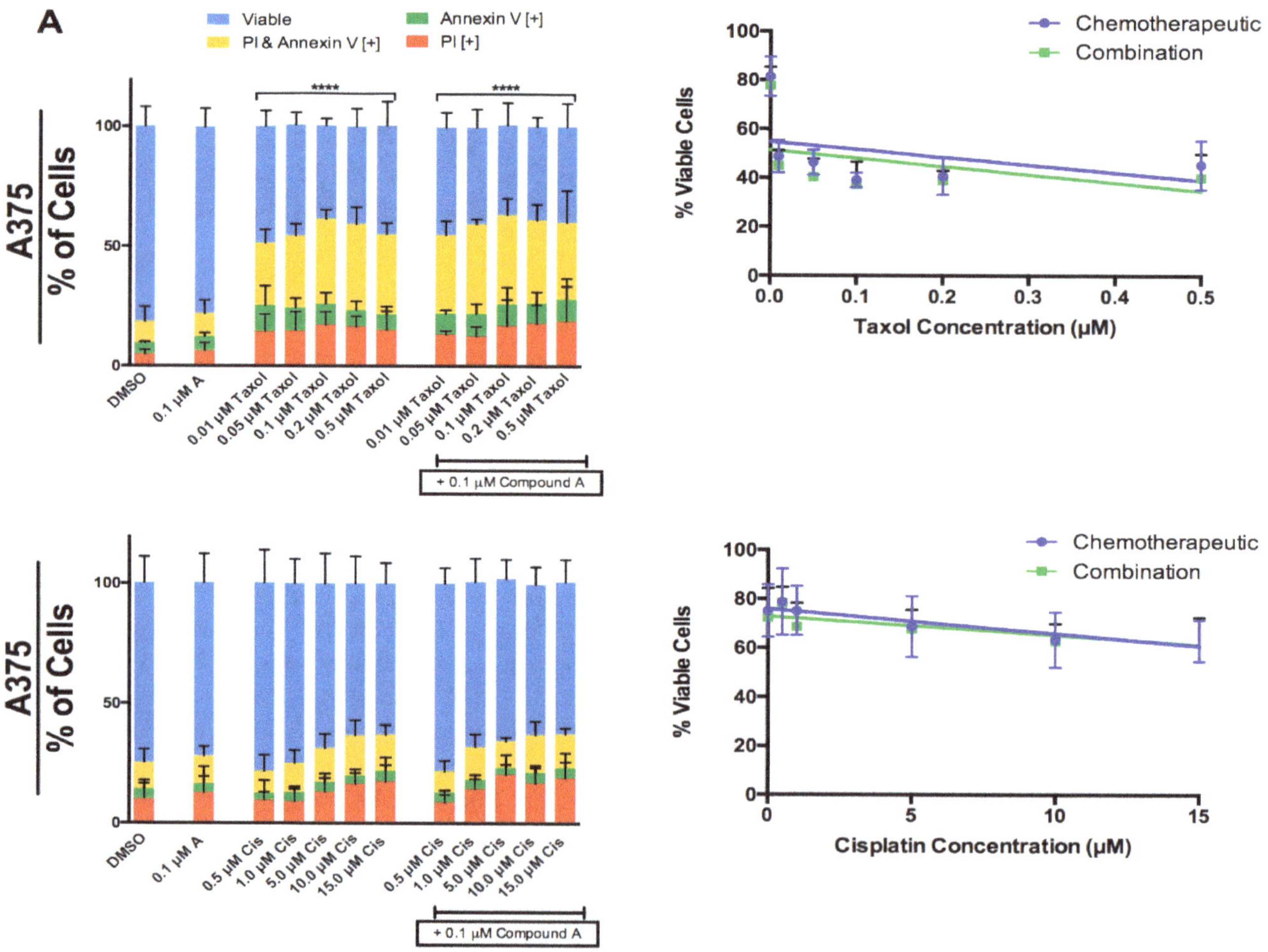

Figure 5. *Cont.*

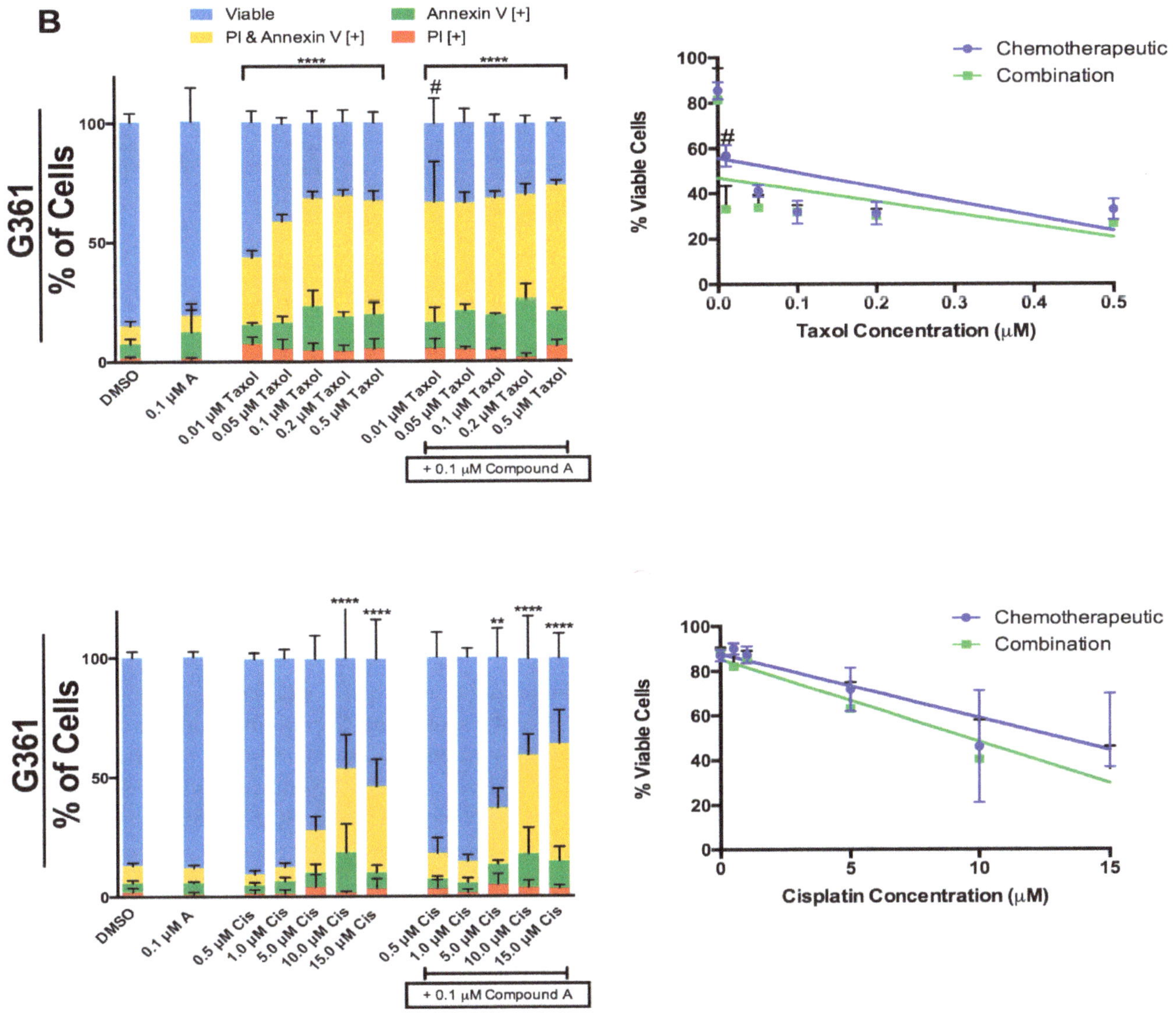

Figure 5. The interaction of Compound A with taxol and cisplatin in two melanoma cell lines. (**A**) A375 and (**B**) G361 melanoma cells were treated with a range of taxol (top panel) and cisplatin concentrations (bottom panel) alone and in combination with a sub lethal dose of Compound A (0.1 μM). Following 48 h of treatment the cells were stained with Annexin V and PI to distinguish early apoptosis and late stage apoptosis, respectively. Image based cytometry was utilized to assess apoptosis. The *y*-axis represents the percent of cells positive for Annexin V (green), PI (red), Annexin V and PI (yellow), or negative for both Annexin V and PI (blue). All graphical values are expressed as a mean ± SD from three independent experiments. A line graph was constructed using viability values for individual chemotherapeutics in the absence and presence of Compound A (combination). **$p < 0.01$ vs. DMSO control (comparison of viable cells only); ****$p < 0.0001$ vs. DMSO control (comparison of viable cells only); #$p < 0.0001$ vs. 0.01 μM taxol alone (comparison of viable cells only). Cis = Cisplatin.

2.5. Induction of Apoptosis by Compound A is Dependent on the Production of Oxidative Stress

To investigate the role of oxidative stress in apoptosis induction by Compound A we first measured the production of ROS using H_2DCFDA in G361 cells as indicated in the materials and methods section. Paraquat (PQ) was used as positive control for ROS generation [32]. Overall, Compound A and curcumin exhibited pro-oxidant effects and induced ROS production in G361 cells after 3 h of treatment. This was indicated by a significant increase in the percent of cells positive for DCF relative to the control (Figure 6A). Subsequently, we used the antioxidant N-Acetyl-L-cysteine (NAC) to determine if the observed increase in oxidative stress was essential for the induction of apoptosis by

Compound A and curcumin. G361 cells pre-treated with NAC demonstrated a reduction in apoptotic markers indicating that ROS played a critical role in the induction of apoptosis of Compound A and curcumin (Figure 6B).

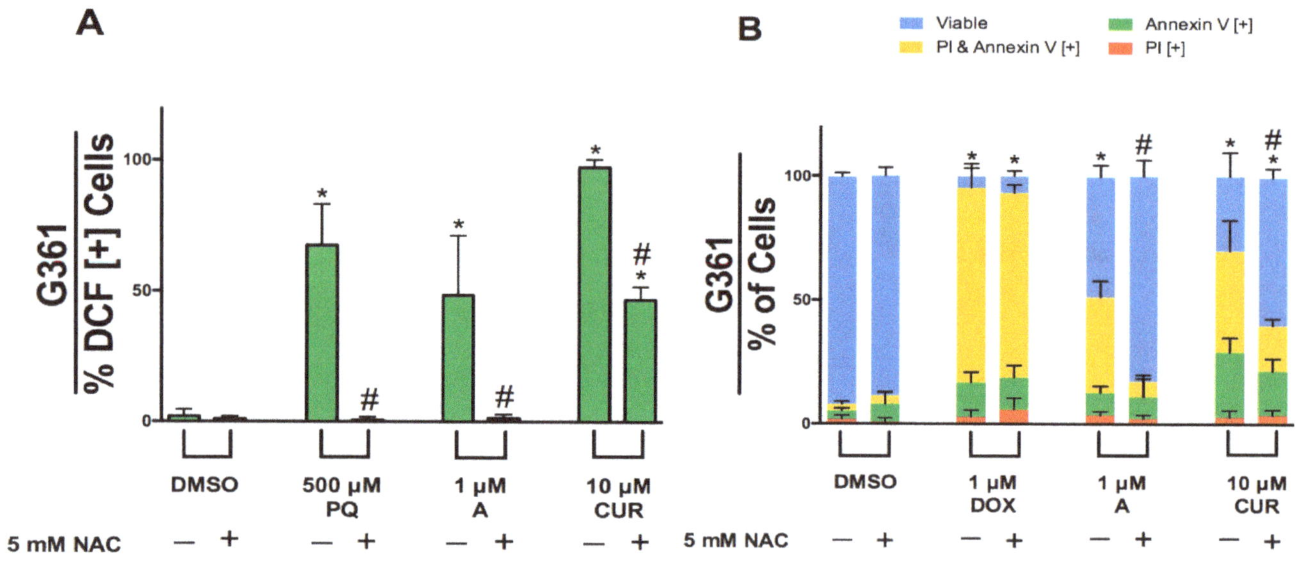

Figure 6. Induction of apoptosis by Compound A is dependent on the production of reactive oxygen species. (**A**) G361 cells were pre-treated with H_2DCFDA and treated with Compound A and curcumin with or without the antioxidant N-Acetyl-L-cysteine (NAC) for 3 h, as described in the materials and methods section. Production of ROS was evaluated through image-based cytometry with the *y*-axis indicative of the percent of DCF positive cells. *$p < 0.05$ vs. DCF [+] cells of DMSO control; #$p < 0.05$ vs. DCF [+] cells of groups treated without NAC. (**B**) G361 cells were treated with the Compound A and curcumin with or without NAC for 48 h. Subsequently, cells were stained with Annexin V and PI, as described in the materials and methods. Image based cytometry was utilized to assess apoptosis. The *y*-axis represents the percent of cells positive for Annexin V (green), PI (red), Annexin V and PI (yellow), or negative for both Annexin V and PI (blue). All graphical values are expressed as a mean ± SD from three independent experiments. Doxorubicin (DOX) was used as a positive control. *$p < 0.05$ vs. DMSO control (comparison of viable cells only); #$p < 0.05$ vs. groups treated without NAC (comparison of viable cells only). PQ = Paraquat, A = Compound A, CUR = Curcumin.

2.6. *Compound A and Curcumin Induce Mitochondrial Destabilization in Human Melanoma Cells*

Increased production of ROS could lead to the collapse of mitochondrial membrane potential in cells undergoing apoptosis. We investigated if G361 cells undergoing apoptosis induced by Compound A and curcumin exhibited mitochondrial destabilization. G361 cells were treated with Compound A and curcumin for 48 h then stained with tetramethylrhodamine methyl ester (TMRM), an indicator of intact mitochondria, as described in the materials and methods. Compound A and curcumin induced mitochondrial collapse as indicated by a decrease in TMRM positive cells (Figure 7).

2.7. *Apoptosis Induction by Compound A is Caspase Dependent*

Caspases have been shown to be involved in the initiation and execution phases of apoptosis. To determine if Compound A-induced apoptosis is dependent on caspase activity, G361 cells were pre-treated with or without the broad spectrum caspase inhibitor Z-VAD FMK. Subsequently, the cells were treated with Compound A for 48 h then stained with Annexin V and propidium iodide to characterize apoptosis. A decrease in apoptotic indicators was observed in cells treated with Z-VAD FMK (Figure 8). These results indicate that caspase activity is critical for Compound A induced apoptosis.

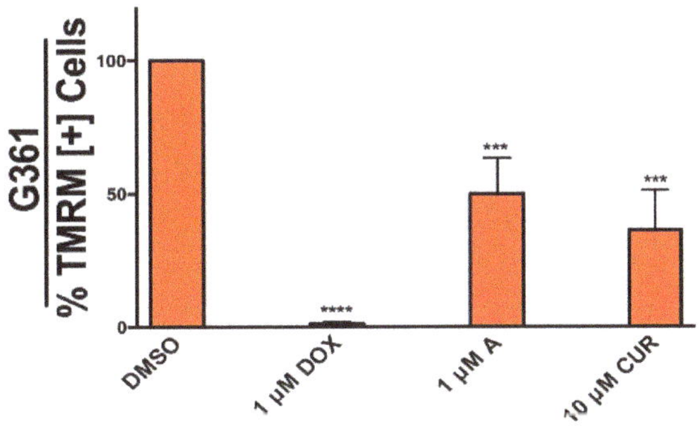

Figure 7. Mitochondrial depolarization in G361 cells undergoing apoptosis. G361 cells were treated with Compound A and curcumin for 48 h followed by incubation with TMRM for 45 min to quantify mitochondrial membrane potential (MMP), as described in the materials and methods section. Results were obtained using image-based cytometry with the y-axis representative of percent of cells positive for TMRM expressed as a mean ± SD from three independent experiments. Doxorubicin (DOX) was used as a positive control. A = Compound A, CUR = Curcumin. ***$p < 0.001$ vs. TMRM [+] cells of DMSO control; ****$p < 0.0001$ vs. TMRM [+] cells of DMSO control.

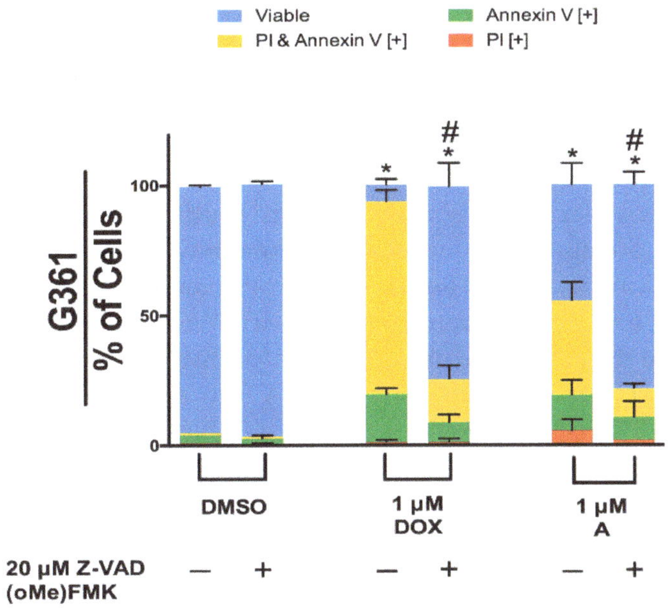

Figure 8. Induction of apoptosis by Compound A is caspase dependent. G361 melanoma cells were pre-treated with or without the caspase inhibitor Z-VAD-FMK for 30 min, followed by treatment with Compound A for 48 h. Cells were stained with Annexin V and propidium iodide to quantify apoptosis. Image based cytometry was utilized to assess apoptosis. The y-axis represents the percent of cells positive for Annexin V (green), PI (red), Annexin V and PI (orange), or cells negative for Annexin V and PI (blue). Values are expressed as mean ± SD from three independent experiments. *$p < 0.05$ vs. DMSO control (comparison of viable cells only); #$p < 0.05$ vs. individual chemotherapeutic treatment (comparison of viable cells only). Doxorubicin (DOX) was used as a positive control. A = Compound A, CUR = Curcumin.

3. Discussion

In this study, we evaluated the anti-cancer efficacy of synthetic derivatives of curcumin against chemo-resistant human melanoma cells. Out of the ten analogs we screened, Compounds A and I (for structures see Figure 1) were the most effective in reducing cell viability. These analogs induced apoptosis effectively and selectively in melanoma cells. We evaluated the interaction of Compound A with tamoxifen and demonstrated a positive interaction on the apoptosis-inducing activity of

Compound A (Figure 4C). We also determined that the induction of apoptosis in cancer cells by Compound A was dependent on the increased production of ROS and caspase activity. Compound A did not interact negatively with taxol and cisplatin in two melanoma cell lines. Overall, we have shown that a novel derivative of natural curcumin, Compound A, targets oxidative vulnerabilities to induce cell death selectively in melanoma cells.

Both melanoma cell lines (A375 and G361) were derived from a primary tumor in malignant melanoma patients. Compounds A and I were found to be very effective at lower doses compared to natural curcumin. Apoptosis is a physiological process important for maintaining homeostasis [30]. Common indicators of apoptosis include DNA condensation or fragmentation, membrane blebbing, and externalization of phosphatidylserine from the inner plasma membrane [30,31]. Analysis of phostatidylserine externalization and permeabilization using the Annexin V binding assay and propidium iodide staining, respectively revealed that these analogs were able to induce apoptosis effectively in A375 cells and at significantly lower concentrations compared to native curcumin. In parallel we tested these compounds on normal human fibroblasts (NHF), a non-transformed noncancerous cell line to investigate the selectivity of Compounds A and I. Importantly, the effective doses of Compounds A and I did not induce apoptosis significantly in NHF cells relative to the DMSO control. Hence, Compounds A and I selectively induce apoptosis in melanoma cells.

Apoptosis can be induced by the extrinsic and intrinsic pathway, which are caused by the activation of a signaling cascade upon binding of an extracellular ligand or a stimulus within the cell, respectively [32]. Both pathways may involve the cleavage and activation of cysteine proteases known as caspases. The intrinsic pathway may be triggered by internal stress, including damage of DNA and oxidative stress [32]. This further causes the mitochondria to lose integrity resulting in the release of apoptogenic factors into the cytoplasm, consequently triggering the induction of apoptosis [33]. Curcumin is a pleiotropic compound with multiple targets and has been characterized to have anti-inflammatory effects [21]. Several researchers have investigated induction of apoptosis targeting mitochondria in cancer cells [34–40]. Curcumin has been shown to induce apoptosis in a caspase dependent [41–43] and independent [44] pathway. We investigated if Compound A induced apoptosis through caspase dependent or independent pathways. Furthermore, the broad caspase inhibitor Z-VAD FMK was able to inhibit Compound A induced apoptosis, indicating a critical role of caspases.

Interestingly, in this study we observed an increased production of ROS following the treatment of melanoma cells with curcumin and Compound A. When curcumin and Compound A were co-treated with the antioxidant NAC, we indeed saw a reduction in ROS generation leading to the inhibition of apoptosis. Thus, Compound A must be targeting oxidative vulnerabilities to induce cell death in melanoma cells. Mitochondrial membrane potential collapse happens at the later stage of apoptosis. Indeed, we observed the collapse of mitochondrial membrane potential (MMP) in melanoma cells following treatment with Compound A and curcumin.

Chemotherapeutic drugs with different targets have the potential to be more effective when combined with a lower chance of resistance [45]. It is integral that we investigate the combined effect of non-toxic, anti-cancer compounds to improve the efficacy of cancer treatments. Tamoxifen is a well-tolerated ER antagonist used for ER positive breast cancer patients and has also been shown to target the mitochondria and induce autophagy [36]. A synergistic induction of apoptosis and autophagy was observed when tamoxifen was combined with an analog of pancratistatin, another mitochondria targeting compound [14]. Likewise, when tamoxifen was combined with curcumin, a synergistic induction of apoptosis and autophagy was observed [29]. We have demonstrated a clear enhancement of Compound A-induced apoptosis by tamoxifen. Importantly, this combination did not exhibit similar toxicity to noncancerous normal human fibroblasts. To our knowledge this is the first time Compound A and tamoxifen have been studied in melanoma cells.

We investigated whether Compound A could be used in conjugation with taxol and cisplatin. Taxol targets the microtubules and causes mitotic arrest [46]. It is used to treat a variety of cancers including melanoma, however is cytotoxic to normal cells [47]. Cisplatin induces apoptosis through DNA damage and is also nonspecific [48]. To determine the drug–drug interactions, we treated A375 and G361 cells with taxol and cisplatin alone or in combination with Compound A. The combination could reveal a positive or negative effect, or no interaction. We did not observe any negative interaction of Compound A with taxol or cisplatin in A375 and G361 cells. However, an enhancement was established at 0.01 μM taxol combined with 0.1 μM Compound A in G361 cells. Overall, Compound A could potentially be combined with taxol and cisplatin, and is safe to use as an adjuvant. Since it is non-toxic compared to other treatments, it could be given over a longer period of time without any adverse side effects.

In conclusion, Compound A is able to induce apoptosis effectively in drug resistant melanoma cells with ten times more efficacy than natural curcumin by targeting oxidative vulnerabilities. The anti-cancer activity of Compound A is enhanced by tamoxifen and the combination treatment was well tolerated by normal cells. Compound A did not interact negatively with taxol and cisplatin. In fact, a positive interaction was observed in G361 cells treated with taxol and Compound A. Compound A could potentially be developed as a safe and effective treatment alone or in combination with tamoxifen. Future work may focus on elucidating the mechanism and targets of Compound A induced cell death, and in vivo models of melanoma should be tested to determine efficacy and stability.

4. Materials and Methods

4.1. Chemical Synthesis of Curcumin Analogs

All chemical reagents were obtained from Sigma–Aldrich, Fluka, and Aladdin (Beijing, China). Synthesis of Compounds A-J has been described previously [24].

4.2. Cell Culture

Malignant melanoma cell line A375 (ATCC, Cat. No. CRL-1619, Manassas, VA, USA) was cultured in RPMI-1640 medium (Sigma–Aldrich Canada, Mississauga, ON, Canada) supplemented with 10% (v/v) fetal bovine serum (FBS) standard (Thermo Scientific, Waltham, MA, USA) and 40 μg/mL gentamicin (Gibco BRL, VWR, Mississauga, ON, Canada).

Malignant melanoma cell line G361 (ATCC, Cat. No. CRL-1424, Manassas, VA, USA) was cultured in McCoy's 5A Medium supplemented with 2 mM L-glutamine, 10% (v/v) FBS (Thermo Scientific, Waltham, MA, USA), and 40 μg/mL gentamicin (Gibco BRL, VWR, Mississauga, ON, Canada).

The noncancerous cell line, normal human skin fibroblast cells (NHF; Coriell Institute for Medical120 Research, Cat. No. AG09309, Camden, NJ, USA) were cultured in Dulbecco's Modified Eagle's Medium (DMEM; ATCC® 30-2002TM) supplemented with 10% (v/v) fetal bovine serum (FBS) and 40 μg/mL gentamicin (Catalog No. 15710-064, Gibco BRL, VWR, Mississauga, ON, CA).

All cultured cells were maintained in an incubator at 37 °C, 5% CO_2, and 95% humidity. The cells were passaged for less than six months.

4.3. Chemicals and Cell Treatment

Human melanoma cells and NHF cells were grown to roughly 70% confluence and then treated with curcumin (CUR; Sigma-Aldrich Canada, Cat. No. 8511, Mississauga, ON, Canada), Compound A and other curcumin analogs (e.g., Compound I) all dissolved in dimethylsulfoxide (DMSO) to make the stock solutions. In parallel, these cells were treated with taxol (Sigma–Aldrich Canada, Cat. No. T7402, Mississauga, ON, Canada), cisplatin (Sigma–Aldrich Canada, Mississauga, ON, Canada), doxorubicin (DOX; Sigma–Aldrich Canada, Cat. No. D1515, Mississauga, ON, Canada), and Z-VAD-FMK (Sigma–Aldrich Canada, Cat. No. V116, Mississauga, ON, Canada). These agents were also dissolved in dimethylsulfoxide (DMSO) to make the stock solutions. *N*-Acetyl-L-cysteine (NAC; Sigma–Aldrich Canada, Cat. No. A7250) and paraquat (PQ; Sigma–Aldrich Canada, Cat. No.856177, Mississauga, ON, Canada) were dissolved in double distilled water.

4.4. WST-1 Assay for Cell Viability

A WST-1 colorimetric assay was used to quantify cell viability of cells treated with curcumin and its analogs (compound A-J), following a previously published protocol [15]. Briefly, A375 and NHF cells were seeded in ninety-six well clear bottom tissue culture plates then treated with the indicated compounds for 48 h. The cells were then incubated with the WST-1 reagent (Roche Applied Sciences, Indianapolis, IN, USA) for 4 h at 37 °C, 5% CO2, and 95% humidity. The WST-1 reagent is cleaved by viable cells to formazan through its enzymes. Absorbance was read at 450 nm on a Wallac Victor3 1420 Multilabel Counter (PerkinElmer, Waltham, MA, USA) to determine cell viability.

4.5. Analysis of Cell Death

Annexin V binding assay and propidium iodide staining were used to determine early apoptosis and cell permeabilization (found in late apoptotic cells), respectively as described previously [15]. Briefly, melanoma and NHF cells were seeded in six-well plates and after 24 h they were treated with different compounds at various concentrations for 48 h. Cells were washed with phosphate buffer saline (PBS), and then Annexin V Binding buffer (10 mM HEPES, 140 mM NaCl, 2.5 mM CaCl2, pH 7.4) was added, followed by the Annexin V AlexaFluor-488 dye, which fluoresces a green color (1:20; Life Technologies Inc., Cat. No. A13201, Burlington, ON, Canada). Afterwards, 0.01 mg/mL of propidium iodide dye (red fluorescent color) was added (Life Technologies Inc, Cat. No. P3566, Burlington, ON, Canada). Afterwards, the cells were incubated for 15 min at 37 degrees Celsius, 5% CO2, and 95% humidity in the absence of light. A Tali Image-Based Cytometer (Life Technologies Inc., Cat. No. T10796, Burlington, ON, Canada) was used to quantify the percentage of cells stained green (early apoptotic), green and red (late apoptotic), and red (necrotic). Cells from 18 random fields were used to analyze the green (ex. 458 nm; em. 525/20 nm) and red (ex. 530 nm; em. 585 nm) channels. In order to visualize cellular death and apoptosis, a similar protocol was carried out. Cells were stained with propidium iodide and Hoechst 3342 (Molecular Probes, Eugene, OR, USA) at 10 μM during the 15 min incubation. Fluorescent and Brightfield micrographs were taken at 400× magnification using a Leica DMI6000 fluorescent microscope with the LAS AF6000 software.

4.6. Tetramethylrhodamine Methyl Ester Staining

Tetramethylrhodamine methyl ester (TMRM; Thermo Fisher Scientific) stain was used to determine mitochondrial membrane potential (MMP) as outlined in a previously published protocol [24]. G361 cells were cultured and then treated with doxorubicin, Compound A, and curcumin for 48 h. Subsequently, the cells were incubated with 100 nM TMRM for 45 min at 37 °C. Cells were washed with PBS, and then a Tali Image-Based Cytometer (Life Technologies Inc., Cat. No. T10796, Burlington, ON, Canada) was then used to quantify the percentage of red stain from TMRM (stable mitochondrial membrane potential). Cells from 18 random fields were used to analyze the red (ex. 530 nm; em. 585 nm) channel.

4.7. Quantification of Reactive Oxygen Species

The molecule 2′,7′-dicholorofluorescin diacetate (H_2DCFDA) was used to determine whole-cell reactive oxygen species (ROS) generation as outlined in a previously published protocol [24]. The molecule is deacetylated by esterases and oxidized by ROS into a fluorescent green 2′,7′-dicholorofluorescein (DCF; ex. 495 nm; em. 529 nm) once inside the cell. G361 cells were pretreated with a final concentration of 20 μM H_2DCFDA (D6883; Sigma-Aldrich) and then incubated for 30 min at 37 °C and 5% CO_2 in the absence of light. Afterwards, the cells were treated with various drug concentrations for 3 h. The cells were centrifuged at 3000 rpm for 5 min and then suspended in PBS. A Tali Image-Based Cytometer (Life Technologies Inc., Cat. No. T10796, Burlington, ON, Canada) was then used to quantify the percentage of green fluorescent cells from the presence of DCF-positive stain. Cells from 18 random fields were used to analyze the green (ex. 458 nm; em. 525/20 nm) channel. In order to determine the mechanism of action of Compound A and curcumin, G361 cells were pretreated with or without *N*-Acetyl-L-cysteine (NAC; final concentration 5 mM; Sigma–Aldrich Canada, Cat. No. A7250) and incubated for 30 min. NAC acts as an antioxidant which inhibits the presence of ROS in the cell. H_2DCFDA was utilized to determine ROS generation as mentioned above. Subsequently, the cells were treated with DMSO, paraquat, Compound A, and curcumin. The cells were then read for the presence of green fluorescence at a time point of 3 h following incubation using a Tali Image-Based Cytometer (Life Technologies Inc., Cat. No. T10796, Burlington, ON, Canada).

4.8. Caspase Inhibition

Cell treatment with or without general caspase inhibitor Z-VAD-FMK was used to determine if the apoptotic mechanism of Compound A was caspase dependent or independent. Cells were pretreated with 4 μL Z-VAD-FMK (final concentration 20 μM) for 30 min at 37 °C at 5% CO_2. Cells were then treated with DMSO, doxorubicin (DOX), and Compound A. After incubation for 48 h, cells were collected, washed with phosphate buffer saline (PBS), and apoptosis was quantified using the Annexin V Binding Assay protocol as previously described.

4.9. Statistical Analysis

Statistical analysis was conducted by the GraphPad Prism 6 software. Significance was considered when the *p*-value was less than 0.05. The type of statistical analysis depended on the experimental variable. Single variable measurements, including quantification of mitochondrial membrane potential, and whole cell ROS, were analyzed by the one-way ANOVA (nonparametric) and the mean of each sample was compared to the mean of the negative control (DMSO) unless otherwise specified. Multi-variable experiments such as the quantification of early and late apoptosis, were analyzed by two-way ANOVA (nonparametric) and the sample of each mean was compared to the mean of the negative control (DMSO) unless otherwise specified.

Author Contributions: K.P. was responsible for the conceptualization, design, and execution of experiments, analysis of data, and preparation of the report. S.S. contributed to the execution of experiments, analysis of data, and preparation of the report. A.M., C.C., C.V., C.N., and C.P. contributed to the execution of the experiments, and analysis of data. Pandey contributed to the conceptualization and design of experiments, analysis of data, preparation and review of the manuscript. J.W. aided in the synthesis of the curcumin analogs. G.L., and Y.W. synthesized and provided the curcumin analogs, provided the chemical stability of curcumin and Compound A.

Acknowledgments: The authors would like to acknowledge Richa Parashar for revising the paper and providing feedback.

References

1. Erdei, E.; Torres, S.M. A new understanding in the epidemiology of melanoma. *Expert Rev. Anticancer* **2011**, *10*, 1811–1823. [CrossRef] [PubMed]
2. Langley, A.; Levesque, L.; Baetz, T.; Asai, Y. Brief Report: Increase in Melanoma Incidence in Ontario. *J. Cutan. Med. Surg.* **2018**, *22*, 476–478. [CrossRef] [PubMed]
3. Linos, E.; Swetter, S.M.; Cockburn, M.G.; Colditz, G.A.; Clarke, C.A. Increasing Burden of Melanoma in the United States. *J. Investig. Derm.* **2009**, *129*, 1666–1674. [CrossRef] [PubMed]
4. Erdmann, F.; Lortet-Tieulent, J.; Schuz, J.; Zeeb, H.; Greinert, R.; Breitbart, E.W.; Bray, F. International trends in the incidence of malignant melanoma 1953–2008—Are recent generations at higher or lower risk? *Int. J. Cancer* **2013**, *132*, 385–400. [CrossRef] [PubMed]
5. Balch, C.M.; Buzaid, A.C.; Soong, S.J.; Atkins, M.B.; Cascinelli, N.; Coit, D.G.; Fleming, I.D.; Gershenwald, J.E.; Houghton, A., Jr.; Kirkwood, J.M.; et al. Final version of the American Joint Committee on Cancer staging system for cutaneous melanoma. *J. Clin. Oncol.* **2001**, *19*, 3635–3648. [CrossRef] [PubMed]
6. Vijuk, G.; Coates, A. Survival of patients with visceral metastatic melanoma from an occult primary lesion: A retrospective matched cohort study. *Ann. Oncol.* **1998**, *9*, 419–422. [CrossRef] [PubMed]
7. Soengas, M.S.; Lowe, S.W. Apoptosis and melanoma chemoresistance. *Oncogene* **2003**, *22*, 3138–3151. [CrossRef]

8. Debatin, K.-M. Apoptosis pathways in cancer and cancer therapy. *Cancer Immunol. Immunother.* **2004**, *53*, 153–159. [CrossRef]
9. Martinez-Outschoorn, U.E.; Peiris-Pagés, M.; Pestell, R.G.; Sotgia, F.; Lisanti, M.P. Cancer metabolism: A therapeutic perspective. *Nat. Rev. Clin. Oncol.* **2017**, *14*, 11–31. [CrossRef]
10. Heiden, M.G.V.; Cantley, L.C.; Thompson, C.B. Understanding the Warburg Effect: The Metabolic Requirements of Cell Proliferation. *Science* **2009**, *324*, 1029–1033. [CrossRef]
11. DeBerardinis, R.J.; Lum, J.J.; Hatzivassiliou, G.; Thompson, C.B. The Biology of Cancer: Metabolic Reprogramming Fuels Cell Growth and Proliferation. *Cell Metab.* **2008**, *7*, 11–20. [CrossRef] [PubMed]
12. Gogvadze, V.; Zhivotovsky, B.; Orrenius, S. The Warburg effect and mitochondrial stability in cancer cells. *Mol. Asp. Med.* **2010**, *31*, 60–74. [CrossRef] [PubMed]
13. Plas, D.R.; Thompson, C.B. Cell metabolism in the regulation of programmed cell death. *Trends Endocrinol. Metab.* **2002**, *13*, 75–78. [CrossRef]
14. Ma, D.; Gilbert, T.; Pignanelli, C.; Tarade, D.; Noel, M.; Mansour, F.; Gupta, M.; Ma, S.; Ropat, J.; Curran, C.; et al. Exploiting mitochondrial and oxidative vulnerabilities with a synthetic analog of pancratistatin in combination with piperlongumine for cancer therapy. *FASEB. J.* **2018**, *32*, 417–430. [CrossRef] [PubMed]
15. Ma, D.; Pignanelli, C.; Tarade, D.; Gilbert, T.; Noel, M.; Mansour, F.; Adams, S.; Dowhayko, A.; Stokes, K.; Vshyvenko, S.; et al. Cancer Cell Mitochondria Targeting by Pancratistatin Analogs is Dependent on Functional Complex II and III. *Sci. Rep.* **2017**, *7*, 42957. [CrossRef] [PubMed]
16. Trachootham, D.; Alexandre, J.; Huang, P. Targeting cancer cells by ROS-mediated mechanisms: A radical therapeutic approach? *Nat. Rev. Drug Discov.* **2009**, *8*, 579–591. [CrossRef] [PubMed]
17. Storz, P. Reactive oxygen species in tumor progression. *Front. Biosci.* **2005**, *10*, 1881–1896. [CrossRef] [PubMed]
18. Reuter, S.; Gupta, S.C.; Chaturvedi, M.M.; Aggarwal, B.B. Oxidative stress, inflammation, and cancer: How are they linked? *Free Radic. Biol. Med.* **2010**, *49*, 1603–1616. [CrossRef] [PubMed]
19. Aoki, H.; Takada, Y.; Kondo, S.; Sawaya, R.; Aggarwal, B.B.; Kondo, Y. Evidence That Curcumin Suppresses the Growth of Malignant Gliomas in Vitro and in Vivo through Induction of Autophagy: Role of Akt and Extracellular Signal-Regulated Kinase Signaling Pathways. *Mol. Pharm.* **2007**, *72*, 29–39. [CrossRef]
20. Yoshino, M.; Haneda, M.; Naruse, M.; Htay, H.H.; Tsubouchi, R.; Qiao, S.L.; Li, W.H.; Murakami, K.; Yokochi, T. Prooxidant activity of curcumin: Copper-dependent formation of 8-hydroxy-2′-deoxyguanosine in DNA and induction of apoptotic cell death. *Toxicol. Vitr.* **2004**, *18*, 783–789. [CrossRef]
21. Gupta, S.C.; Patchva, S.; Koh, W.; Aggarwal, B.B. Discovery of curcumin, a component of golden spice, and its miraculous biological activities. *Clin. Exp. Pharm. Physiol.* **2012**, *39*, 283–299. [CrossRef] [PubMed]
22. Kunwar, A.; Jayakumar, S.; Srivastava, A.K.; Priyadarsini, K.I. Dimethoxycurcumin-induced cell death in human breast carcinoma MCF7 cells: Evidence for pro-oxidant activity, mitochondrial dysfunction, and apoptosis. *Arch. Toxicol.* **2012**, *86*, 603–614. [CrossRef] [PubMed]
23. Aggeli, I.-K.; Koustas, E.; Gaitanaki, C.; Aggeli, I.; Beis, I. Curcumin Acts as a Pro–Oxidant Inducing Apoptosis Via JNKs in the Isolated Perfused Rana ridibunda Heart. *J. Exp. Zool. Part A Ecol. Genet. Physiol.* **2013**, *319*, 328–339. [CrossRef] [PubMed]
24. Pignanelli, C.; Ma, D.; Noel, M.; Ropat, J.; Mansour, F.; Curran, C.; Pupulin, S.; Larocque, K.; Wu, J.; Liang, G.; et al. Selective Targeting of Cancer Cells by Oxidative Vulnerabilities with Novel Curcumin Analogs. *Sci. Rep.* **2017**, *7*, 1603. [CrossRef] [PubMed]
25. Howell, A. The endocrine prevention of breast cancer. *Best Pr. Res. Clin. Endocrinol. Metab.* **2008**, *22*, 615–623. [CrossRef] [PubMed]
26. Moreira, P.I.; Custódio, J.; Moreno, A.; Oliveira, C.R.; Santos, M.S. Tamoxifen and Estradiol Interact with the Flavin Mononucleotide Site of Complex I Leading to Mitochondrial Failure. *J. Boil. Chem.* **2006**, *281*, 10143–10152. [CrossRef]
27. Siedlakowski, P.; Mclachlan-Burgess, A.; Griffin, C.; Tirumalai, S.S.; McNulty, J.; Pandey, S. Synergy of pancratistatin and tamoxifen on breast cancer cells in inducing apoptosis by targeting mitochondria. *Cancer Boil.* **2008**, *7*, 376–384. [CrossRef]
28. Chatterjee, S.J.; McNulty, J.; Pandey, S. Sensitization of human melanoma cells by tamoxifen to apoptosis induction by pancratistatin, a nongenotoxic natural compound. *Melanoma Res.* **2011**, *21*, 1–11. [CrossRef]
29. Chatterjee, S.J.; Pandey, S. Chemo-resistant melanoma sensitized by tamoxifen to low dose curcumin treatment through induction of apoptosis and autophagy. *Cancer Boil.* **2011**, *11*, 216–228. [CrossRef]

30. Kroemer, G.; Mariño, G.; Levine, B. Autophagy and the integrated stress response. *Mol. Cell* **2010**, *40*, 280–293. [CrossRef]
31. Dalby, K.N.; Tekedereli, I.; Lopez-Berestein, G.; Ozpolat, B. Targeting the prodeath and prosurvival functions of autophagy as novel therapeutic strategies in cancer. *Autophagy* **2010**, *6*, 322–329. [CrossRef] [PubMed]
32. Cochemé, H.M.; Murphy, M.P. Complex I is the major site of mitochondrial superoxide production by paraquat. *J. Biol. Chem.* **2008**, *283*, 1786–1798. [CrossRef] [PubMed]
33. Canta, A.; Pozzi, E.; Carozzi, V.A. Mitochondrial Dysfunction in Chemotherapy-Induced Peripheral Neuropathy (CIPN). *Toxics* **2015**, *3*, 198–223. [CrossRef] [PubMed]
34. Naksuriya, O.; Okonogi, S.; Schiffelers, R.M.; Hennink, W.E. Curcumin nanoformulations: A review of pharmaceutical properties and preclinical studies and clinical data related to cancer treatment. *Biomaterials* **2014**, *35*, 3365–3383. [CrossRef] [PubMed]
35. Tonnesen, H.H.; Másson, M.; Loftsson, T. Studies of curcumin and curcuminoids. XXVII. Cyclodextrin complexation: Solubility, chemical and photochemical stability. *Int. J. Pharm.* **2002**, *244*, 127–135. [CrossRef]
36. Gupta, S.C.; Patchva, S.; Aggarwal, B.B. Therapeutic roles of curcumin: Lessons learned from clinical trials. *AAPS J.* **2013**, *15*, 195–218. [CrossRef] [PubMed]
37. Kerr, J.F.R.; Wyllie, A.H.; Currie, A.R. Apoptosis: A Basic Biological Phenomenon with Wide-ranging Implications in Tissue Kinetics. *Br. J. Cancer* **1972**, *26*, 239–257. [CrossRef]
38. Fadok, V.A.; Bratton, D.L.; Frasch, S.C.; Warner, M.L.; Henson, P.M. The role of phosphatidylserine in recognition of apoptotic cells by phagocytes. *Cell Death Differ.* **1998**, *5*, 551–562. [CrossRef]
39. Fulda, S.; Debatin, K.-M. Extrinsic versus intrinsic apoptosis pathways in anticancer chemotherapy. *Oncogene* **2006**, *25*, 4798–4811. [CrossRef]
40. Debatin, K.-M.; Poncet, D.; Kroemer, G. Chemotherapy: Targeting the mitochondrial cell death pathway. *Oncogene* **2002**, *21*, 8786–8803. [CrossRef]
41. Mukhopadhyay, A.; Bueso-Ramos, C.; Chatterjee, D.; Pantazis, P.; Aggarwal, B.B. Curcumin downregulates cell survival mechanisms in human prostate cancer cell lines. *Oncogene* **2001**, *20*, 7597–7609. [CrossRef] [PubMed]
42. Gogada, R.; Amadori, M.; Zhang, H.; Jones, A.; Verone, A.; Pitarresi, J.; Jandhyam, S.; Prabhu, V.; Black, J.D.; Chandra, D. Curcumin induces Apaf-1-dependent, p21-mediated caspase activation and apoptosis. *Cell Cycle* **2011**, *10*, 4128–4137. [CrossRef] [PubMed]
43. Sikora, E. Curcumin induces caspase-3-dependent apoptotic pathway but inhibits DNA fragmentation factor 40/caspase-activated DNase endonuclease in human Jurkat cells. *Mol. Cancer* **2006**, *5*, 927–934. [CrossRef] [PubMed]
44. Hilchie, A.L.; Furlong, S.J.; Sutton, K.; Richardson, A.; Robichaud, M.R.J.; Giacomantonio, C.A.; Ridgway, N.D.; Hoskin, D.W. Curcumin-Induced Apoptosis in PC3 Prostate Carcinoma Cells Is Caspase-Independent and Involves Cellular Ceramide Accumulation and Damage to Mitochondria. *Nutr. Cancer* **2010**, *62*, 379–389. [CrossRef] [PubMed]
45. Mokhtari, R.B.; Homayouni, T.S.; Baluch, N.; Morgatskaya, E.; Kumar, S.; Das, B.; Yeger, H. Combination therapy in combating cancer. *Oncotarget* **2017**, *8*, 38022–38043. [CrossRef] [PubMed]
46. Cunha, K.S.; Reguly, M.L.; Graf, U.; Helena, H. Taxanes: The genetic toxicity of paclitaxel and docetaxel in comatic cells of Drosophila melanogaster. *Mutagenesis* **2001**, *16*, 79–84. [CrossRef] [PubMed]
47. Weaver, B.A. How Taxol/paclitaxel kills cancer cells. *Mol. Biol. Cell* **2014**, *25*, 2677–2681. [CrossRef] [PubMed]
48. Dasari, S.; Tchounwou, P.B. Cisplatin in cancer therapy: Molecular mechanisms of action. *Eur. J. Pharm.* **2014**, *740*, 364–378. [CrossRef]

6

Relating Advanced Electrospun Fiber Architectures to the Temporal Release of Active Agents to Meet the Needs of Next-Generation Intravaginal Delivery Applications

Kevin M. Tyo [1,2,†], Farnaz Minooei [3,†], Keegan C. Curry [4], Sarah M. NeCamp [5], Danielle L. Graves [5], Joel R. Fried [3] and Jill M. Steinbach-Rankins [1,2,5,6,*]

1. Department of Pharmacology and Toxicology, School of Medicine, University of Louisville, Louisville, KY 40202, USA; kevin.tyo@louisville.edu
2. Center for Predictive Medicine, Louisville, KY 40202, USA
3. Department of Chemical Engineering, University of Louisville, Louisville, KY 40292, USA; farnaz.minooei@louisville.edu (F.M.); joel.fried@louisville.edu (J.R.F.)
4. Department of Biology, University of Louisville, Louisville, KY 40292, USA; keegan.curry@louisville.edu
5. Department of Bioengineering, Speed School of Engineering, University of Louisville, Louisville, KY 40292, USA; sarah.necamp@louisville.edu (S.M.N.); danielle.graves@louisville.edu (D.L.G.)
6. Department of Microbiology and Immunology, School of Medicine, University of Louisville, Louisville, KY 40292, USA

* Correspondence: jmstei01@louisville.edu
† Co-first authors.

Abstract: Electrospun fibers have emerged as a relatively new delivery platform to improve active agent retention and delivery for intravaginal applications. While uniaxial fibers have been explored in a variety of applications including intravaginal delivery, the consideration of more advanced fiber architectures may offer new options to improve delivery to the female reproductive tract. In this review, we summarize the advancements of electrospun coaxial, multilayered, and nanoparticle-fiber architectures utilized in other applications and discuss how different material combinations within these architectures provide varied durations of release, here categorized as either transient (within 24 h), short-term (24 h to one week), or sustained (beyond one week). We seek to systematically relate material type and fiber architecture to active agent release kinetics. Last, we explore how lessons derived from these architectures may be applied to address the needs of future intravaginal delivery platforms for a given prophylactic or therapeutic application. The overall goal of this review is to provide a summary of different fiber architectures that have been useful for active agent delivery and to provide guidelines for the development of new formulations that exhibit release kinetics relevant to the time frames and the diversity of active agents needed in next-generation multipurpose applications.

Keywords: electrospun fibers; fiber architecture; drug delivery; intravaginal delivery; delivery vehicle

---

1. Introduction

Intravaginal delivery is an effective strategy to improve the localization of antiviral, antibacterial, antifungal, chemotherapeutic, and contraceptive agents within the female reproductive tract (FRT) [1,2]. Relative to oral administration routes, intravaginal delivery localizes agents to the FRT, avoiding both the harsh gastrointestinal environment and hepatic first pass effect. This results in an increase in drug bioavailability within target tissue and corresponding functional activity by decreasing off-target effects and systemic exposure [3]. The inherent characteristics of the FRT, including its large surface area and low enzymatic activity, additionally make the FRT a favorable site for localized active agent administration and targeting [4,5].

Although intravaginal delivery offers a variety of advantages to enhance the delivery of active agents [6], challenges unique to the FRT must be overcome to provide efficacious prophylaxis and treatment. One of the most important components of the FRT is the mucus layer, which protects the epithelium and lamina propria from incoming pathogens (Figure 1). However, it can also act as a barrier, impeding therapeutic transport to underlying epithelial and immune cells [7,8]. In addition to these challenges, the frequent shedding and production of cervicovaginal mucus can decrease active agent retention, while bacterial flora, enzymes, and the acidic environment created by beneficial bacteria can contribute to metabolization and degradation of active agents, reducing efficaciousness.

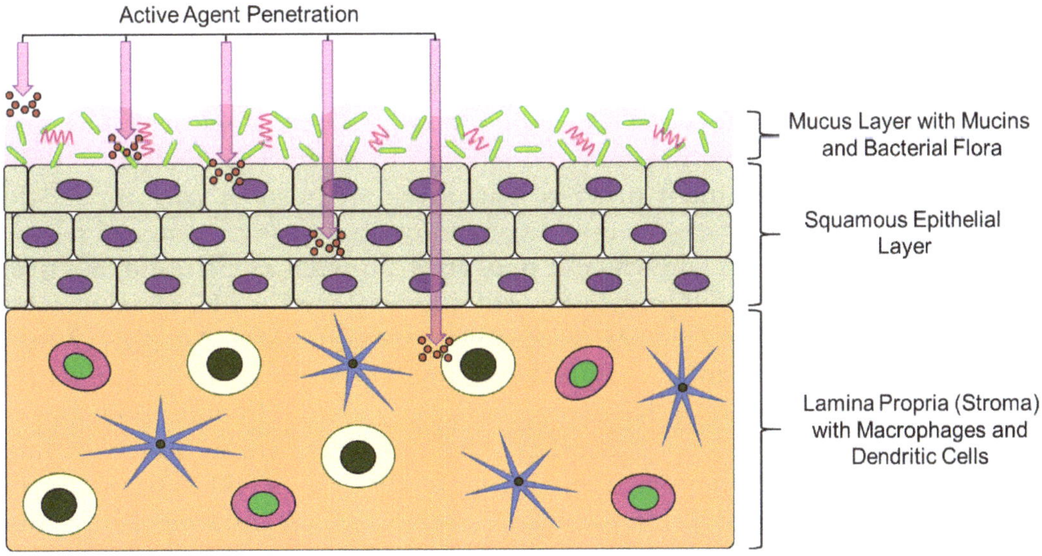

Figure 1. Schematic depicting the structure and specific layers of the vaginal mucosa that can act as a barrier to active agent transport (not to scale). The mucus layer of the female reproductive tract (FRT) frequently sheds and can immobilize active agents (shown in red), leading to decreased efficacy of the administered agents. The bacterial flora normally present within the FRT can also metabolize and degrade agents, further contributing to decreased efficacy. Last, the squamous epithelium can hinder transport to underlying immune cells present near the epithelial surface and/or in the lamina propria.

To address these challenges, intravaginal delivery platforms have been formulated as solid or semi-solid dosage forms that include suppositories, tablets, capsules, gels, rings, and creams to enhance delivery to and retention in the FRT [9–13]. While these dosage forms have enabled high levels of active agent incorporation and localization, these traditionally used delivery platforms still face significant challenges, including difficulty of self-administration, economic feasibility, poor user-compliance, vaginal irritation, the need for frequent administration, and low residence times [14]. Of these platforms, intravaginal rings have provided the "gold standard" for long-term delivery due to their ability to sustain the release of one or multiple active agents for weeks to months, avoid leakage and loss of active agent, and improve drug stability [15–19]. However, some biological agents have difficulty withstanding the high temperature and solvent processes often required for fabrication, limiting their incorporation [20].

More recently, nanoparticles (NPs) have been developed for topical intravaginal delivery due to their ability to encapsulate both hydrophilic and hydrophobic agents and to provide encapsulant stability while enhancing cell specific targeting, transport, and internalization [21–29]. However, NPs can experience low intravaginal retention due to mucus shedding, or conversely experience immobilization within the mucus layer, resulting in inadequate transport to underlying tissue [29]. To improve retention and to maximize transport, NPs have been surface-modified [30,31], while carrier solutions with different osmolarities have been explored to increase retention within and penetration of the vaginal lumen [32–34]. Despite these efforts, hurdles including low encapsulation efficiency and rapid release of hydrophilic agents have hindered the ability to achieve long-term delivery and retention [35]. Given these issues, other delivery platforms have been investigated that may increase the longevity of active agents within the FRT and improve user adherence while also offering a new dosage form alternative to women.

Electrospun fibers have recently gained attention for intravaginal delivery due to their ease of use, ability to be fabricated into various geometries and sizes, and tunable release properties [36,37]. They have been considered for sustained-delivery, a characteristic that is often desirable for intravaginal applications, due to their high surface area-to-volume ratio, degree of interconnected porosity, tunable pore sizes, surface-modification potential, interchangeable polymer options, and diverse fiber architectures that enable finer control over the rate, duration, and site of agent release [38]. Electrospun fibers have the additional advantage that they can be fabricated using a variety of natural or synthetic polymers to tailor release properties [39], and these polymer types are typically selected based on their biocompatibility, hydrophobicity, and related degradation properties.

One of the most significant factors that contributes to active agent release from fibers is the relative hydrophobicity of the selected polymer material [40,41]. In addition to polymer hydrophobicity, the medium (in vitro) or environment (in vivo) surrounding the fiber can impact drug release. Simulated vaginal and seminal fluids, often used to preliminarily assess intravaginal release, may alter the release of agents relative to testing in water or phosphate buffered saline (PBS) (in vitro) or in vivo, due to differences in viscosity, salt, and protein concentrations, as well as pH. Therefore, depending on the degree of polymer hydrophobicity and the environment release it is tested in, the same encapsulated active agent can have distinctly different release profiles, in some cases ranging from hours to months [42,43]. Usually, independent of these conditions, the use of hydrophilic polymers often results in the immediate release of both hydrophilic and hydrophobic active agents due to the high solubility and degradation rate of hydrophilic polymers in aqueous environments [44]. Natural polymers such as collagen, gelatin, chitosan, elastin, and laminin, and synthetic polymers including poly(ethylene oxide) (PEO), polyvinyl alcohol (PVA), and polyvinylpyrrolidone (PVP) are examples of hydrophilic materials that have been fabricated into fibers with micron- and nanometer-scaled properties. In contrast, synthetic hydrophobic polymers including polycaprolactone (PCL), poly(lactic-*co*-glycolic acid) (PLGA), and polyurethane (PU) have demonstrated burst or sustained-release kinetics depending on the hydrophobicity of the incorporated active agent [45–49]. Moreover, synthetic hydrophobic polymers can also serve as a mechanical and structural basis for different fiber architectures in which the release of single or multiple encapsulants may be tailored by using more complex fiber designs or composites. Fiber release rates can also be optimized by adjusting the polymer molecular weight or hydrophilicity, for example, by adding hydrophilic groups such as aliphatic poly(phosphoester) to the polymer structure [50]. Together, these features have enabled the incorporation and release of a variety of antiviral, antimicrobial, and biological agents from fiber scaffolds [51–53].

Active agent release from polymeric fibers typically occurs via diffusion, polymer degradation, and erosion [41]. When fibers are first administered, solvent or solution diffuses through the porous fiber matrix. Once in contact with the solvent or solution, the polymer matrix swells, loosening polymer chains and enabling the diffusion of active agents, dependent in part on molecular size. Concurrently, the fiber surface may undergo bulk erosion at a rate corresponding to polymer hydrophilicity. These features in combination with the large surface-to-volume ratio of the fibers allows for the increased diffusion of encapsulants relative to diffusion from non-porous bulk materials [54]. Traditionally, fibers have been electrospun as uniaxial fibers or fibers that comprise a single polymer or polymer blend and exhibit homogeneous morphology. Diffusion of active agents from more traditional uniaxial fibers is dependent upon the compatibility of the encapsulant, polymer, and surrounding eluant. In contrast with diffusion, polymer degradation is observed when fibers are exposed to aqueous environments, and polymer bonds are cleaved by either passive hydrolysis or enzymatic reaction [55], resulting in slow degradation of the fiber scaffold. This degradation alters the distance between and size of interconnected pores, thereby impacting the diffusion and release of incorporated active agents. For most synthetic polymers, hydrolysis is the most common mechanism of degradation, although hydrolysis-resistant polymers have been utilized [56], which significantly impact active agent release. As the fibers degrade, they can also undergo surface or bulk erosion, which is dependent upon solvent diffusivity into the fiber, polymer solubility, and overall fiber matrix dimensions [57].

As a result of these mechanisms and the materials selected, electrospun fibers can tailor the release of encapsulated agents within different durations to achieve immediate (transient or rapid), short-term, or sustained-release. Within this review, we defined release as transient, when the complete release of active agents occurs within 24 h of administration; short-term, when the release occurs from one day to one week; or sustained, when the release of the active agent occurs over a duration of weeks to months. A schematic showing an example of these different potential release profiles is provided in Figure 2. Factors including the electrospinning parameters, polymer materials, fiber architecture, the resulting structure and morphology, and the distribution and amount of incorporated active agent each contribute to the resulting release kinetics and efficacy of delivery [37].

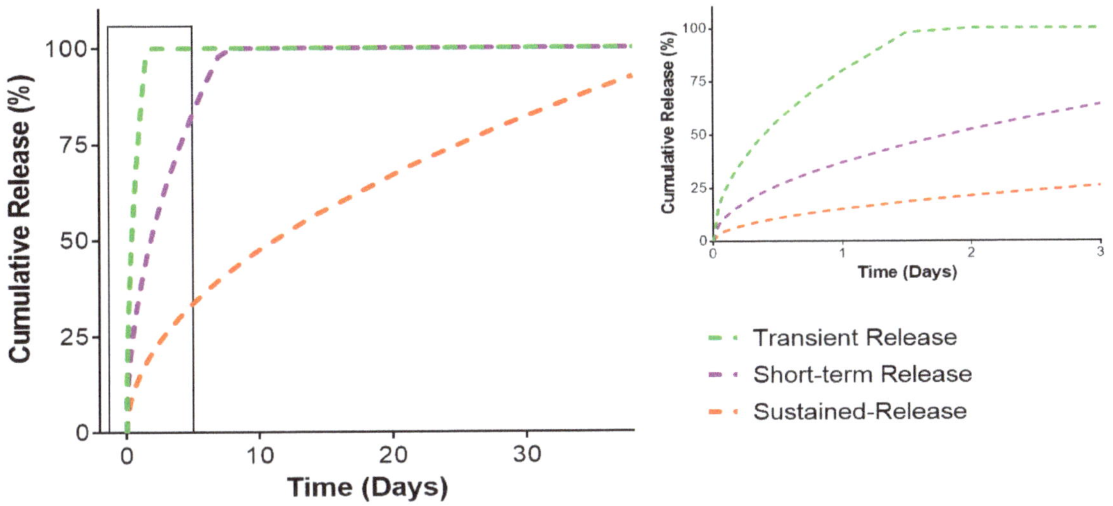

Figure 2. Schematic depicting examples of transient, short-term, and sustained-release profiles.

Traditional uniaxial electrospun fibers in which each individual fiber is composed of a single cohesive polymer layer were the first fiber architectures to be fabricated [58] and have been utilized in a variety of drug delivery applications over the past decade [36,37,59–61]. While uniaxial fibers offer high encapsulation efficiencies, cost-effectiveness, and ease of use, they have suffered from burst release and challenges in tailoring release properties [37,42,62]. These challenges are most evident in achieving the sustained-release of hydrophilic agents, often necessitating hydrophilic polymers to attain high encapsulation efficacy as well as hydrophobic polymers for sustained-release. More complex fiber architectures offer alternative options to address these limitations by combining different polymer types in distinct layers to modulate the release.

While the release characteristics of traditional uniaxial electrospun fibers have been thoroughly reviewed in literature [63–68], to our knowledge, there has not yet been a review of the more advanced fiber architectures used to deliver active agents, nor a review that considers the impact these architectures may have on intravaginal delivery applications. Here, we seek to provide an overview of different polymer architectures including coaxial, multilayered, and nanoparticle-fiber composites (Figure 3) as a function of the materials used to construct these architectures that have been utilized in a diversity of health applications. We seek to present different material combinations in these architectures to systematically relate material type and fiber architecture to active agent release kinetics. Last, we explore how lessons derived from these different architectures might be applied in the context of intravaginal delivery to address the needs of future topical sustained-release platforms for a given prophylactic or therapeutic application. The overall goal of this review is to provide a summary of different fiber architectures that have been useful for active agent delivery and to provide guidelines for the development of new formulations based on the knowledge obtained from previous work across other applications. While some of these more complex architectures have only recently been investigated relative to uniaxial fibers, they have demonstrated promise in enabling greater tunability of release and may be useful to apply as new dosage forms for intravaginal delivery and other similar applications.

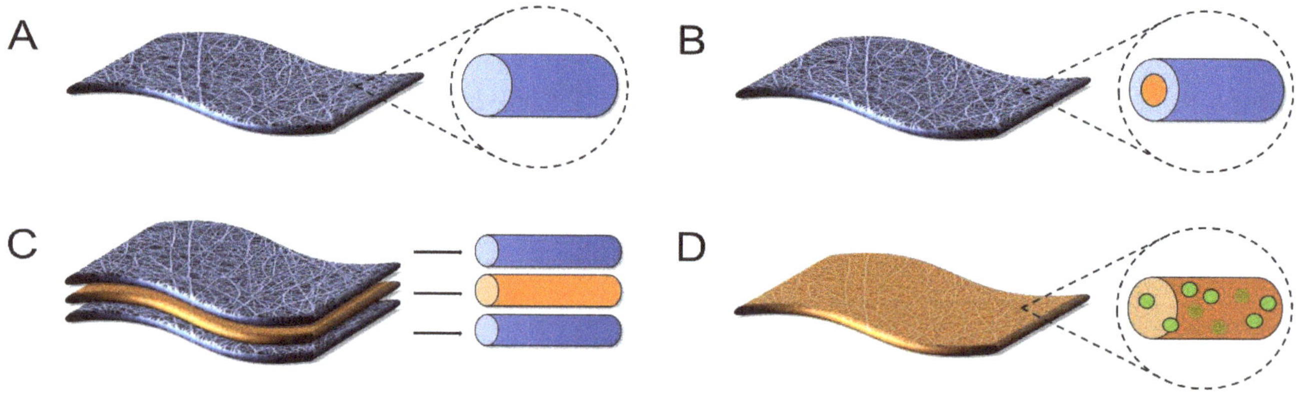

Figure 3. Schematic of different electrospun fiber composites. Diagrams representing (**A**) traditional uniaxial fibers, (**B**) coaxial fibers, (**C**) multilayered fibers, and (**D**) nanoparticle-fiber composites. (**A**) Uniaxial fibers are comprised of a single polymer or polymer blend (shown in blue) that is distributed homogenously throughout the fiber structure. (**B**) In contrast, coaxial fibers contain both core (orange) and shell (blue) layers that are chemically distinct. (**C**) Multilayered fibers result from sequentially electrospinning different fiber layers together or integrating individual layers post-fabrication. (**D**) Finally, nanoparticle-fiber composites consist of hydrophilic or hydrophobic fibers (orange) that encapsulate nanoparticles (green).

2. Coaxial Electrospun Fibers

2.1. Coaxial Architectures and Properties

Coaxial electrospinning, adapted from uniaxial or single axial electrospinning, provides a multicomponent fiber scaffold that easily allows the tunable release of active agents [69,70]. Coaxial fibers are usually comprised of two parts, an outer protective layer or shell and an inner layer or core [71], where encapsulants are typically localized (Figures 3B and 4). Coaxial fibers can provide several advantages relative to uniaxially spun fibers. First, electrospinning the core and shell polymer solutions simultaneously through a coaxial spinneret allows for the design of unique fiber architectures. The thickness and ratios of the core and shell layers can be modulated, providing more reproducible fiber properties with a greater ability to alter encapsulant release relative to other fabrication methods. Additionally, coaxial electrospinning ensures that the active agent in the core phase is protected within harsh physiological environments, such as the female reproductive tract [53]. Furthermore, a variety of materials can be used as either the core or shell to finely regulate encapsulant release (Figure 4) [69,72].

Despite these advantages, the added complexity of simultaneously electrospinning two or more polymer phases and the additional interactions between the core and shell solutions requires additional optimization relative to uniaxial electrospinning in terms of selecting compatible polymers and solvents. In addition to the core-shell architecture itself, the release profiles of active agents from coaxial fibers are impacted by solvent choice, polymer-solvent miscibility, the miscibility between core and shell solvents/solutions, solvent volatility, and layer thicknesses [73,74]. Solvent choice has been shown to alter fiber diameter and structure [75], thereby impacting active agent release [76]. Additionally, miscible core and shell solvents/solutions may lead to the partial dissolution of core encapsulants in the shell, whereas, immiscible core and shell solvents may promote material delamination at the core-shell interface, facilitating burst release of the core encapsulant. Therefore, the polymers and solvents for both core and shell layers must be selected based on their individual properties as well as their anticipated interactions [77,78]. In addition, solvent volatility and evaporation rate can affect the distribution and subsequent release of active agents, while the thickness of the polymer shell, polymer composition, and spinning conditions influence encapsulant diffusion rates [79]. Here, we discuss coaxial fibers as a function of their core-shell design, composition, and incorporated active agents to help relate these considerations to the resulting transient, short-term, or sustained-release characteristics.

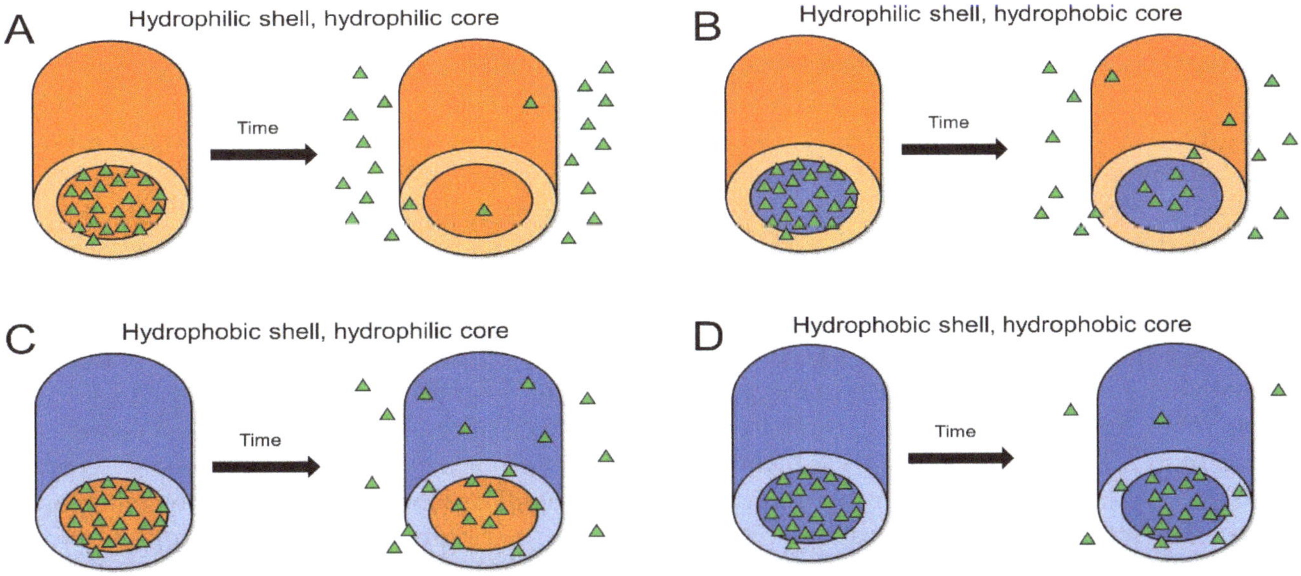

Figure 4. Schematic of anticipated release profiles from different coaxial fiber architectures. Generally, the release of encapsulants from coaxial fibers is dependent on the core and shell hydrophobicity. The release of active agents from coaxial fibers with (**A**) hydrophilic core and shell, (**B**) hydrophobic core and hydrophilic shell, (**C**) hydrophilic core and hydrophobic shell, and (**D**) hydrophobic core and shell are shown. Hydrophilic polymers (shown in orange) typically promote transient release, while more hydrophobic polymers (blue) are typically used to provide short-term or sustained-release.

2.2. Release Kinetics from Coaxial Fibers

2.2.1. Transient Release (within 24 h)

Hydrophobic Shell—Hydrophilic Core

Electrospun fibers can be designed to release the active agent immediately or within 24 h of administration if a rapid onset of action is needed for a given application [80]. Moreover, multiple active agents can be incorporated into different layers of a coaxial fiber (core or shell) to provide transient release.

For application to infectious diseases, coaxially spun fibers that demonstrate burst release followed by lower levels of short-term release may provide on-demand protection against incoming pathogens, increasing the immediate efficaciousness of agents by releasing initially high (burst) concentrations. This type of release can be achieved by employing coaxial fibers comprised of hydrophobic shells and hydrophilic cores. In one study, coaxial and triaxial fiber multi-drug delivery platforms that used PCL as the outermost shell released ~15% and ~80% of two different hydrophilic dyes, keyacid blue and keyacid uranine (KAB and KAU), from the PVP core and PCL shell fibers, respectively, within one hour [69]. In both the coaxial and triaxial fibers, the PVP core containing KAB was protected by the surrounding PCL layer containing KAU, which helped to extend the release of the remaining

KAB to 24 h. For the triaxial fibers, a blank PCL layer was electrospun between the outer PCL shell and the inner PEO core. In both the coaxial and triaxial fibers, KAU was released from the shell within 3 h; however, the triaxial fibers better modulated the release of KAB from the core, releasing 50% less during the first hour. The burst release of the KAU dye, observed from both coaxial and triaxial fibers, was attributed to water penetrating the porous fiber shell, allowing transient release. In another example of coaxial fiber design, water-soluble PVP was used as a core with a hydrophobic ethyl cellulose (EC) shell to encapsulate hydrophobic compounds of either quercetin or ketoprofen. Using this architecture, ~75% of both hydrophobic encapsulants were released within 24 h.

Hydrophilic Shell—Hydrophobic or Hydrophilic Cores

Similarly, coaxial fibers that have hydrophilic shells can facilitate the rapid release of encapsulated agents with an initial burst release of 1 to 4 h followed by continued transient release within 24 h of administration. One architecture that has been adopted to achieve rapid- or on-demand release from coaxial fibers is a hydrophilic shell in combination with a hydrophilic or hydrophobic core. In one study, zein-PVP core-shell fibers were developed that incorporated the active agent in both the core (zein) and the shell (PVP) layers [81]. Zein, a natural, moderately hydrophobic polymer was used to achieve immediate and transient release of the hydrophobic drug, ketoprofen. A burst release of 43% was observed within the first hour, followed by transient release of the remaining ketoprofen over 10 h. The initial burst release was correlated with rapid dissolution of the hydrophilic shell, while the more transient 10 h release was attributed to the hydrophobic core. In another study, the release profile of a hydrophobic drug, asiaticoside, was compared between coaxial fibers composed of chitosan cores with either a hydrophilic alginate and PVA-blended polymer shell or a hydrophobic centella triterpenes cream shell [82]. The coaxial fiber with the alginate-PVA shell demonstrated 80% more asiaticoside release relative to the centella control within 10 h, which was attributed to the shell hydrophilicity [82]. Additionally, the trend of burst release followed by more gradual transient release was attributed to rapid degradation of the alginate-PVA shell, followed by subsequent degradation of the chitosan core. While this example incorporated a polymer blend (alginate-PVA) as the hydrophilic shell, to be considered a core-shell structure, it should be noted that the material itself needs to be electrospinnable without other polymers. As this example demonstrates, hydrophilic polymers such as PVP, PVA, or PEO can be electrospun alone or in blends to create hydrophilic core and shell layers.

Core-Shell Architectures with Similar Core-Shell Hydrophobicity

Coaxial fibers comprised of both hydrophilic core and shell layers have also been investigated to provide transient release of active agents. For example, coaxial fibers fabricated with a hydrophilic PVP shell and hydrophilic cellulose acetate core were investigated. These coaxial fibers with both a hydrophilic core and shell released 31% of their hydrophobic encapsulant (epicatechin) within 10 min, followed by 80% release after 4 h [83].

In addition to the utilization of materials with similar hydrophobicities, coaxial fibers consisting of identical core-shell materials have been fabricated to provide the rapid release of active agents. In one study, fibers with PVP shells and cores were investigated to provide rapid release of the hydrophobic drug, quercetin. The PVP shell-PVP core fibers released quercetin within one minute [84], and this burst release was similarly observed in a separate study that used the same fiber formulation to deliver acyclovir [85]. In another study, the hydrophobic antibiotic, allyltriphenylphosphonium bromide, was incorporated within the core of coaxial fibers, and the volumetric ratios of core-shell solutions were varied to study release. Fibers comprised of zein-zein with core-shell volume ratios greater than 1:2 were found to suppress the burst release of the antibiotic, only releasing 15% within the first hour. In contrast, 35% and 45% of the antibiotic were released from fibers with a 1:1 core:shell volumetric ratio or blended fiber controls over the same duration [86]. In a separate study, a triaxial fiber in which all three layers were comprised of ethyl cellulose provided zero-order release of ketoprofen over 20 h due to the gradual increase in the drug content moving from shell to the core [87]. These studies highlight the role of the active agent distribution within the fiber layers, suggesting that encapsulant localization within the fiber core may enhance release.

Finally, the release of fluorescently labeled bovine serum albumin (BSA) from core-shell hydrogel nanofilaments composed of a poly(lactide-*co*-ε-caprolactone) (PLCL) shell and *N*,*N*-isopropylacrylamide (NIPAAm)/*N*,*N*′-methylene bisacrylamide crosslinked core was studied. The crosslinker, *N*,*N*′-methylene bisacrylamide, was used to polymerize NIPAAm during the electrospinning process. This study showed that by changing the NIPAAm-crosslinker (*w*/*w*) ratio from 4:1 to 37:1, the release of BSA increased from 0.15 to 0.7 ug/mg over 24 h. However, in the absence of a hydrogel within the core, BSA showed nearly complete release over the same duration. This study demonstrated that the mechanical and corresponding drug release properties could be more finely tailored by altering the NIPAAm-crosslinker (*w*/*w*) ratio [88].

Stimuli-Responsive Coaxial Architectures

Another method to modulate the release of active agents from coaxial fibers is to integrate stimuli-responsive layers to precisely release agents in response to surrounding physiological conditions [89]. Unlike stimuli-responsive uniaxial fibers, the more complex interactions between the core and shell layers in coaxial fibers can provide increased control of active agent release via pH- or other stimuli-based mechanisms. A variety of natural and synthetic materials have been investigated for their use in pH-responsive applications. In one example, a coaxial fiber comprised of a lecithin-diclofenac sodium core and a Eudragit S100 shell provided the pH-responsive release of ferulic acid for 10 h [90]. Ferulic acid release was facilitated under conditions of neutral pH (pH 7), with minimal release occurring in a more acidic (pH 2) environment. Another pH-sensitive polymethacrylate-based copolymer [90–92], Eudragit EPO, was used to fabricate pH-responsive antibacterial fibers. Here, Eudragit EPO cores, which dissolve below pH 5, were used in combination with Eudragit L100 shells, which dissolve at a pH greater than 6. These coaxial fibers provided pH-responsive release for an hour under slightly acidic conditions (pH 6) while demonstrating attenuated release in very acidic conditions (pH 2) [93]. Additionally, two separate studies investigated coaxial fibers comprised of Eudragit S100 shells and PEO cores to stimulate pH-responsive release within the gastrointestinal tract [94,95]. In both studies, the release of hydrophobic indomethacin and hydrophilic mebeverine hydrochloride agents was minimal (~10%) after 2 h under acidic conditions, followed by rapid release for 6 h when switched to neutral conditions (pH 7.4). Coaxial fibers comprised of cellulose acetate phthalate shells with polyurethane cores, as well as gelatin-sodium bicarbonate shells with PLCL cores have also been used to provide similarly rapid pH-responsive release of ciprofloxacin and rhodamine B (Rhd B). These studies demonstrated the potential of coaxial fibers as pH-sensitive delivery systems [96,97].

Coaxial fibers with other stimuli-responsive properties have been investigated for on-demand, rapid release applications. Although studies with other stimuli-responsive systems have been limited, one study investigated the use of self-immolative polymers, or polymers that depolymerize when exposed to specific external stimuli, for rapid stimuli-responsive release [98]. In this study, self-immolative fibers comprised of dibutyltin dilaurate and phenyl (4-(hydroxymethyl)phenyl) carbamate were blended with polyacrylonitrile and used as shells to surround PVP cores. The fibers provided minimal release of KAB dye when incubated in water; however, the fibers depolymerized when exposed to trifluoroacetic acid, resulting in zero-order release of ~40% dye within a week.

2.2.2. Short-Term Release (One Day to One Week)

Hydrophobic Shell—Hydrophilic Core

A key advantage of short-term release specifically for intravaginal delivery is that the burden of frequent or daily administration may decrease, thereby increasing user adherence of prophylactics and therapeutics. Traditionally, hydrophobic materials have been well-suited to provide longer durations of release (depending on the encapsulant) due to their decreased degradation rates in aqueous environments. For more traditional uniaxial hydrophobic fiber platforms, most hydrophobic small molecule drugs or larger macromolecules achieve release for up to one week due to the similar hydrophobic properties of the polymer and encapsulant [6]. This compatibility allows for hydrophobic encapsulants to partition more evenly within and distribute throughout hydrophobic polymers. However, hydrophilic agents, which have low solubility in nonpolar polymers, often partition to the fiber surface, resulting in burst release and suboptimal short-term and/or sustained-release properties. To address this challenge, coaxial fibers in which hydrophilic agents are encapsulated within a hydrophilic core and surrounded by a protective hydrophobic shell can prolong and adjust the release of hydrophilic molecules.

The use of coaxial fibers with hydrophobic shells and hydrophilic cores has been shown to extend the release of many encapsulants [71,99,100]. In one study, a coaxial fiber comprised of a hydrophobic ethyl cellulose shell with a hydrophilic PVP core was investigated for short-term release. These fibers released maraviroc over a duration of hours to days depending on the thickness of the hydrophobic shell, which was modulated via flow rate and total electrospun volume. The increased thickness of the hydrophobic shell extended encapsulant release from 24 h to five days by increasing the shell-to-core volume ratio from 0.5 to 4 [99]. In another study, a PCL fiber shell surrounding a PVP-graphene oxide blended core was studied. These fibers released 65% of hydrophilic vancomycin hydrochloride within 4 h and attained full release of vancomycin after 96 h [101]. Although this coaxial fiber provided short-term release, the long-term safety of graphene oxide within the FRT is unknown, and further studies are required to assess its safety in intravaginal delivery applications. Finally, a coaxial fiber composed of a synthetic hydrophilic poly-cyclodextrin core and hydrophobic poly(methacrylic acid) shell reduced the burst release of a hydrophilic drug, propranolol hydrochloride, by 50%, and extended release to 180 h relative to the 140 hour release obtained from uniaxial fibers [102].

Hydrophobic Shell—Hydrophobic Core

In addition to the widely used hydrophobic shell-hydrophilic core coaxial architectures, the use of hydrophobic materials in both the core and the shell layers has also been investigated to provide the short-term release of active agents. In one study, a PCL core surrounded by an outer PCL shell was used to prolong the release of the antibiotic ampicillin. Ampicillin, a hydrophilic compound, normally localizes to the surface of PCL when spun as a uniaxial fiber, resulting in burst release [103]. As an alternative, a 4% (w/v) PCL solution was used to fabricate an ultra-thin shell to delay release. In addition, the parameters for coaxial electrospinning were modified using dilute sheath solutions to improve the control of fiber diameter and morphology. The resulting coaxial fiber efficiently encapsulated ampicillin and provided short-term release for ~80 h [103]. In another study, coaxial fibers comprised of a zein shell with a PCL core reduced the burst release of the hydrophilic antibiotic, metronidazole, achieving short-term release for more than four days [78].

Stimuli-Responsive Coaxial Architectures

Coaxial fibers exhibiting stimuli-responsive properties have also been investigated to provide short-term release of active agents. As one example, poly(*N*-isopropylacrylamide), a thermoresponsive polymer, was used as a core layer in combination with an ethyl cellulose and anhydrous ethanol shell solution. At room temperature, poly(*N*-isopropylacrylamide) exhibits hydrophilic properties; however, at temperatures above 32 °C, the polymer demonstrates more hydrophobic characteristics. At room temperature and after 55 h, the fibers released 65% of ketoprofen in PBS, while only 40% of the same drug was released at 37 °C [104].

Blended Polymers in Coaxial Architectures

Another method of prolonging release is to use blended polymers to formulate coaxial fibers, which can decrease fiber wettability. One study combined gelatin, a natural hydrophilic protein, with the hydrophobic polymer, PCL, to create coaxial fibers with increased hydrophobicity and mechanical stability relative to gelatin alone [105]. In one study, the release of hydrophilic doxycycline was measured from three different fiber architectures—a uniaxial PCL-gelatin blended fiber, coaxial fibers with three different cores (PCL, gelatin, or a PCL-gelatin blend) and a PCL-gelatin blended shell, and a triaxial fiber with both a PCL-gelatin blended core and outer shell and an intermediate gelatin layer. Among these five designs, uniaxial PCL-gelatin blended fibers released the most doxycycline within 24 h (90%), while coaxial fibers with a PCL-gelatin core and shell released the least (50%). Additionally, only coaxial fibers with either a PCL-gelatin or gelatin core prolonged release over five days. Furthermore, the other architectures including the uniaxial PCL-gelatin blend, coaxial fiber with PCL core, and triaxial fibers failed to release doxycycline for more than 30 h. The burst release observed in fibers with PCL cores was attributed to the lack of compatibility between the hydrophobic PCL cores and hydrophilic encapsulant, which caused doxycycline to localize on the core surface. Additionally, the subsequent suboptimal encapsulant release was attributed to low water penetration into the hydrophobic core. These studies demonstrate that utilization of both hydrophobic and hydrophilic polymers alone or as blends can modulate the short-term release of hydrophilic encapsulants due to the variation in the permeability of different layers and core-encapsulant interactions.

2.2.3. Sustained-Release (One Week to Multiple Months)

Hydrophobic Shell—Hydrophilic Core

Similar to fibers that provide short-term release, fibers designed for sustained-release commonly use hydrophobic polymers as the outer shell to prevent the fiber from undergoing rapid hydrolysis. Studies have demonstrated that the most promising coaxial architecture to achieve sustained-delivery utilizes a hydrophobic shell and hydrophilic core [6]. A polymer that is frequently used in coaxial fibers to provide sustained-release is poly(lactic-*co*-glycolic acid) (PLGA). In one study, a coaxial fiber composed of a PLGA shell was used to shield a hydrophilic core consisting of tragacanth gum. The encapsulant, tetracycline hydrochloride, served as a model hydrophilic agent. Investigators observed that PLGA (shell)-tragacanth gum (core) coaxial fibers diminished burst release and provided sustained-release of tetracycline hydrochloride for 75 days, releasing 68% of tetracycline hydrochloride during this period [106]. In another study, a PLGA (shell)-polyethylenimine (PEI, core) architecture was used to prolong the release and stability of bone morphogenetic protein-2 plasmid (pBMP2-2). The hydrophilic PEI core was used to encapsulate and retain the bioactivity of pBMP2-2, while the hydrophobic PLGA shell was used as a protective barrier to prolong release. When compared to uniaxial PLGA-PEI blended fibers, the PLGA (shell)-PEI (core) coaxial fiber exhibited both improved bioactivity and prolonged release of the pBMP2-2 plasmid. The coaxial fiber released 80% of the plasmid over 20 days, while the uniaxial fibers released the same amount over seven days [107].

Polymers other than PLGA have been used as hydrophobic shells to sustain the release of active agents from coaxial fibers. One study formulated coaxial fibers containing a hydrophilic dextran core and hydrophobic PCL shell. The addition of polyethylene glycol (PEG) to the PCL shell increased the release of the encapsulated BSA by forming pores in the shell layer. Although all fibers released ~20% BSA within the first 24 h, increasing the PEG concentration increased the amount of BSA released over extended durations. Interestingly, all fibers demonstrated sustained-release regardless of PEG concentration; coaxial fibers fabricated with 5% PEG shells released ~60% BSA, while fibers containing 40% PEG shells released 90% BSA over 27 days [108]. In another study, the relationship between PEG (core):PCL (shell) molar ratio and the release of BSA or lysozyme was investigated. The thinnest shell layers with a core:shell molar ratio of 1.59 and a core flow rate of 2 mL/h provided complete release of both encapsulants within 24 days, compared to only 50% release from thicker fibers with a core:shell molar ratio of 0.32 and a core flow rate of 0.6 mL/h. Moreover, the fibers preserved the bioactivity of lysozyme and released BSA over 29 days, with no noticeable differences between BSA and lysozyme release rates [109]. In addition to conventional coaxial spinning, the use of emulsion electrospinning has also been investigated to fabricate coaxial fibers, which can be electrospun using a uniaxial spinneret [70]. One study that used emulsion electrospinning fabricated core-shell fibers composed of a PEG-poly(D,L-lactic acid) shell and methyl cellulose core to minimize the burst release of lysozyme [110]. The release of lysozyme from the core was achieved over 15 days and was dependent on the percent of lysozyme loaded, while the structural integrity and bioactivity of lysozyme was protected by the shell. A later study compared these same coaxial fibers to blended uniaxial fibers composed of PCL and PEG and showed that the coaxial fibers improved sustained-release by releasing ~50% of BSA over 35 days relative to blended fibers, which released ~75% BSA [111].

Another study explored the effects of multiple processing parameters, including PEG and PCL concentrations, PEG molecular weight, encapsulant concentration, and fiber diameter, in modulating the release of plasmid DNA (pDNA). Plasmid DNA was encapsulated in a PEI core, and a non-viral gene delivery vector (r-PEI-HA) was incorporated within a PCL shell [112]. An increase in fiber diameter was observed with an increase in all of the three other parameters, while the loading and release of r-PEI-HA were correlated to pDNA concentration in the fiber core and PEG molecular weight. The fibers formulated with high PEG molecular weight and low pDNA concentration exhibited ~30% release of r-PEI-HA over 60 days, while the fibers with high pDNA concentration and low molecular weight PEG completely released pDNA within 60 days.

Core-Shell Architectures with the Same Core-Shell Hydrophobicity

Although coaxial architectures with similar core and shell hydrophobicities have been utilized to obtain transient and short-term release, coaxial fibers that use the same materials have been less frequently investigated to provide sustained-release. In one study, PLGA was utilized in both the core and shell layers to investigate the effect on vancomycin and ceftazidime delivery [113]. Both hydrophilic drugs were encapsulated within the core PLGA layer and exhibited similar burst release kinetics within the first day, followed by a second phase of more gradual release over five to ten days. Ninety percent of the antibiotics were released after 11 days, followed by complete release after 25 days, with the more gradual release attributed to the PLGA barrier layer.

2.3. Applications for Intravaginal Delivery

The enhanced tunability and versatility provided by the core and shell layers of coaxial fibers make them excellent candidates for intravaginal delivery applications. While uniaxial fibers have been studied for sustained- and stimuli-responsive release of active agents in the FRT [6,114–119], they have faced challenges in providing the sustained-release of therapeutically relevant concentrations of individual active agents and effectively modulating the release of multiple agents core [6]. Often, compatibility between the polymer and encapsulant can pose challenges to achieving sustained-release with uniaxial fibers, while coaxial fibers may circumvent this issue by integrating two different polymers, enabling the separation of agents within a compatible polymer formulation (core or shell). Moreover, the additional outer shell can help to modulate release. One can envision that with a coaxial architecture, multiple agents may be delivered against a particular infection to provide a synergistic effect or to provide protection against multiple types of viral or bacterial infections. Together, these features allow for enhanced tunability with the option of providing immediate to short-term release for on-demand applications while also providing long-term release that may be particularly useful in prophylactic or contraceptive applications.

A variety of release kinetics can be attained from coaxial fibers by using different combinations of materials in the core and shell layers. Transient or rapid release of active agents is often accomplished with the use of hydrophilic polymers due to their rapid dissolution in aqueous environments. To achieve short-term release extending to one week, a hydrophilic core in combination with a hydrophobic shell is the most frequently used architecture, enabling the slow dissolution of the shell layer, which acts as a barrier to encapsulant diffusion from the core. For sustained-release applications that require delivery on the order of weeks to months, hydrophobic polymers such as

PLGA and PCL are often selected as shell polymers due to their slower degradation kinetics and biocompatibility. Yet, due to the number of parameters involved in the synthesis of coaxial fibers, two similar architectures may still be tailored to perform very differently by altering physical versus chemical properties. An example may be seen in which fibers composed of similar or even the same polymers display very different release rates due to the modulation of shell thickness. In these cases, thinner shells have been shown to provide more transient release, while increasing the shell thickness delays or alters the trend to more gradual release.

Coaxial fibers have been investigated previously for intravaginal delivery [96,99]. In one study, maraviroc release from coaxial fibers was adjusted by varying the drug loading and solution flow rates to provide release over five days [99]. In addition, pH-responsive coaxial fibers have been fabricated to react in the presence of semen by utilizing the pH-sensitive polymer cellulose acetate phthalate as a shell. The outer shell dissolved immediately after exposure to PBS, promoting pH-responsive release of Rhd B [96].

Although coaxial fibers have shown promise in general drug and initial intravaginal delivery applications, further refinements are required to expand their overall utility. First, compatibility between the solvents of the two polymer electrospinning solutions may limit the potential combinations of core-shell materials and encapsulated agents to achieve successful electrospinning. Additionally, residual solvents from the electrospinning process may interact with and inactivate encapsulated active agents in the core layer. Therefore, while research in coaxial fiber design is still ongoing, other fiber architectures such as multilayered fibers may offer additional advantages to advance intravaginal delivery.

3. Multilayered Electrospun Fibers

3.1. *Multilayered Fiber Architectures and Properties*

Multilayered fibers can provide layer-by-layer delivery platforms that are relatively simple and inexpensive to fabricate while allowing for the encapsulation of different active agents within the individual layers. The topology, thickness, and composition of each individual layer can be easily tuned to provide different release properties based on the envisioned application. Moreover, multilayered fibers have been shown to have increased mechanical stability and flexibility compared to coaxial fibers [120]. While the interactions between two or more polymer solution interfaces must be considered for coaxial fibers, multilayered fibers can be fabricated from normally incompatible polymers due to their sequential versus simultaneous fabrication process.

Electrospun multilayered fibers can be fabricated by sequential layering, stacking, or interweaving fibers [121–123]. In sequential layering, the first layer of polymer is electrospun onto a collector, followed by electrospinning additional polymer layers directly onto the same collector. In comparison, "stacking" fibers refers to individually electrospinning each layer separately and subsequently adhering individual layers together post-spin. Stacked fibers share similar physical properties with sequentially-layered fibers, enabling temporally-programmed or spatially-specific delivery of active agents [124]. Finally, the fabrication of interwoven fibers utilizes dual or multiple-syringes to simultaneously electrospin two or more different polymer solutions (usually one hydrophilic and hydrophobic) onto the same collector. In contrast to fibers produced using the sequential layering and stacking processes, which have distinct, separate layers of polymeric fibers, interwoven fibers result from the blending of these different polymer solutions from syringes placed opposite of or adjacent to each other into one integrated layer [125–127]. This technique seamlessly integrates both hydrophilic and hydrophobic polymers in a way that prevents unwanted interactions between the electrospun polymer solutions [127,128] while enabling the porosity of the hydrophilic fibers to be altered to more finely tune fiber degradation [129]. Although interwoven fibers do not have a shell layer, the interwoven architecture has been beneficial in promoting cell adhesion and growth and has the potential to more finely modulate active agent release via porosity-based mechanisms for drug delivery applications [130,131].

Regardless of fabrication technique, multilayered fibers are beneficial in that they can temporally modulate the release of multiple agents from a single delivery platform and can provide additional tunability by modulating the barrier or discrete layers of the multilayered structure (Figure 5). In addition, the ability to impart spatially-specific release—where specific layers of the multilayered fiber possess distinct release profiles—is a key advantage of this architecture. This advantage may be envisioned for intravaginal delivery applications where one layer provides rapid active agent release to the mucus while another layer enables sustained-delivery specific to underlying epithelial or immune cells [121,123]. For interwoven multilayered fibers, studies have shown that the incorporation of a hydrophilic polymer can alter the overall porosity and wettability [129,132,133], while using a hydrophobic outer layer in multilayered fibers (similar to coaxial fibers) can decrease surface wettability and corresponding active agent release [134].

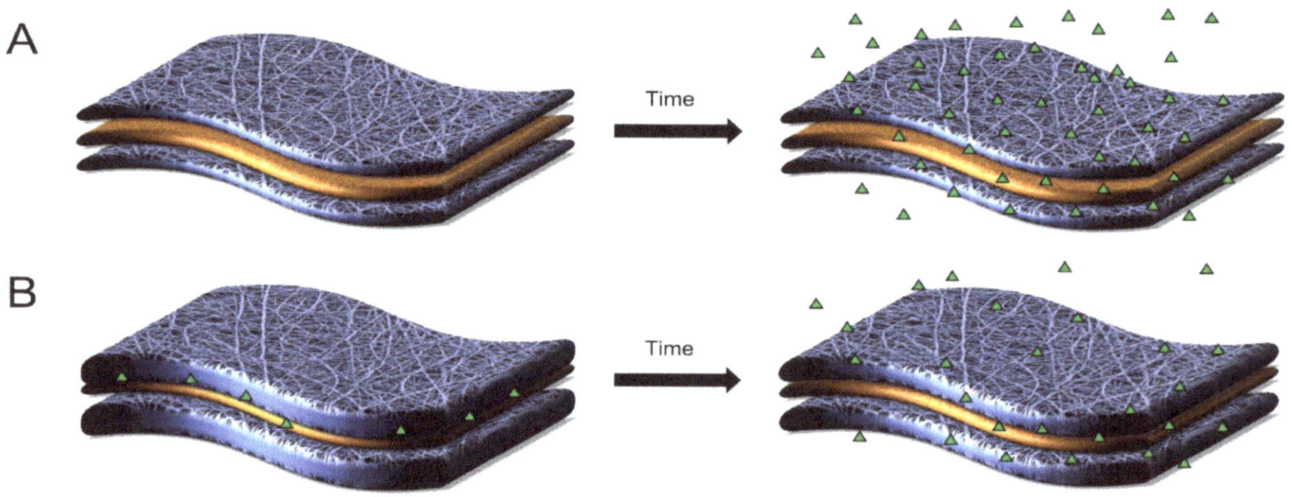

Figure 5. Schematic of anticipated active agent release from multilayered fibers. One method to modulate the release of active agents (shown in green) is to vary the thickness of the outer layer (shown in blue). (**A**) A thin outer layer provides both rapid burst release and limited sustained-release of encapsulants. (**B**) In contrast, increased outer layer thickness can delay the release of some active agents.

While the process of creating multilayered fibers is well established, more work is required to elucidate how each polymer layer impacts release kinetics. Physical properties including the pore size, fiber diameter, and thickness of traditional uniaxial fibers are known to impact the delivery kinetics of active agents from individual layers. Thus, the presence of one or more fiber layers can contribute to the complexity in establishing and predicting the release kinetics of diverse active agents from differently layered architectures. Despite these considerations and complexities, the adoption of different layering techniques to create multilayered fibers can achieve diverse patterns of release for transient, short-term, and sustained-release applications.

3.2. Release Kinetics from Multilayered Fibers

3.2.1. Transient and Short-Term Release

Multilayered fibers have shown promise in providing transient and short-term release of active agents. Conventionally, a hydrophilic layer serves as a reservoir for active agents, while hydrophobic materials provide an outer shell layer to prolong release. One study utilized a multilayered fabrication approach to encapsulate the hydrophobic antibiotic, gentamicin, in a hydrophilic PVA center layer and utilized a PU outer layer to envelop the inner PVA fiber [135]. Three separate fibers were fabricated by altering the thickness of the PU outer layer between 3.4 and 8.1 μm. The release of gentamicin was modulated with the thinnest PU layer (3.4 μm) demonstrating complete release within 1 h, relative to 10% release obtained from the thickest layer (8.1 μm). Furthermore, the thickest PU layer continued to release gentamicin for 24 h. Another study using interwoven electrospun fibers containing PEO and PCL demonstrated that by adjusting the ratio of the two polymers, tunable fiber degradation could be achieved from the resulting changes in pore size and porosity [127]. Although this study investigated interwoven fibers to enhance cell infiltration through the pores, the use of sacrificial fiber layers may be applied to modulate active agent release from the fibers for intravaginal delivery applications [127].

In addition to modulating the outer layer thickness and overall fiber composition, alterations to the number of layers have been shown to impact active agent release. In one study, fibroin-gelatin blended uniaxial fibers exhibited release of trypan blue, fluorescein isothiocyanate (FITC)-inulin, and FITC-BSA within minutes [136]. In contrast, multilayered fibers composed of the same materials extended the release of all three model compounds to 28 days [136]. In another study, dual-release, multilayered electrospun fibers containing the model dyes, 5,10,15,20-tetraphenyl-21*H*,23*H*-porphinetetrasulfonic acid disulfuric acid (TPPS) and chromazurol B, were encapsulated in four-layered PLCL (75:25) fibers. The release rate and duration of the dyes were controlled by the fiber diameter and individual fiber layer thicknesses. Minimal release of both dyes was observed for the first 15 min, followed by a quasi-linear release profile for up to 4 h. However, increasing the thickness of dye-loaded layers resulted in higher quasi-linear release rates due to the reduced density of the fiber surface [137]. In another study, the transient release of ketoprofen was achieved using trilayer fibers composed of two EC outer layers surrounding a center PVP fiber. These fibers provided nearly complete release of ketoprofen within 24 h [121]. Last, asymmetric multilayered polylactide fibers with different designs on each side were fabricated to prevent liver cancer recurrence by promoting one-sided prolonged chemotherapeutic release [138]. The fiber was composed of five poly(lactic acid) (PLA) layers, with each layer serving as either a barrier to release or a drug encapsulating reservoir. In vivo studies in a murine model demonstrated tumor suppression for at least four days, indicating that the multilayered fiber may provide localized chemotherapy for short-term durations [138].

Multilayered fibers with stimuli-responsive properties have also been investigated for transient and short-term release applications. In one of the first studies to investigate multilayered architectures, the pH-responsive polymers, poly(acrylic acid) (PAA) and poly(allylamine hydrochloride) (PAH), were electrospun together to create a blended fiber. These fibers were loaded with a low molecular weight cationic molecule, methylene blue, and demonstrated rapid release of methylene blue (~10 min) at a neutral pH (7.4). However, by gradually adjusting the pH from 6 to 2 in aqueous solutions, the step-wise pH-responsive release of methylene blue was achieved over three and a half days. Building upon this work, the effect of coating the fibers with a thermoresponsive polymer blend, poly(*N*-isopropylacrylamide)-PAA, or perfluorosilane was assessed. The addition of the thermoresponsive poly(*N*-isopropylacrylamide)-PAA coating modulated methylene blue release via temperature. Above a critical temperature, the thermoresponsive polymer became insoluble and formed intramolecular hydrogen bonds, which led to the release of methylene blue within 50 min (PBS, pH 7.4). In comparison, coating with perfluorosilane modulated release for up to 20 h at neutral pH. When both the pH-responsive and multiple layers of thermoresponsive polymers were integrated and evaluated at 25 and 40 °C, dye released for a maximum of 10 h regardless of layer thickness [139].

3.2.2. Sustained-Release

The ability of multilayered fibers to provide long-term release has been demonstrated in a variety of studies [66,67,140]. In one study, the release of a hydrophobic chemotherapeutic agent, 7-ethyl-10-hydroxycamptothecin (SN-38), was prolonged to 30 days by using a triple-layered fiber in which SN-38 was encapsulated in the center layer and surrounded by two superhydrophobic outer layers consisting of PCL and poly(glycerol monostearate-*co*-ε-caprolactone) [134]. Similar to the trends seen for transient and short-term release from multilayered fibers, increasing the thickness of the outer fiber substantially improved the longevity and amount of drug released. In another study, multilayered fibers comprised of a PCL shell and a PEO/Rhd B core were fabricated to assess the effect of increasing the outer layer thicknesses between 46.1, 68.9, and 186.1 μm [141]. While the thinnest 46 μm layers released 85% of Rhd B in one day, the 68.9 and 186.1 μm layers increased release to 15 and 25 days, respectively. Moreover, the release from the two fibers with the thicker outer layers demonstrated zero-order kinetics, producing gradual, even release of drug with respect to time.

3.3. Applications for Intravaginal Delivery

Multilayered fibers have shown promise as a platform to co-deliver or prolong the release of active agents in different environments. The process of creating multilayered fibers is relatively simple, eliminating the more complex set-up and considerations of polymer-solvent interactions between the adjacent, simultaneously spun layers present in coaxial spinning. By removing this complexity of interactions, multilayered fibers can achieve "programmed release" by simply modulating the thickness of each layer.

Multilayered fibers possess other unique features that make them excellent candidates for intravaginal delivery applications. One of the unique strengths of multilayered fibers is that they can provide spatially-specific release in that, unlike other architectures, the individual layers of multilayered fibers can be designed for specific and discrete purposes. For example, one layer may be designed to improve mucoadhesion for enhanced longevity and biocompatibility within the FRT, while another layer may provide release of active agents dependent on its location within the multilayered matrix. Compared to coaxial fibers, the optimization of multilayered fibers is not limited by solvent compatibility, as they can be sequentially spun and assembled post-fabrication. Moreover, multiple individually spun layers can increase the ease of encapsulating multiple types of active agents, which serve mechanistically different roles against a single type of viral infection or as a multipurpose viral-contraceptive or viral-bacterial dosage form. Finally, each fiber layer can be adjusted to have distinct mechanical properties that include tensile strength, porosity, and elasticity, important for comfort and user preference [142].

To date, the use of multilayered fibers for intravaginal delivery has been briefly explored [56,99,123]. In one study, circular sheets of pre-spun PVP and PVP-EC fibers were stacked and annealed via a pressed metal die that was dipped in solvent. The die annealed the edges of the stacked fibers, creating a multilayered fiber with a PVP inner layer surrounded by blended PVP-EC sheaths. Other multilayered fibers were also constructed by folding the outer layers and pressing the seams. Both types of multilayered fibers encapsulated the hydrophilic compound maraviroc and provided biphasic release, exhibiting an initial burst release followed by short-term release for up to five days. Another study from the same group examined tenofovir (TFV) localization within stacked PCL/PLGA fibers. It was found that TFV localization within the multilayered fiber could be predicted by considering the changes in polymer crystalline structure caused by encapsulant-polymer interactions and correlating drug-polymer hydrophilicity [56].

Both multilayered and coaxial fibers have the potential to provide tunable and sustained-release; however, each architecture still faces the challenges surrounding FRT delivery. For example, the interplay between two polymer solutions still needs to be considered for interwoven multilayered (and coaxial) fibers, which may result in challenges to altering active agent release. Additionally, as stated previously, the most significant obstacles to intravaginal delivery are providing a dosage form that can facilitate active agent penetration of mucus and retention and release of therapeutically relevant agent concentrations within the FRT. To improve retention, fibers can be fabricated using polymers or polymer blends that have mucoadhesive properties. However, this longevity is rarely translated to active agents once they have been released from fibers. Thus, new measures may be considered to provide efficacious and sustained-delivery from fibers.

4. Composite Nanoparticle-Fiber Delivery Vehicles

4.1. Nanoparticle-Fiber Architectures and Properties

Over the past two decades, polymeric NPs have been extensively studied as efficacious drug delivery platforms for a variety of applications. Polymeric nanoparticles are an attractive option for intravaginal delivery relative to traditional delivery platforms such as gels and films due to the tunability of active agent release, ability for surface modification, potential for targeted delivery, enhanced distribution potential, and the often resulting enhanced efficacy of encapsulated agents. Additionally, polymeric NPs have been shown to elicit minimal immune response and to improve the delivery and bioactivity of biologics [29,143,144]. Although metallic nanoparticles have also been explored for use in many drug delivery applications, they have been less commonly administered within the FRT, hence, a more comprehensive review of their applications may be found in [145,146].

Many physicochemical characteristics of NPs can be altered, such as particle size, surface charge, and hydrophobicity, which contribute to their success in achieving sustained-release and localization to target sites [147]. Although NPs have proven to be effective delivery platforms, as discussed in previous reviews [148,149], achieving the prolonged release of active agents can be difficult due to the natural clearance mechanisms of the FRT. In particular, NPs are challenged with retention in the vaginal cavity due to mucus clearance and transport through mucus to underlying tissue [28,150,151]. These challenges may be overcome by incorporating NPs into electrospun fibers, thereby creating a composite delivery vehicle that complements the capabilities of both technologies. One might envision that fibers may act as a reservoir for NPs, improving NP and active agent retention, while the innate fiber porosity can help to more finely tune encapsulant release from NPs relative to the release observed from freely administered NPs or fibers.

Nanoparticle-fiber composites are dual-component systems that have the ability to alter the release kinetics of active agents from NPs or NPs themselves [152,153]. Often, the active agent of interest is encapsulated within the NPs, which are then preloaded into polymer solutions for subsequent electrospinning. While a variety of inorganic NPs have been incorporated into fibers [154–156], concerns still persist regarding the safety of their use relative to polymeric NPs, particularly for intravaginal applications. By utilizing biocompatible polymeric materials for both nanoparticles and fibers, composites may provide safe and prolonged release for clinical applications.

4.2. Release Kinetics from Nanoparticle-Fiber Composites

4.2.1. Transient Release

Nanoparticle-fiber composites have been used to rapidly release NPs and their encapsulated agents. A study was conducted with hydrophilic PVA and PEO fibers that incorporated PLGA NPs that contained the dye, Coumarin 6 [157]. PEO fibers released 90% of NPs within 30 min when immersed in a 50:50 ethanol:PBS solution, followed by additional release (5%) after 3.5 h. In comparison, PVA fibers released approximately 70% of PLGA NPs within 30 min, followed by a decrease in NP release (15%) over 8 h. Slightly slower release over 24 h was observed when PVA fibers were crosslinked prior to NP incorporation. This study highlights that nanoparticle-fiber composites can be used to successfully incorporate NPs and to modulate the transient release of NPs from these composites within aqueous solutions [157].

4.2.2. Short-Term Release

Several studies have utilized nanoparticle-fiber composites to provide the short-term release of active agents. One group explored a composite drug delivery system that encapsulated the antibiotic, erythromycin, in gelatin NPs and free lidocaine hydrochloride within PVA-chitosan blended fibers [158]. Eighty percent of the lidocaine hydrochloride was released from the fibers within 54 h, while 70% of the erythromycin was released after 70 h. In contrast, free gelatin NPs released 90% of erythromycin within the same duration. In a separate study, chitosan-PEO blended fibers containing methoxypolyethylene glycol (mPEG)-b-PLA micelles demonstrated a low initial burst release (15%) of 5-fluorouracil (5-FU), followed by prolonged release (91%) for 109 h [159]. In another study, the release of free hydrophobic naproxen and chitosan nanoparticles containing Rhd B was studied from PCL fiber scaffolds [160]. Rhodamine B exhibited low levels (5%) of burst release, while 30–40% of naproxen was released within the first 2 h.

Moreover, after 72 h, only 20% of Rhd B was released, while 60% of naproxen was released. The rapid release of naproxen was achieved via incorporation within the fiber scaffold, while the extended release of Rhd B was obtained and enhanced through nanoparticle-fiber encapsulation. These results demonstrate the utility of nanoparticle-fiber composites in providing the short-term release of multiple agents.

4.2.3. Sustained-Release

Nanoparticle-fiber composites have also demonstrated long-term release capabilities in several studies. In one study, dual-release nanoparticle-fiber composites were used to mend and treat critically sized calvarial defects in rats [161]. These composites, consisting of PCL-*co*-PEG fibers encapsulating dexamethasone and BSA NPs and loaded with bone morphogenic protein-2 (BMP-2), demonstrated sustained-release of both molecules over 35 days. Another study explored the incorporation of siRNA into chitosan NPs and PLGA fiber composites [153]. In these composites, the release of active siRNA was sustained in vitro, with 95% of siRNA released from the fibers over 32 days, while gene silencing activity was maintained. Sustained-release from nanoparticle-fiber composites was also demonstrated in another study with chitosan-PEO electrospun fibers that were loaded with PLGA NPs encapsulating phenytoin. Nearly complete release of phenytoin from the composite scaffold was achieved over nine days [162]. Lastly, PLA fibers encapsulating chitosan particles provided sustained-release of BSA (45%) for 27 days, while chitosan particles alone released 80% BSA in 14 days [163].

In addition to NP incorporation within traditional uniaxial or blended fibers, NPs have been incorporated in more complex fiber architectures to prolong the release of active agents. For instance, the effect of combining a multilayered fiber architecture with nanoparticle-fiber composites was investigated by fabricating alternating layers of poly-L-lactic acid (PLLA) and PCL fibers with layers of PCL fibers encapsulating positively-charged chitosan BSA NPs [164]. The multilayered composite released 80% of the BSA in approximately eight days, whereas the monolayer control released the same concentration of BSA within 24 h.

4.3. Applications for Intravaginal Delivery

Composite delivery vehicles containing nanoparticles and fibers have thus far been primarily studied in wound healing and tissue engineering to fabricate scaffolds for tissue regeneration and bone remodeling [86,165–167]. However, these platforms may be promising candidates for intravaginal delivery applications due to their structural stability and ability to sustain the release of active agents. In such systems, the fibers may be utilized as a reservoir for NPs to aid in intravaginal retention by helping to decrease NP clearance during shedding. In addition, it is envisioned that, depending on fiber formulation and, importantly, NP size and charge, NP (and active agent) release may be modulated, enabling NPs to traverse mucus and deliver agents to target cells that reside in the epithelium or underlying lamina propria. Similar to other architectures, fiber parameters such as polymer composition and size can be tailored to impact release in combination with altering NP composition, size, and loading within the fiber.

For intravaginal delivery applications, NPs can impart cell specificity, cell internalization, as well as mucoadhesive or mucopenetrative properties to their encapsulated active agents [14]. Numerous studies have demonstrated the ability of NPs to enhance cell targeting via surface modification [168,169]. Additionally, surface modification can increase cell internalization, which may enhance the transport, subcellular localization, and corresponding efficacy of drugs like tenofovir disoproxil fumarate (TDF), which require cell internalization. Furthermore, the NP surface charge can be modulated to provide either mucoadhesive or mucopenetrative properties that further enhance active agent delivery. Additionally, fibers can be fabricated to encapsulate NPs for sustained-release as well as free agents for rapid release, providing both on-demand and sustained-release in one platform. Finally, nanoparticle-fiber composites, when coupled with coaxial or multilayered fiber architectures, provide an attractive strategy to retain and sustain the release of active agents within the FRT (Figure 6).

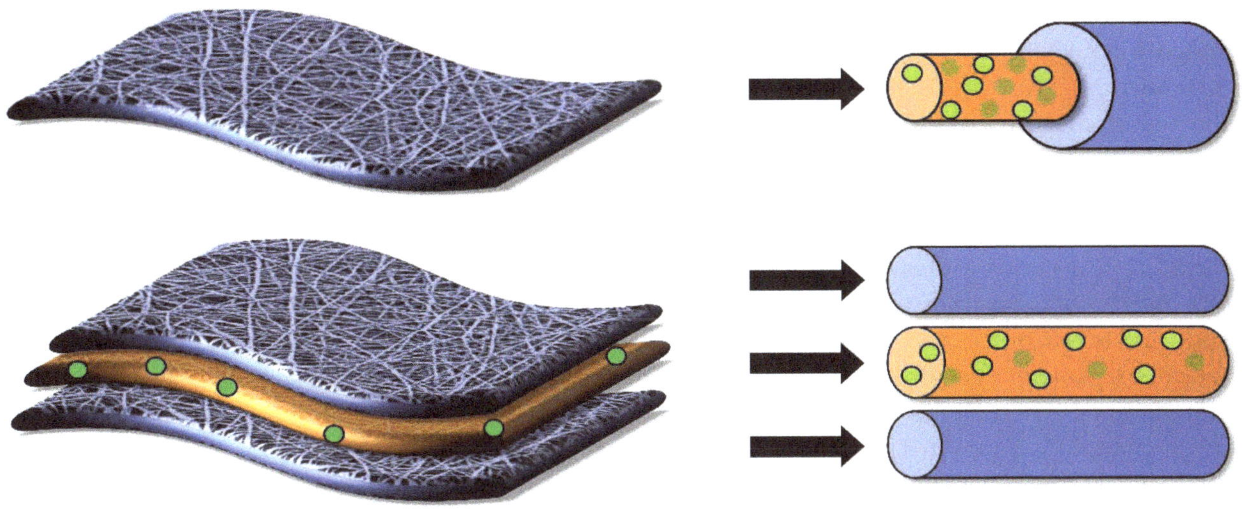

Figure 6. Schematic of electrospun nanoparticle-fiber composites that integrate coaxial and multilayered fiber architectures. (**A**) Coaxial fibers can be fabricated to encapsulate nanoparticles (NPs) within the core fiber, conferring sustained- or delayed-release of active agents that are encapsulated in NPs (shown in green). (**B**) Multilayered fibers that encapsulate NPs can also act as reservoirs for either NP or active agent release.

As with multilayered fibers, the use of nanoparticle-fiber composites has only recently been investigated for intravaginal delivery. In a proof-of-concept study, rapid-release PEO, PVA, or PVP fibers encapsulated PLGA NPs containing C6 dye or etravirine drug [23]. In this study, composites and free NPs were administered within murine FRTs and assessed for retention and release. The encapsulated nanoparticles exhibited a 30-fold increase in retention in the mouse FRTs relative to free NPs. Furthermore, nanoparticles alone provided transient release of etravirine, while all nanoparticle-fiber composites demonstrated release for up to seven days. To date, this is the only investigation of nanoparticle-fiber composites for use in intravaginal delivery. However, the significant difference in retention and release rate achieved with nanoparticle-fiber composites highlights the immense potential of this architecture for sustained-delivery in the FRT.

Although combining nanoparticles and electrospun fibers into one delivery vehicle has demonstrated potential, challenges exist for this platform. The major concern is related to the concentration of nanoparticles that can be effectively encapsulated within fibers without hindering the ability of the polymer solution to be electrospun [170]. Furthermore, the concentration of active agent may decrease with the use of a coaxial or multilayered architecture, as only specific layers of the fiber will encapsulate NPs. Finally, polymeric NPs are often comprised of the same or similar polymers as electrospun fibers, thus care must be taken to prevent polymer solvents from dissolving the NPs prior to or during the electrospinning process [171]. Moreover, the morphology of NPs may also be adversely affected by electrospinning voltage. These factors limit the combinations of fiber and nanoparticle materials available for composite fabrication. Thus, for composite delivery applications to succeed, polymer choice and electrospinning conditions must be taken into consideration.

5. Future Directions and Discussion

Within the past decade, electrospun fibers have been explored as a multipurpose delivery platform to prevent and treat sexually transmitted infections (STIs). For intravaginal applications, fibers have typically been uniaxially electrospun to release active agents targeted to HIV-1/HSV-2 infections and contraceptive applications. However, other electrospun architectures have been developed that may provide more finely-tuned active agent release, the encapsulation of multiple agents, and longer release durations, desirable for next-generation vehicles. Given this, the goal of this review was to summarize the advancements in electrospun fiber architectures including coaxial, multilayered, and nanoparticle-fiber composites, to meet these needs, and to review their use in other drug delivery applications. We sought to relate different temporal regimens of delivery, including transient (occurring within hours), short-term (spanning hours to one week), and sustained (extending from one week to months), to architectural design and materials selection to help guide the design of future platforms that meet the unique temporal needs of intravaginal delivery.

One of the major challenges facing intravaginal delivery is the lack of user adherence surrounding the administration of current delivery platforms. Several clinical trials have highlighted how a lack of user adherence contributes to decreased efficacy in clinical trials. In both the FACTS-001 and VOICE trials, South African women deemed high risk for HIV-1 exposure were given antiretroviral TFV gels to administer prior to intercourse [93,172]. Despite the known efficaciousness of TFV, the gels provided suboptimal protection against HIV-1 infection, which was attributed to low user adherence of the gels prior to intercourse. Another study examined the efficacy of gels that incorporated the antiviral polysaccharide, carrageenan, in women in Thailand. This study demonstrated similarly disappointing clinical outcomes, with low user adherence considered the most significant reason for the lack of clinical efficacy [173]. Negative outcomes in other trials such as PRO-2000 and cellulose sulfate gel studies, which examined the efficacy of anti-HIV gels in female populations, further validated these studies, highlighting that both user preference and adherence regimens must be considered during product design rather than at the clinical trial stage. As a result of these studies, there has been an increased emphasis to design vehicles that decrease the administration frequency by prolonging active agent release after a single topical application.

In conjunction with improving user adherence, the development of multipurpose delivery vehicles that offer long-term protection against the various stages of a single infection or a diversity of different types of infections is highly desirable [174]. For single infections, a delivery platform may administer multiple agents with different mechanisms of action that target different stages of the viral or bacterial life cycle. However, the increased likelihood of viral co-infections, such as HSV-2 and HIV, as well as bacterial and fungal infections will likely require co-administration of antiviral and antimicrobial agents to be successful. Furthermore, applications that seek to meet both antiviral and contraceptive needs in the same dosage form will require the incorporation of multiple types of agents to expand a platform's effectiveness. Therefore, a delivery platform that has the capability to release multiple active agents, each over time frames relevant to the application or active agent, will have greater utility and enable more convenient administration schedules based on specific user needs.

Despite these needs, tailoring the delivery of multiple types of active agents for viral, bacterial, fungal, and contraceptive applications is an ambitious goal given the unique chemical properties of each agent. For example, the antiretroviral TFV and its pro-drug TDF have similar structures and both work as nucleoside reverse transcriptase inhibitors yet possess markedly different hydrophobicities. As such, a delivery platform designed to prolong TFV release may result in different release kinetics of TDF, requiring the formulation of distinct delivery vehicles specific to the selected active agents [56,116,118,175,176]. Furthermore, each active agent may necessitate specific temporal dosing regimens to provide protection or treatment. For example, it may be desirable to administer viral entry inhibitors, which inactivate virions prior to cell entry, over a different time frame than active agents that work inside of cells and need to transport through and localize to target tissue. Several studies have investigated this and have found that more complex and specialized architectures may be useful to achieve temporal delivery goals by tuning the release properties of multiple encapsulants for multiple targets [177,178]. Similarly, for contraceptive applications, on-demand and/or zero-order release with equivalent daily dosing may be desirable for spermicides and hormonal/non-hormonal contraceptives, respectively. Conversely, it may be desirable to deliver active agents such as hormones and small hydrophilic drugs (e.g., etonogestrel and acyclovir) within the same time frame for simultaneous long-term contraception and prevention. However, the drastically different chemical properties of these agents will require more complex solutions to achieve similar release profiles. Given this, multipurpose intravaginal delivery platforms must be tailored to maximize the efficacy of individual active agents, including small molecule drugs, proteins, antibiotics, hormones, and live organisms (e.g., probiotics), to meet the needs of these diverse applications.

While providing distinct release profiles of different active agents is an important criterion for the development of future intravaginal platforms, to date, intravaginal rings (IVRs) are the only platforms that provide delivery over a duration of weeks to months [179–183]. Furthermore, IVR studies indicate that more complex dosage forms, such as rings with drug-encapsulating pods, may more likely succeed, particularly in challenging delivery scenarios, e.g., achieving the sustained-release of small hydrophilic molecules [177]. These and other studies [177,178,184,185] emphasize the need to offer alternative delivery vehicles for women, with the key lesson that platform architecture must be designed to consider the hydrophobicity and chemical compatibility of the encapsulants in combination with its surrounding materials.

In addition to the development of fibers with more complex architectures, active agent release and transport from these platforms must be assessed. Tissue mimetics and ex vivo tissues have been used to assess these parameters within the context of intravaginal delivery applications [116,186–191]. One of the most common ways in which to assess intravaginal delivery is by using human ectocervical tissue explants derived from patients [187–191]. These explants provide a representative environment in which to measure transport by accounting for the three-dimensional structure of patient tissue. However, patient-specific variations and tissue availability can limit the use of vaginal explants. Given this, organotypic three-dimensional vaginal tissue models such as Epivaginal™ tissue have been created to help evaluate the safety, transport, and efficacy of active agents within an FRT mimetic [192,193]. Other in vitro models have also been developed to explore bacteria and host cell interactions in the reproductive environment [194]. Moreover, within the past decade, new biomarkers and assay endpoints have been identified and studied in different models to more fully assess microbicide interactions with the FRT [195]. The use of tissue models promises to streamline the assessment of future fiber platforms as viable intravaginal delivery platforms.

To date, a variety of studies have developed uniaxial electrospun fibers for intravaginal applications, including HIV prevention [56,115–119,175,176,196–199]. In these studies, electrospun fibers have demonstrated promising potential for intravaginal applications due to their mucoadhesive characteristics, mechanical properties, and ability to be fabricated in different shapes and sizes [53]. Depending upon the polymer hydrophilicity, traditional uniaxial fibers have been formulated as transient, short-term, or long-term delivery platforms. For the purposes of on-demand and short-term release, many of these studies use hydrophilic fibers, which dissolve or degrade quickly. In contrast, fibers consisting of more hydrophobic materials are expected to persist within the FRT, acting as reservoirs to sustain the release of active agents. We envision (and have observed) that long-term delivery vehicles maintain their structure during the delivery duration of interest and may require physical removal from the FRT, similar to current IVRs. However, one of the key challenges for intravaginal delivery has been to sustain the release of small hydrophilic antiretrovirals due to their rapid diffusion through the porous fiber matrix, solubility in aqueous solutions, and chemical incompatibility with hydrophobic polymer cores [6]. Many of these uniaxial fibers demonstrated burst release of hydrophilic agents followed by short-term release [59,200], partially attributed to the localization of hydrophilic agents on the fiber surface. Compounding this, concerns exist that the subsequent release of active agents may be insufficient to provide complete protection against future infections. While blended uniaxial fibers have been moderately successful in addressing these challenges, more work is required [119].

The primary parameters that impact release from uniaxial fibers are the choice of solvent and polymer. Other factors such as polymer concentration and electrospinning parameters also play a role in attaining different release profiles; however, it is unlikely that these factors alone are sufficient to overcome the challenge of delivering sustained and therapeutically-relevant concentrations of hydrophilic agents. Furthermore, it is difficult to utilize traditional uniaxial fibers for the encapsulation of multiple diverse agents such as large proteins and small drugs. Due to these issues, other electrospinning architectures may be better suited to meet the diverse challenges of intravaginal delivery.

As discussed previously, coaxial fibers have shown promise for the encapsulation and release of small hydrophilic and hydrophobic molecules, which may be useful for intravaginal delivery applications. The different goals of transient, short-term and long-term release can be achieved by changing the composition and hydrophobicity of core and shell materials as well as by modulating the shell thickness and core:shell ratio. As described, the shell layer can help regulate active agent release, while the core layer is designed to provide optimal compatibility with an encapsulant. For instance, by using pH-responsive polymer shells, an immediate stimuli-responsive release of agents can be achieved when the fiber is in contact with semen. In this scenario, the core layer may be tailored to encapsulate multiple agents, while the shell, comprised of pH-sensitive polymers, retains encapsulants until needed. Another advantage of coaxial fibers is that they can be fabricated to exploit drug-polymer hydrophilicities. For example, a coaxial fiber comprised of a hydrophobic shell and hydrophilic core can be utilized to provide long-term release of hydrophilic compounds. Agent encapsulation into both layers would allow for both transient burst release from the shell due to surface localization and high loading and sustained-release from the core layer. Finally, coaxial fibers can provide release of biological agents such as large proteins. Coaxial cores may be engineered to achieve high protein encapsulation and biocompatibility, while shells can be constructed with porous surfaces, allowing tunable release. This is particularly significant given that many biologics are being investigated as future viral prophylaxes and therapeutics. Although coaxial electrospinning is a more complex process that requires additional optimization, relative to uniaxial spinning, it may enable a versatile platform for transient, short-term, and long-term release [119].

Multilayered fibers combine different polymer layers via sequential or post-spinning to incorporate multiple and chemically distinct drugs within specific layers, thereby tailoring the release kinetics for each encapsulated agent. Multilayered interwoven fibers can be utilized to provide transient release using sacrificial layers to encapsulate agents for on-demand applications. The sacrificial layers comprised of hydrophilic polymers would provide on-demand release of agents based on their immediate degradation when exposed to physiological fluids. Active agent release can be further modulated by the number, thickness, and porosity of each fiber layer [201]. Moreover, blank fibers may be incorporated within the multilayers to either act as a physical barrier for sustained-release or for contraceptive purposes. The layer thickness and level of porosity of blank fibers can be conveniently modulated to delay the release of small hydrophilic molecules from the drug-loaded layers, serving to prolong release. Additionally, multilayered fibers have the potential to deliver biologics and non-hormonal contraceptives. These agents, although efficacious, may degrade when exposed to harsh solvents during the electrospinning process. By incorporating these active agents in distinct layers and integrating barrier layers, multilayered fibers can provide long-term release of drugs and biologics while retaining their activities.

While each of these strategies offers advantages relative to uniaxial spinning, the delivery of active agents may be further enhanced by integrating nanoparticles with fibers. A composite platform may offer a new alternative to address the challenges of intravaginal delivery, such as the maintaining active agent stability, providing cell-specific targeting (via NPs), and enhancing cell internalization. Like electrospun fibers, nanoparticles can be designed to encapsulate virtually any compound. The limitations of nanoparticle-fiber composites mentioned earlier may be overcome by utilizing fibers as a reservoir for both active agents and nanoparticles to release multiple therapeutics. Furthermore, the release rates of encapsulants from both nanoparticles and fibers may be modulated by adjusting the composition of the polymeric scaffold. For on-demand transient release, hydrophilic polymers may be used to enable rapid release of NPs for immediate distribution through and enhanced retention within tissue. In contrast, more hydrophobic fibers may be used to delay the release of NPs or NP-encapsulated agents. Although drug-polymer hydrophobicity is a major contributor to release, other factors such as polymer choice, molecular weight, and crystallinity, as well as solvent choice and electrospinning parameters, also affect the release of agents from fibers.

The application of advanced fiber architectures has only recently been explored in the context of intravaginal delivery. Advanced fiber architectures demonstrate the potential to provide the sustained-release of individual active agents in addition to concurrently providing both transient and sustained-delivery of multiple active agents. These are key advantages over traditional uniaxial fibers, which are challenged with the long-term delivery of small hydrophilic molecules, in addition to providing transient and sustained-release simultaneously. We envision that future fiber architectures will localize active agents within specific sections of the fiber to tailor the release of individual agents independent of other encapsulants. Moreover, we anticipate that future platforms will combine architectures to maximize or complement the advantages of individual platforms. As previous clinical trials have shown, effective protection will be dependent upon fulfilling user preferences, offering convenience, and providing necessary release profiles from one vehicle, which fibers have the potential to realize.

References

1. Wira, C.R.; Patel, M.V.; Ghosh, M.; Mukura, L.; Fahey, J.V. Innate immunity in the human female reproductive tract: Endocrine regulation of endogenous antimicrobial protection against HIV and other sexually transmitted infections. *Am. J. Reprod. Immunol.* **2011**, *65*, 196–211. [CrossRef]
2. Unnithan, A.R.; Barakat, N.A.; Pichiah, P.T.; Gnanasekaran, G.; Nirmala, R.; Cha, Y.-S.; Jung, C.-H.; El-Newehy, M.; Kim, H.Y. Wound-dressing materials with antibacterial activity from electrospun polyurethane–dextran nanofiber mats containing ciprofloxacin HCl. *Carbohydr. Polym.* **2012**, *90*, 1786–1793. [CrossRef] [PubMed]
3. Tourgeman, D.E.; Gentzchein, E.; Stanczyk, F.Z.; Paulson, R.J. Serum and tissue hormone levels of vaginally and orally administered estradiol. *Am. J. Obstet. Gynecol.* **1999**, *180*, 1480–1483. [CrossRef]
4. Steinbach, J.M. Protein and oligonucleotide delivery systems for vaginal microbicides against viral STIs. *Cell. Mol. Life Sci.* **2015**, *72*, 469–503. [CrossRef] [PubMed]
5. Bernkop-Schnürch, A.; Hornof, M. Intravaginal drug delivery systems. *Am. J. Drug Deliv.* **2003**, *1*, 241–254. [CrossRef]
6. Chou, S.F.; Carson, D.; Woodrow, K.A. Current strategies for sustaining drug release from electrospun nanofibers. *J. Control. Release* **2015**, *220 Pt B*, 584–591. [CrossRef]
7. Hickey, D.K.; Patel, M.V.; Fahey, J.V.; Wira, C.R. Innate and adaptive immunity at mucosal surfaces of the female reproductive tract: Stratification and integration of immune protection against the transmission of sexually transmitted infections. *J. Reprod. Immunol.* **2011**, *88*, 185–194. [CrossRef]
8. Wiggins, R.; Hicks, S.; Soothill, P.; Millar, M.; Corfield, A. Mucinases and sialidases: Their role in the pathogenesis of sexually transmitted infections in the female genital tract. *Sex. Transm. Infect.* **2001**, *77*, 402–408. [CrossRef]
9. Das Neves, J.; Bahia, M.F. Gels as vaginal drug delivery systems. *Int. J. Pharm.* **2006**, *318*, 1–14. [CrossRef]
10. Andrews, G.P.; Donnelly, L.; Jones, D.S.; Curran, R.M.; Morrow, R.J.; Woolfson, A.D.; Malcolm, R.K. Characterization of the rheological, mucoadhesive, and drug release properties of highly structured gel platforms for intravaginal drug delivery. *Biomacromolecules* **2009**, *10*, 2427–2435. [CrossRef]
11. Devlin, B.; Nuttall, J.; Wilder, S.; Woodsong, C.; Rosenberg, Z. Development of dapivirine vaginal ring for HIV prevention. *Antivir. Res.* **2013**, *100*, S3–S8. [CrossRef] [PubMed]
12. Derby, N.; Zydowsky, T.; Robbiani, M. In search of the optimal delivery method for anti-HIV microbicides: Are intravaginal rings the way forward? *Expert Rev. Anti-Infect. Ther.* **2013**, *11*, 5–8. [CrossRef]
13. Ho, E.A. Intravaginal rings as a novel platform for mucosal vaccination. *J. Mol. Pharm. Org. Process Res.* **2013**, *1*, e103.
14. Mallipeddi, R.; Rohan, L.C. Nanoparticle-based vaginal drug delivery systems for HIV prevention. *Expert Opin. Drug Deliv.* **2010**, *7*, 37–48. [CrossRef] [PubMed]
15. Kiser, P.F.; Johnson, T.J.; Clark, J.T. State of the art in intravaginal ring technology for topical prophylaxis of HIV infection. *Aids Rev.* **2012**, *14*, 62–77.
16. Dieben, T.O.; Roumen, F.J.; Apter, D. Efficacy, cycle control, and user acceptability of a novel combined contraceptive vaginal ring. *Obstet. Gynecol.* **2002**, *100*, 585–593.

17. Malcolm, R.K.; Edwards, K.-L.; Kiser, P.; Romano, J.; Smith, T.J. Advances in microbicide vaginal rings. *Antivir. Res.* **2010**, *88*, S30–S39. [CrossRef] [PubMed]
18. Roumen, F.; Apter, D.; Mulders, T.; Dieben, T. Efficacy, tolerability and acceptability of a novel contraceptive vaginal ring releasing etonogestrel and ethinyl oestradiol. *Hum. Reprod.* **2001**, *16*, 469–475. [CrossRef]
19. Nel, A.; van Niekerk, N.; Kapiga, S.; Bekker, L.-G.; Gama, C.; Gill, K.; Kamali, A.; Kotze, P.; Louw, C.; Mabude, Z. Safety and efficacy of a dapivirine vaginal ring for HIV prevention in women. *N. Engl. J. Med.* **2016**, *375*, 2133–2143. [CrossRef]
20. Kim, S.; Traore, Y.L.; Chen, Y.; Ho, E.A.; Liu, S. Switchable On-Demand Release of a Nanocarrier from a Segmented Reservoir Type Intravaginal Ring Filled with a pH-Responsive Supramolecular Polyurethane Hydrogel. *ACS Appl. Bio Mater.* **2018**, *1*, 652–662. [CrossRef]
21. Vanić, Ž.; Škalko-Basnet, N. Nanopharmaceuticals for improved topical vaginal therapy: Can they deliver? *Eur. J. Pharm. Sci.* **2013**, *50*, 29–41. [CrossRef] [PubMed]
22. Zhang, T.; Sturgis, T.F.; Youan, B.-B.C. pH-responsive nanoparticles releasing tenofovir intended for the prevention of HIV transmission. *Eur. J. Pharm. Biopharm.* **2011**, *79*, 526–536. [CrossRef] [PubMed]
23. Krogstad, E.A.; Ramanathan, R.; Nhan, C.; Kraft, J.C.; Blakney, A.K.; Cao, S.; Ho, R.J.; Woodrow, K.A. Nanoparticle-releasing nanofiber composites for enhanced in vivo vaginal retention. *Biomaterials* **2017**, *144*, 1–16. [CrossRef]
24. Martínez-Pérez, B.; Quintanar-Guerrero, D.; Tapia-Tapia, M.; Cisneros-Tamayo, R.; Zambrano-Zaragoza, M.L.; Alcalá-Alcalá, S.; Mendoza-Muñoz, N.; Piñón-Segundo, E. Controlled-release biodegradable nanoparticles: From preparation to vaginal applications. *Eur. J. Pharm. Sci.* **2018**, *115*, 185–195. [CrossRef] [PubMed]
25. Marciello, M.; Rossi, S.; Caramella, C.; Remuñán-López, C. Freeze-dried cylinders carrying chitosan nanoparticles for vaginal peptide delivery. *Carbohydr. Polym.* **2017**, *170*, 43–51. [CrossRef]
26. Leyva-Gómez, G.; Piñón-Segundo, E.; Mendoza-Muñoz, N.; Zambrano-Zaragoza, M.; Mendoza-Elvira, S.; Quintanar-Guerrero, D. Approaches in Polymeric Nanoparticles for Vaginal Drug Delivery: A Review of the State of the Art. *Int. J. Mol. Sci.* **2018**, *19*, 1549. [CrossRef]
27. Sims, L.B.; Frieboes, H.B.; Steinbach-Rankins, J.M. Nanoparticle-mediated drug delivery to treat infections in the female reproductive tract: Evaluation of experimental systems and the potential for mathematical modeling. *Int. J. Nanomed.* **2018**, *13*, 2709–2727. [CrossRef]
28. El-Hammadi, M.M.; Arias, J.L. Nanotechnology for Vaginal Drug Delivery and Targeting. In *Nanotechnology and Drug Delivery, Volume Two: Nano-Engineering Strategies and Nanomedicines against Severe Diseases*; CRC Press: Boca Raton, FL, USA, 2016; p. 191.
29. Ensign, L.M.; Tang, B.C.; Wang, Y.Y.; Tse, T.A.; Hoen, T.; Cone, R.; Hanes, J. Mucus-penetrating nanoparticles for vaginal drug delivery protect against herpes simplex virus. *Sci. Transl. Med.* **2012**, *4*, 138ra79. [CrossRef] [PubMed]
30. Maisel, K.; Reddy, M.; Xu, Q.; Chattopadhyay, S.; Cone, R.; Ensign, L.M.; Hanes, J. Nanoparticles coated with high molecular weight PEG penetrate mucus and provide uniform vaginal and colorectal distribution in vivo. *Nanomedicine* **2016**, *11*, 1337–1343. [CrossRef] [PubMed]
31. Henry, C.E.; Wang, Y.-Y.; Yang, Q.; Hoang, T.; Chattopadhyay, S.; Hoen, T.; Ensign, L.M.; Nunn, K.L.; Schroeder, H.; McCallen, J. Anti-PEG antibodies alter the mobility and biodistribution of densely PEGylated nanoparticles in mucus. *Acta Biomater.* **2016**, *43*, 61–70. [CrossRef] [PubMed]
32. Mohideen, M.; Quijano, E.; Song, E.; Deng, Y.; Panse, G.; Zhang, W.; Clark, M.R.; Saltzman, W.M. Degradable bioadhesive nanoparticles for prolonged intravaginal delivery and retention of elvitegravir. *Biomaterials* **2017**, *144*, 144–154. [CrossRef] [PubMed]
33. Ensign, L.; Cone, R.; Hanes, J. Nanoparticle Formulations with Enhanced Mucosal Penetration. U.S. Patent 9,415,020, 16 August 2016.
34. Lai, S.K.; O'Hanlon, E.D.; Man, S.T.; Cone, R.; Hanes, J. Real-time transport of polymer nanoparticles in cervical vaginal mucus. In Proceedings of the 05AIChE: 2005 AIChE Annual Meeting and Fall Showcase, Cincinnati, OH, USA, 30 October–4 November 2005.
35. Meng, J.; Agrahari, V.; Ezoulin, M.J.; Zhang, C.; Purohit, S.S.; Molteni, A.; Dim, D.; Oyler, N.A.; Youan, B.-B.C. Tenofovir containing thiolated chitosan core/shell nanofibers: In vitro and in vivo evaluations. *Mol. Pharm.* **2016**, *13*, 4129–4140. [CrossRef]

36. Zamani, M.; Prabhakaran, M.P.; Ramakrishna, S. Advances in drug delivery via electrospun and electrosprayed nanomaterials. *Int. J. Nanomed.* **2013**, *8*, 2997–3017.
37. Hu, X.; Liu, S.; Zhou, G.; Huang, Y.; Xie, Z.; Jing, X. Electrospinning of polymeric nanofibers for drug delivery applications. *J. Control. Release* **2014**, *185*, 12–21. [CrossRef]
38. Jain, K.K. *Drug Delivery Systems*; Springer Science & Business Media: Berlin, Germany, 2008.
39. Sharma, R.; Singh, H.; Joshi, M.; Sharma, A.; Garg, T.; Goyal, A.K.; Rath, G. Recent advances in polymeric electrospun nanofibers for drug delivery. *Crit. Rev. Ther. Drug Carr. Syst.* **2014**, *31*, 187–217. [CrossRef]
40. Repanas, A.; Andriopoulou, S.; Glasmacher, B. The significance of electrospinning as a method to create fibrous scaffolds for biomedical engineering and drug delivery applications. *J. Drug Deliv. Sci. Technol.* **2016**, *31*, 137–146. [CrossRef]
41. Fu, Y.; Kao, W.J. Drug release kinetics and transport mechanisms of non-degradable and degradable polymeric delivery systems. *Expert Opin. Drug Deliv.* **2010**, *7*, 429–444. [CrossRef] [PubMed]
42. Kim, T.G.; Lee, D.S.; Park, T.G. Controlled protein release from electrospun biodegradable fiber mesh composed of poly(ε-caprolactone) and poly(ethylene oxide). *Int. J. Pharm.* **2007**, *338*, 276–283. [CrossRef]
43. Qi, H.; Hu, P.; Xu, J.; Wang, A. Encapsulation of drug reservoirs in fibers by emulsion electrospinning: Morphology characterization and preliminary release assessment. *Biomacromolecules* **2006**, *7*, 2327–2330. [CrossRef] [PubMed]
44. Nair, L.S.; Laurencin, C.T. Biodegradable polymers as biomaterials. *Prog. Polym. Sci.* **2007**, *32*, 762–798. [CrossRef]
45. Liu, H.; Leonas, K.K.; Zhao, Y. Antimicrobial properties and release profile of ampicillin from electrospun poly (ε-caprolactone) nanofiber yarns. *J. Eng. Fabr. Fiber.* **2010**, *5*, 10–19. [CrossRef]
46. Yoshimoto, H.; Shin, Y.; Terai, H.; Vacanti, J. A biodegradable nanofiber scaffold by electrospinning and its potential for bone tissue engineering. *Biomaterials* **2003**, *24*, 2077–2082. [CrossRef]
47. Luu, Y.; Kim, K.; Hsiao, B.; Chu, B.; Hadjiargyrou, M. Development of a nanostructured DNA delivery scaffold via electrospinning of PLGA and PLA–PEG block copolymers. *J. Control. Release* **2003**, *89*, 341–353. [CrossRef]
48. Puppi, D.; Zhang, X.; Yang, L.; Chiellini, F.; Sun, X.; Chiellini, E. Nano/microfibrous polymeric constructs loaded with bioactive agents and designed for tissue engineering applications: A review. *J. Biomed. Mater. Res. B* **2014**, *102*, 1562–1579. [CrossRef]
49. Cipitria, A.; Skelton, A.; Dargaville, T.; Dalton, P.; Hutmacher, D. Design, fabrication and characterization of PCL electrospun scaffolds—A review. *J. Mater. Chem. A* **2011**, *21*, 9419–9453. [CrossRef]
50. Uhrich, K.E.; Cannizzaro, S.M.; Langer, R.S.; Shakesheff, K.M. Polymeric systems for controlled drug release. *Chem. Rev.* **1999**, *99*, 3181–3198. [CrossRef]
51. Ulery, B.D.; Nair, L.S.; Laurencin, C.T. Biomedical applications of biodegradable polymers. *J. Polym. Sci. Part B Polym. Phys.* **2011**, *49*, 832–864. [CrossRef] [PubMed]
52. Chen, D.W.-C.; Liu, S.-J. Nanofibers used for delivery of antimicrobial agents. *Nanomedicine* **2015**, *10*, 1959–1971. [CrossRef] [PubMed]
53. Blakney, A.K.; Ball, C.; Krogstad, E.A.; Woodrow, K.A. Electrospun fibers for vaginal anti-HIV drug delivery. *Antivir. Res.* **2013**, *100*, S9–S16. [CrossRef] [PubMed]
54. Ramakrishna, S.; Fujihara, K.; Teo, W.-E.; Yong, T.; Ma, Z.; Ramaseshan, R. Electrospun nanofibers: Solving global issues. *Mater. Today* **2006**, *9*, 40–50. [CrossRef]
55. Göpferich, A. Mechanisms of polymer degradation and erosion. *Biomaterials* **1996**, *17*, 103–114. [CrossRef]
56. Chou, S.F.; Woodrow, K.A. Relationships between mechanical properties and drug release from electrospun fibers of PCL and PLGA blends. *J. Mech. Behav. Biomed. Mater.* **2017**, *65*, 724–733. [CrossRef] [PubMed]
57. von Burkersroda, F.; Schedl, L.; Göpferich, A. Why degradable polymers undergo surface erosion or bulk erosion. *Biomaterials* **2002**, *23*, 4221–4231. [CrossRef]
58. Doshi, J.; Reneker, D.H. Electrospinning process and applications of electrospun fibers. *J. Electrostat.* **1995**, *35*, 151–160. [CrossRef]
59. Zeng, J.; Xu, X.; Chen, X.; Liang, Q.; Bian, X.; Yang, L.; Jing, X. Biodegradable electrospun fibers for drug delivery. *J. Control Release* **2003**, *92*, 227–231. [CrossRef]
60. Sill, T.J.; von Recum, H.A. Electrospinning: Applications in drug delivery and tissue engineering. *Biomaterials* **2008**, *29*, 1989–2006. [CrossRef]

61. Kenawy, E.-R.; Abdel-Hay, F.I.; El-Newehy, M.H.; Wnek, G.E. Processing of polymer nanofibers through electrospinning as drug delivery systems. In *Nanomaterials: Risks and Benefits*; Springer: Dordrecht, The Netherlands, 2009; pp. 247–263.
62. Ji, W.; Sun, Y.; Yang, F.; van den Beucken, J.J.; Fan, M.; Chen, Z.; Jansen, J.A. Bioactive electrospun scaffolds delivering growth factors and genes for tissue engineering applications. *Pharm. Res.* **2011**, *28*, 1259–1272. [CrossRef]
63. Pillay, V.; Dott, C.; Choonara, Y.E.; Tyagi, C.; Tomar, L.; Kumar, P.; du Toit, L.C.; Ndesendo, V.M. A review of the effect of processing variables on the fabrication of electrospun nanofibers for drug delivery applications. *J. Nanomater.* **2013**, *2013*, 789289. [CrossRef]
64. Xie, J.; Li, X.; Xia, Y. Putting electrospun nanofibers to work for biomedical research. *Macromol. Rapid Commun.* **2008**, *29*, 1775–1792. [CrossRef]
65. Subbiah, T.; Bhat, G.; Tock, R.; Parameswaran, S.; Ramkumar, S. Electrospinning of nanofibers. *J. Appl. Polym. Sci.* **2005**, *96*, 557–569. [CrossRef]
66. Hadjiargyrou, M.; Chiu, J.B. Enhanced composite electrospun nanofiber scaffolds for use in drug delivery. *Expert Opin. Drug Deliv.* **2008**, *5*, 1093–1106. [CrossRef]
67. Zhang, Y.; Lim, C.T.; Ramakrishna, S.; Huang, Z.-M. Recent development of polymer nanofibers for biomedical and biotechnological applications. *J. Mater. Sci. Mater. Med.* **2005**, *16*, 933–946. [CrossRef]
68. Verreck, G.; Chun, I.; Rosenblatt, J.; Peeters, J.; van Dijck, A.; Mensch, J.; Noppe, M.; Brewster, M.E. Incorporation of drugs in an amorphous state into electrospun nanofibers composed of a water-insoluble, nonbiodegradable polymer. *J. Control. Release* **2003**, *92*, 349–360. [CrossRef]
69. Han, D.; Steckl, A.J. Triaxial electrospun nanofiber membranes for controlled dual release of functional molecules. *ACS Appl. Mater. Interfaces* **2013**, *5*, 8241–8245. [CrossRef]
70. Yarin, A. Coaxial electrospinning and emulsion electrospinning of core–shell fibers. *Polym. Adv. Technol.* **2011**, *22*, 310–317. [CrossRef]
71. He, C.L.; Huang, Z.M.; Han, X.J.; Liu, L.; Zhang, H.S.; Chen, L.S. Coaxial electrospun poly (L-lactic acid) ultrafine fibers for sustained drug delivery. *J. Macromol. Sci. B* **2006**, *45*, 515–524. [CrossRef]
72. Lu, Y.; Huang, J.; Yu, G.; Cardenas, R.; Wei, S.; Wujcik, E.K.; Guo, Z. Coaxial electrospun fibers: Applications in drug delivery and tissue engineering. *Wiley Interdiscip. Rev. Nanomed. Nanobiotechnol.* **2016**, *8*, 654–677. [CrossRef]
73. Yu, D.G.; Branford-White, C.; Bligh, S.A.; White, K.; Chatterton, N.P.; Zhu, L.M. Improving Polymer Nanofiber Quality Using a Modified Co-axial Electrospinning Process. *Macromol. Rapid Commun.* **2011**, *32*, 744–750. [CrossRef]
74. Nezarati, R.M.; Eifert, M.B.; Cosgriff-Hernandez, E. Effects of humidity and solution viscosity on electrospun fiber morphology. *Tissue Eng. Part C Methods* **2013**, *19*, 810–819. [CrossRef]
75. Wang, J.; Jákli, A.; West, J.L. Morphology tuning of electrospun liquid crystal/polymer fibers. *ChemPhysChem* **2016**, *17*, 3080–3085. [CrossRef]
76. Yang, J.-M.; Zha, L.-S.; Yu, D.-G.; Liu, J. Coaxial electrospinning with acetic acid for preparing ferulic acid/zein composite fibers with improved drug release profiles. *Colloids Surf. B Biointerfaces* **2013**, *102*, 737–743. [CrossRef]
77. Tang, C.; Ozcam, A.E.; Stout, B.; Khan, S.A. Effect of pH on protein distribution in electrospun PVA/BSA composite nanofibers. *Biomacromolecules* **2012**, *13*, 1269–1278. [CrossRef]
78. He, M.; Jiang, H.; Wang, R.; Xie, Y.; Zhao, C. Fabrication of metronidazole loaded poly (ε-caprolactone)/zein core/shell nanofiber membranes via coaxial electrospinning for guided tissue regeneration. *J. Colloid Interface Sci.* **2017**, *490*, 270–278. [CrossRef]
79. Wang, C.; Yan, K.-W.; Lin, Y.-D.; Hsieh, P.C. Biodegradable core/shell fibers by coaxial electrospinning: Processing, fiber characterization, and its application in sustained drug release. *Macromolecules* **2010**, *43*, 6389–6397. [CrossRef]
80. Perrie, Y.; Rades, T. *FASTtrack Pharmaceutics: Drug Delivery and Targeting*; Pharmaceutical Press: London, UK, 2012.
81. Jiang, Y.-N.; Mo, H.-Y.; Yu, D. Electrospun drug-loaded core-sheath PVP/zein nanofibers for biphasic drug release. *Int. J. Pharm.* **2012**, *438*, 232–239. [CrossRef]
82. Zhu, L.; Liu, X.; Du, L.; Jin, Y. Preparation of asiaticoside-loaded coaxially electrospinning nanofibers and their effect on deep partial-thickness burn injury. *Biomed. Pharmacother.* **2016**, *83*, 33–40. [CrossRef]

83. Castillo-Ortega, M.; Montaño-Figueroa, A.; Rodríguez-Félix, D.; Prado-Villegas, G.; Pino-Ocaño, K.; Valencia-Córdova, M.; Quiroz-Castillo, J.; Herrera-Franco, P. Preparation by coaxial electrospinning and characterization of membranes releasing (−) epicatechin as scaffold for tissue engineering. *Mater. Sci. Eng. C* **2015**, *46*, 184–189. [CrossRef] [PubMed]
84. Li, X.-Y.; Li, Y.-C.; Yu, D.-G.; Liao, Y.-Z.; Wang, X. Fast disintegrating quercetin-loaded drug delivery systems fabricated using coaxial electrospinning. *Int. J. Mol. Sci.* **2013**, *14*, 21647–21659. [CrossRef]
85. Yu, D.-G.; Zhu, L.-M.; Branford-White, C.J.; Yang, J.-H.; Wang, X.; Li, Y.; Qian, W. Solid dispersions in the form of electrospun core-sheath nanofibers. *Int. J. Nanomed.* **2011**, *6*, 3271–3280. [CrossRef]
86. Fu, L.; Zhang, J.; Yang, G. Present status and applications of bacterial cellulose-based materials for skin tissue repair. *Carbohydr. Polym.* **2013**, *92*, 1432–1442. [CrossRef]
87. Yu, D.-G.; Li, X.-Y.; Wang, X.; Yang, J.-H.; Bligh, S.A.; Williams, G.R. Nanofibers fabricated using triaxial electrospinning as zero order drug delivery systems. *ACS Appl. Mater. Interfaces* **2015**, *7*, 18891–18897. [CrossRef]
88. Nakielski, P.; Pawłowska, S.; Pierini, F.; Liwińska, W.; Hejduk, P.; Zembrzycki, K.; Zabost, E.; Kowalewski, T.A. Hydrogel nanofilaments via core-shell electrospinning. *PLoS ONE* **2015**, *10*, e0129816.
89. Zhu, Y.J.; Chen, F. pH-Responsive Drug-Delivery Systems. *Chem.—Asian J.* **2015**, *10*, 284–305. [CrossRef]
90. Yang, C.; Yu, D.-G.; Pan, D.; Liu, X.-K.; Wang, X.; Bligh, S.A.; Williams, G.R. Electrospun pH-sensitive core–shell polymer nanocomposites fabricated using a tri-axial process. *Acta Biomater.* **2016**, *35*, 77–86. [CrossRef]
91. Thakral, S.; Thakral, N.K.; Majumdar, D.K. Eudragit®: A technology evaluation. *Expert Opin. Drug Deliv.* **2013**, *10*, 131–149. [CrossRef]
92. Yoshida, T.; Lai, T.C.; Kwon, G.S.; Sako, K. pH-and ion-sensitive polymers for drug delivery. *Expert Opin. Drug Deliv.* **2013**, *10*, 1497–1513. [CrossRef] [PubMed]
93. Marrazzo, J.M.; Ramjee, G.; Richardson, B.A.; Gomez, K.; Mgodi, N.; Nair, G.; Palanee, T.; Nakabiito, C.; van der Straten, A.; Noguchi, L.; et al. Tenofovir-based preexposure prophylaxis for HIV infection among African women. *N. Engl. J. Med.* **2015**, *372*, 509–518. [CrossRef] [PubMed]
94. Jin, M.; Yu, D.-G.; Geraldes, C.F.; Williams, G.R.; Bligh, S.A. Theranostic fibers for simultaneous imaging and drug delivery. *Mol. Pharm.* **2016**, *13*, 2457–2465. [CrossRef] [PubMed]
95. Jia, D.; Gao, Y.; Williams, G.R. Core/shell poly (ethylene oxide)/Eudragit fibers for site-specific release. *Int. J. Pharm.* **2017**, *523*, 376–385. [CrossRef]
96. Hua, D.; Liu, Z.; Wang, F.; Gao, B.; Chen, F.; Zhang, Q.; Xiong, R.; Han, J.; Samal, S.K.; de Smedt, S.C.; et al. pH responsive polyurethane (core) and cellulose acetate phthalate (shell) electrospun fibers for intravaginal drug delivery. *Carbohydr. Polym.* **2016**, *151*, 1240–1244. [CrossRef]
97. Sang, Q.; Li, H.; Williams, G.; Wu, H.; Zhu, L.-M. Core-shell poly (lactide-co-ε-caprolactone)-gelatin fiber scaffolds as pH-sensitive drug delivery systems. *J. Biomater. Appl.* **2018**, *32*, 1105–1118. [CrossRef] [PubMed]
98. Han, D.; Yu, X.; Chai, Q.; Ayres, N.; Steckl, A.J. Stimuli-responsive self-immolative polymer nanofiber membranes formed by coaxial electrospinning. *ACS Appl. Mater. Interfaces* **2017**, *9*, 11858–11865. [CrossRef] [PubMed]
99. Ball, C.; Chou, S.-F.; Jiang, Y.; Woodrow, K.A. Coaxially electrospun fiber-based microbicides facilitate broadly tunable release of maraviroc. *Mater. Sci. Eng. C* **2016**, *63*, 117–124. [CrossRef] [PubMed]
100. Zhang, Y.; Wang, X.; Feng, Y.; Li, J.; Lim, C.; Ramakrishna, S. Coaxial electrospinning of (fluorescein isothiocyanate-conjugated bovine serum albumin)-encapsulated poly (ε-caprolactone) nanofibers for sustained release. *Biomacromolecules* **2006**, *7*, 1049–1057. [CrossRef]
101. Yu, H.; Yang, P.; Jia, Y.; Zhang, Y.; Ye, Q.; Zeng, S. Regulation of biphasic drug release behavior by graphene oxide in polyvinyl pyrrolidone/poly (ε-caprolactone) core/sheath nanofiber mats. *Colloids Surf. B Biointerfaces* **2016**, *146*, 63–69. [CrossRef] [PubMed]
102. Oliveira, M.F.; Suarez, D.; Rocha, J.C.B.; de Carvalho Teixeira, A.V.N.; Cortés, M.E.; De Sousa, F.B.; Sinisterra, R.D. Electrospun nanofibers of polyCD/PMAA polymers and their potential application as drug delivery system. *Mater. Sci. Eng. C* **2015**, *54*, 252–261. [CrossRef]
103. Sultanova, Z.; Kaleli, G.; Kabay, G.; Mutlu, M. Controlled release of a hydrophilic drug from coaxially electrospun polycaprolactone nanofibers. *Int. J. Pharm.* **2016**, *505*, 133–138. [CrossRef]

104. Lv, Y.; Pan, Q.; Bligh, S.W.; Li, H.; Wu, H.; Sang, Q.; Zhu, L.M. Core-Sheath Nanofibers as Drug Delivery System for Thermoresponsive Controlled Release. *J. Pharm. Sci.* **2017**, *106*, 1258–1265. [CrossRef] [PubMed]
105. Khalf, A.; Madihally, S.V. Modeling the permeability of multiaxial electrospun poly (ε-caprolactone)-gelatin hybrid fibers for controlled doxycycline release. *Mater. Sci. Eng. C* **2017**, *76*, 161–170. [CrossRef] [PubMed]
106. Ranjbar-Mohammadi, M.; Zamani, M.; Prabhakaran, M.P.; Bahrami, S.H.; Ramakrishna, S. Electrospinning of PLGA/gum tragacanth nanofibers containing tetracycline hydrochloride for periodontal regeneration. *Mater. Sci. Eng. C Mater. Biol. Appl.* **2016**, *58*, 521–531. [CrossRef]
107. Xie, Q.; Jia, L.-N.; Xu, H.-Y.; Hu, X.-G.; Wang, W.; Jia, J. Fabrication of core-shell PEI/pBMP2-PLGA electrospun scaffold for gene delivery to periodontal ligament stem cells. *Stem Cells Int.* **2016**, *2016*, 5385137. [CrossRef]
108. Jiang, H.; Hu, Y.; Zhao, P.; Li, Y.; Zhu, K. Modulation of protein release from biodegradable core-shell structured fibers prepared by coaxial electrospinning. *J. Biomed. Mater. Res. B Appl. Biomater.* **2006**, *79*, 50–57. [CrossRef]
109. Jiang, H.; Hu, Y.; Li, Y.; Zhao, P.; Zhu, K.; Chen, W. A facile technique to prepare biodegradable coaxial electrospun nanofibers for controlled release of bioactive agents. *J. Control. Release* **2005**, *108*, 237–243. [CrossRef]
110. Yang, Y.; Li, X.; Qi, M.; Zhou, S.; Weng, J. Release pattern and structural integrity of lysozyme encapsulated in core–sheath structured poly (DL-lactide) ultrafine fibers prepared by emulsion electrospinning. *Eur. J. Pharm. Biopharm.* **2008**, *69*, 106–116. [CrossRef]
111. Ji, W.; Yang, F.; van den Beucken, J.J.; Bian, Z.; Fan, M.; Chen, Z.; Jansen, J.A. Fibrous scaffolds loaded with protein prepared by blend or coaxial electrospinning. *Acta Biomater.* **2010**, *6*, 4199–4207. [CrossRef]
112. Saraf, A.; Baggett, L.S.; Raphael, R.M.; Kasper, F.K.; Mikos, A.G. Regulated non-viral gene delivery from coaxial electrospun fiber mesh scaffolds. *J. Control. Release* **2010**, *143*, 95–103. [CrossRef]
113. Hsu, Y.-H.; Lin, C.-T.; Yu, Y.-H.; Chou, Y.-C.; Liu, S.-J.; Chan, E.-C. Dual delivery of active antibactericidal agents and bone morphogenetic protein at sustainable high concentrations using biodegradable sheath-core-structured drug-eluting nanofibers. *Int. J. Nanomed.* **2016**, *11*, 3927–3937. [CrossRef]
114. Aniagyei, S.E.; Sims, L.B.; Malik, D.A.; Tyo, K.M.; Curry, K.C.; Kim, W.; Hodge, D.A.; Duan, J.; Steinbach-Rankins, J.M. Evaluation of poly(lactic-co-glycolic acid) and poly(dl-lactide-co-ε-caprolactone) electrospun fibers for the treatment of HSV-2 infection. *Mater. Sci. Eng. C* **2017**, *72*, 238–251. [CrossRef]
115. Ball, C.; Woodrow, K.A. Electrospun Solid Dispersions of Maraviroc for Rapid Intravaginal Preexposure Prophylaxis of HIV. *Antimicrob. Agents Chemother.* **2014**, *58*, 4855–4865. [CrossRef]
116. Tyo, K.M.; Vuong, H.R.; Malik, D.A.; Sims, L.B.; Alatassi, H.; Duan, J.; Watson, W.H.; Steinbach-Rankins, J.M. Multipurpose tenofovir disoproxil fumarate electrospun fibers for the prevention of HIV-1 and HSV-2 infections in vitro. *Int. J. Pharm.* **2017**, *531*, 118–133. [CrossRef]
117. Grooms, T.N.; Vuong, H.R.; Tyo, K.M.; Malik, D.A.; Sims, L.B.; Whittington, C.P.; Palmer, K.E.; Matoba, N.; Steinbach-Rankins, J.M. Griffithsin-Modified Electrospun Fibers as a Delivery Scaffold To Prevent HIV Infection. *Antimicrob. Agents Chemother.* **2016**, *60*, 6518–6531. [CrossRef]
118. Tyo, K.M.; Duan, J.; Kollipara, P.; Cerna, M.V.C.D.; Lee, D.; Palmer, K.E.; Steinbach-Rankins, J.M. pH-responsive delivery of Griffithsin from electrospun fibers. *Eur. J. Pharm. Biopharm.* **2018**. [CrossRef] [PubMed]
119. Carson, D.; Jiang, Y.H.; Woodrow, K.A. Tunable Release of Multiclass Anti-HIV Drugs that are Water-Soluble and Loaded at High Drug Content in Polyester Blended Electrospun Fibers. *Pharm. Res.* **2016**, *33*, 125–136. [CrossRef] [PubMed]
120. Liu, L.; Kamei, K.-i.; Yoshioka, M.; Nakajima, M.; Li, J.; Fujimoto, N.; Terada, S.; Tokunaga, Y.; Koyama, Y.; Sato, H. Nano-on-micro fibrous extracellular matrices for scalable expansion of human ES/iPS cells. *Biomaterials* **2017**, *124*, 47–54. [CrossRef] [PubMed]
121. Huang, L.-Y.; Branford-White, C.; Shen, X.-X.; Yu, D.-G.; Zhu, L.-M. Time-engineeringed biphasic drug release by electrospun nanofiber meshes. *Int. J. Pharm.* **2012**, *436*, 88–96. [CrossRef]
122. Meinel, A.J.; Germershaus, O.; Luhmann, T.; Merkle, H.P.; Meinel, L. Electrospun matrices for localized drug delivery: Current technologies and selected biomedical applications. *Eur. J. Pharm. Biopharm.* **2012**, *81*, 1–13. [CrossRef]
123. Blakney, A.K.; Krogstad, E.A.; Jiang, Y.H.; Woodrow, K.A. Delivery of multipurpose prevention drug combinations from electrospun nanofibers using composite microarchitectures. *Int. J. Nanomed.* **2014**, *9*, 2967–2978. [CrossRef]

124. Mehrotra, S.; Lynam, D.; Maloney, R.; Pawelec, K.M.; Tuszynski, M.H.; Lee, I.; Chan, C.; Sakamoto, J. Time controlled protein release from layer-by-layer assembled multilayer functionalized agarose hydrogels. *Adv. Funct. Mater.* **2010**, *20*, 247–258. [CrossRef]
125. Pan, H.; Li, L.; Hu, L.; Cui, X. Continuous aligned polymer fibers produced by a modified electrospinning method. *Polymer* **2006**, *47*, 4901–4904. [CrossRef]
126. Shin, J.-W.; Shin, H.; Heo, S.; Lee, Y.; Hwang, Y.; Kim, D.; Kim, J.; Shin, J. Hybrid nanofiber scaffolds of polyurethane and poly (ethylene oxide) using dual-electrospinning for vascular tissue engineering. In *3rd Kuala Lumpur International Conference on Biomedical Engineering 2006*; Springer: Berlin/Heidelberg, Germany, 2007; pp. 692–695.
127. Baker, B.M.; Gee, A.O.; Metter, R.B.; Nathan, A.S.; Marklein, R.A.; Burdick, J.A.; Mauck, R.L. The potential to improve cell infiltration in composite fiber-aligned electrospun scaffolds by the selective removal of sacrificial fibers. *Biomaterials* **2008**, *29*, 2348–2358. [CrossRef]
128. Tijing, L.D.; Ruelo, M.T.G.; Amarjargal, A.; Pant, H.R.; Park, C.-H.; Kim, C.S. One-step fabrication of antibacterial (silver nanoparticles/poly(ethylene oxide))—Polyurethane bicomponent hybrid nanofibrous mat by dual-spinneret electrospinning. *Mater. Chem. Phys.* **2012**, *134*, 557–561. [CrossRef]
129. Wulkersdorfer, B.; Kao, K.; Agopian, V.; Ahn, A.; Dunn, J.; Wu, B.; Stelzner, M. Bimodal porous scaffolds by sequential electrospinning of poly (glycolic acid) with sucrose particles. *Int. J. Polym. Sci.* **2010**, *2010*, 436178. [CrossRef]
130. Wan, A.C.; Ying, J.Y. Nanomaterials for in situ cell delivery and tissue regeneration. *Adv. Drug Deliv. Rev.* **2010**, *62*, 731–740. [CrossRef]
131. Dvir, T.; Timko, B.P.; Kohane, D.S.; Langer, R. Nanotechnological strategies for engineering complex tissues. *Nat. Nanotechnol.* **2011**, *6*, 13–22. [CrossRef]
132. Kharaziha, M.; Fathi, M.; Edris, H. Tunable cellular interactions and physical properties of nanofibrous PCL-forsterite: Gelatin scaffold through sequential electrospinning. *Compos. Sci. Technol.* **2013**, *87*, 182–188. [CrossRef]
133. Tan, L.; Hu, J.; Zhao, H. Design of bilayered nanofibrous mats for wound dressing using an electrospinning technique. *Mater. Lett.* **2015**, *156*, 46–49. [CrossRef]
134. Falde, E.J.; Freedman, J.D.; Herrera, V.L.M.; Yohe, S.T.; Colson, Y.L.; Grinstaff, M.W. Layered superhydrophobic meshes for controlled drug release. *J. Control. Release* **2015**, *214*, 23–29. [CrossRef]
135. Sirc, J.; Kubinova, S.; Hobzova, R.; Stranska, D.; Kozlik, P.; Bosakova, Z.; Marekova, D.; Holan, V.; Sykova, E.; Michalek, J. Controlled gentamicin release from multi-layered electrospun nanofibrous structures of various thicknesses. *Int. J. Nanomed.* **2012**, *7*, 5315–5325. [CrossRef] [PubMed]
136. Mandal, B.B.; Mann, J.K.; Kundu, S. Silk fibroin/gelatin multilayered films as a model system for controlled drug release. *Eur. J. Pharm. Sci.* **2009**, *37*, 160–171. [CrossRef] [PubMed]
137. Okuda, T.; Tominaga, K.; Kidoaki, S. Time-programmed dual release formulation by multilayered drug-loaded nanofiber meshes. *J. Control. Release* **2010**, *143*, 258–264. [CrossRef] [PubMed]
138. Liu, S.; Wang, X.; Zhang, Z.; Zhang, Y.; Zhou, G.; Huang, Y.; Xie, Z.; Jing, X. Use of asymmetric multilayer polylactide nanofiber mats in controlled release of drugs and prevention of liver cancer recurrence after surgery in mice. *Nanomed. Nanotechnol. Biol. Med.* **2015**, *11*, 1047–1056. [CrossRef]
139. Chunder, A.; Sarkar, S.; Yu, Y.; Zhai, L. Fabrication of ultrathin polyelectrolyte fibers and their controlled release properties. *Colloids Surf. B Biointerfaces* **2007**, *58*, 172–179. [CrossRef] [PubMed]
140. Son, Y.J.; Kim, W.J.; Yoo, H.S. Therapeutic applications of electrospun nanofibers for drug delivery systems. *Arch. Pharmacal Res.* **2014**, *37*, 69–78. [CrossRef] [PubMed]
141. Yoon, H.; Kim, G.H. Layer-by-layered electrospun micro/nanofibrous mats for drug delivery system. *Macromol. Res.* **2012**, *20*, 402–406. [CrossRef]
142. Park, J.H.; Kim, B.S.; Yoo, Y.C.; Khil, M.S.; Kim, H.Y. Enhanced mechanical properties of multilayer nano-coated electrospun nylon 6 fibers via a layer-by-layer self-assembly. *J. Appl. Polym. Sci.* **2008**, *107*, 2211–2216. [CrossRef]
143. Woodrow, K.A.; Cu, Y.; Booth, C.J.; Saucier-Sawyer, J.K.; Wood, M.J.; Saltzman, W.M. Intravaginal gene silencing using biodegradable polymer nanoparticles densely loaded with small-interfering RNA. *Nat. Mater.* **2009**, *8*, 526–533. [CrossRef] [PubMed]
144. Ensign, L.M.; Cone, R.; Hanes, J. Nanoparticle-based drug delivery to the vagina: A review. *J. Control. Release* **2014**, *190*, 500–514. [CrossRef]

145. Ahmad, M.Z.; Akhter, S.; Jain, G.K.; Rahman, M.; Pathan, S.A.; Ahmad, F.J.; Khar, R.K. Metallic nanoparticles: Technology overview & drug delivery applications in oncology. *Expert Opin. Drug Deliv.* **2010**, *7*, 927–942. [PubMed]
146. Mody, V.V.; Siwale, R.; Singh, A.; Mody, H.R. Introduction to metallic nanoparticles. *J. Pharm. Bioallied Sci.* **2010**, *2*, 282–289. [CrossRef] [PubMed]
147. Singh, R.; Lillard, J.W., Jr. Nanoparticle-based targeted drug delivery. *Exp. Mol. Pathol.* **2009**, *86*, 215–223. [CrossRef]
148. Blanco, E.; Shen, H.; Ferrari, M. Principles of nanoparticle design for overcoming biological barriers to drug delivery. *Nat. Biotechnol.* **2015**, *33*, 941–951. [CrossRef]
149. Peer, D.; Karp, J.M.; Hong, S.; Farokhzad, O.C.; Margalit, R.; Langer, R. Nanocarriers as an emerging platform for cancer therapy. *Nat. Nanotechnol.* **2007**, *2*, 751–760. [CrossRef]
150. Gu, J.; Yang, S.; Ho, E.A. Biodegradable film for the targeted delivery of siRNA-loaded nanoparticles to vaginal immune cells. *Mol. Pharm.* **2015**, *12*, 2889–2903. [CrossRef] [PubMed]
151. Wang, Y.Y.; Lai, S.K.; Suk, J.S.; Pace, A.; Cone, R.; Hanes, J. Addressing the PEG mucoadhesivity paradox to engineer nanoparticles that "slip" through the human mucus barrier. *Angew. Chem. Int. Ed.* **2008**, *47*, 9726–9729. [CrossRef] [PubMed]
152. Wang, S.; Zhao, Y.; Shen, M.; Shi, X. Electrospun hybrid nanofibers doped with nanoparticles or nanotubes for biomedical applications. *Ther. Deliv.* **2012**, *3*, 1155–1169. [CrossRef] [PubMed]
153. Chen, M.; Gao, S.; Dong, M.; Song, J.; Yang, C.; Howard, K.A.; Kjems, J.; Besenbacher, F. Chitosan/siRNA nanoparticles encapsulated in PLGA nanofibers for siRNA delivery. *ACS Nano* **2012**, *6*, 4835–4844. [CrossRef] [PubMed]
154. Sridhar, R.; Lakshminarayanan, R.; Madhaiyan, K.; Barathi, V.A.; Lim, K.H.C.; Ramakrishna, S. Electrosprayed nanoparticles and electrospun nanofibers based on natural materials: Applications in tissue regeneration, drug delivery and pharmaceuticals. *Chem. Soc. Rev.* **2015**, *44*, 790–814. [CrossRef]
155. Mehrasa, M.; Asadollahi, M.A.; Nasri-Nasrabadi, B.; Ghaedi, K.; Salehi, H.; Dolatshahi-Pirouz, A.; Arpanaei, A. Incorporation of mesoporous silica nanoparticles into random electrospun PLGA and PLGA/gelatin nanofibrous scaffolds enhances mechanical and cell proliferation properties. *Mater. Sci. Eng. C* **2016**, *66*, 25–32. [CrossRef]
156. Song, B.; Wu, C.; Chang, J. Controllable delivery of hydrophilic and hydrophobic drugs from electrospun poly (lactic-co-glycolic acid)/mesoporous silica nanoparticles composite mats. *J. Biomed. Mater. Res. B* **2012**, *100*, 2178–2186. [CrossRef]
157. Beck-Broichsitter, M.; Thieme, M.; Nguyen, J.; Schmehl, T.; Gessler, T.; Seeger, W.; Agarwal, S.; Greiner, A.; Kissel, T. Novel 'Nano in Nano'Composites for Sustained Drug Delivery: Biodegradable Nanoparticles Encapsulated into Nanofiber Non-Wovens. *Macromol. Biosci.* **2010**, *10*, 1527–1535. [CrossRef] [PubMed]
158. Fathollahipour, S.; Mehrizi, A.A.; Ghaee, A.; Koosha, M. Electrospinning of PVA/chitosan nanocomposite nanofibers containing gelatin nanoparticles as a dual drug delivery system. *J. Biomed. Mater. Res. Part A* **2015**, *103*, 3852–3862. [CrossRef]
159. Hu, J.; Zeng, F.; Wei, J.; Chen, Y.; Chen, Y. Novel controlled drug delivery system for multiple drugs based on electrospun nanofibers containing nanomicelles. *J. Biomater. Sci. Polym. Ed.* **2014**, *25*, 257–268. [CrossRef]
160. Wang, Y.; Wang, B.; Qiao, W.; Yin, T. A novel controlled release drug delivery system for multiple drugs based on electrospun nanofibers containing nanoparticles. *J. Pharm. Sci.* **2010**, *99*, 4805–4811. [CrossRef]
161. Li, L.; Zhou, G.; Wang, Y.; Yang, G.; Ding, S.; Zhou, S. Controlled dual delivery of BMP-2 and dexamethasone by nanoparticle-embedded electrospun nanofibers for the efficient repair of critical-sized rat calvarial defect. *Biomaterials* **2015**, *37*, 218–229. [CrossRef]
162. Ali, I.H.; Khalil, I.A.; El-Sherbiny, I.M. Single-Dose Electrospun Nanoparticles-in-Nanofibers Wound Dressings with Enhanced Epithelialization, Collagen Deposition, and Granulation Properties. *ACS Appl. Mater. Interfaces* **2016**, *8*, 14453–14469. [CrossRef]
163. Sun, X.; Li, K.; Chen, S.; Yao, B.; Zhou, Y.; Cui, S.; Hu, J.; Liu, Y. Rationally designed particle preloading method to improve protein delivery performance of electrospun polyester nanofibers. *Int. J. Pharm.* **2016**, *512*, 204–212. [CrossRef]
164. Vakilian, S.; Mashayekhan, S.; Shabani, I.; Khorashadizadeh, M.; Fallah, A.; Soleimani, M. Structural stability and sustained release of protein from a multilayer nanofiber/nanoparticle composite. *Int. J. Biol. Macromol.* **2015**, *75*, 248–257. [CrossRef]

165. Nie, H.; Wang, C.-H. Fabrication and characterization of PLGA/HAp composite scaffolds for delivery of BMP-2 plasmid DNA. *J. Control. Release* **2007**, *120*, 111–121. [CrossRef]
166. Cui, W.; Zhou, Y.; Chang, J. Electrospun nanofibrous materials for tissue engineering and drug delivery. *Sci. Technol. Adv. Mater.* **2010**, *11*, 014108. [CrossRef]
167. Shao, W.; He, J.; Sang, F.; Ding, B.; Chen, L.; Cui, S.; Li, K.; Han, Q.; Tan, W. Coaxial electrospun aligned tussah silk fibroin nanostructured fiber scaffolds embedded with hydroxyapatite–tussah silk fibroin nanoparticles for bone tissue engineering. *Mater. Sci. Eng. C* **2016**, *58*, 342–351. [CrossRef]
168. Weissleder, R.; Kelly, K.; Sun, E.Y.; Shtatland, T.; Josephson, L. Cell-specific targeting of nanoparticles by multivalent attachment of small molecules. *Nat. Biotechnol.* **2005**, *23*, 1418–1423. [CrossRef]
169. Kohler, N.; Fryxell, G.E.; Zhang, M. A bifunctional poly (ethylene glycol) silane immobilized on metallic oxide-based nanoparticles for conjugation with cell targeting agents. *JACS* **2004**, *126*, 7206–7211. [CrossRef]
170. Yao, L.; Lin, Y.; Watkins, J.J. Ultrahigh loading of nanoparticles into ordered block copolymer composites. *Macromolecules* **2014**, *47*, 1844–1849. [CrossRef]
171. Zhu, J.; Wei, S.; Chen, X.; Karki, A.B.; Rutman, D.; Young, D.P.; Guo, Z. Electrospun polyimide nanocomposite fibers reinforced with core-shell Fe-FeO nanoparticles. *J. Phys. Chem. C* **2010**, *114*, 8844–8850. [CrossRef]
172. Delany-Moretlwe, S.; Lombard, C.; Baron, D.; Bekker, L.-G.; Nkala, B.; Ahmed, K.; Sebe, M.; Brumskine, W.; Nchabeleng, M.; Palanee-Philips, T.; et al. Tenofovir 1% vaginal gel for prevention of HIV-1 infection in women in South Africa (FACTS-001): A phase 3, randomised, double-blind, placebo-controlled trial. *Lancet Infect. Dis.* **2018**, *18*, 1241–1250. [CrossRef]
173. Skoler-Karpoff, S.; Ramjee, G.; Ahmed, K.; Altini, L.; Plagianos, M.G.; Friedland, B.; Govender, S.; de Kock, A.; Cassim, N.; Palanee, T.; et al. Efficacy of Carraguard for prevention of HIV infection in women in South Africa: A randomised, double-blind, placebo-controlled trial. *Lancet* **2008**, *372*, 1977–1987. [CrossRef]
174. Thurman, A.R.; Clark, M.R.; Doncel, G.F. Multipurpose prevention technologies: Biomedical tools to prevent HIV-1, HSV-2, and unintended pregnancies. *Infect. Dis. Obstet. Gynecol.* **2011**, *2011*, 429403. [CrossRef]
175. Blakney, A.K.; Simonovsky, F.I.; Suydam, I.T.; Ratner, B.D.; Woodrow, K.A. Rapidly Biodegrading PLGA-Polyurethane Fibers for Sustained Release of Physicochemically Diverse Drugs. *ACS Biomater. Sci. Eng.* **2016**, *2*, 1595–1607. [CrossRef]
176. Halwes, M.E.; Tyo, K.M.; Steinbach-Rankins, J.M.; Frieboes, H.B. Computational Modeling of Antiviral Drug Diffusion from Poly(lactic- co-glycolic-acid) Fibers and Multicompartment Pharmacokinetics for Application to the Female Reproductive Tract. *Mol. Pharm.* **2018**, *15*, 1534–1547. [CrossRef]
177. Moss, J.A.; Malone, A.M.; Smith, T.J.; Kennedy, S.; Nguyen, C.; Vincent, K.L.; Motamedi, M.; Baum, M.M. Pharmacokinetics of a Multipurpose Pod-Intravaginal Ring Simultaneously Delivering Five Drugs in an Ovine Model. *Antimicrob. Agents Chemother.* **2013**, *57*, 3994–3997. [CrossRef]
178. Smith, J.M.; Moss, J.A.; Srinivasan, P.; Butkyavichene, I.; Gunawardana, M.; Fanter, R.; Miller, C.S.; Sanchez, D.; Yang, F.; Ellis, S.; et al. Novel multipurpose pod-intravaginal ring for the prevention of HIV, HSV, and unintended pregnancy: Pharmacokinetic evaluation in a macaque model. *PLoS ONE* **2017**, *12*, e0185946. [CrossRef]
179. Morrow, R.J.; Woolfson, A.D.; Donnelly, L.; Curran, R.; Andrews, G.; Katinger, D.; Malcolm, R.K. Sustained release of proteins from a modified vaginal ring device. *Eur. J. Pharm. Biopharm.* **2011**, *77*, 3–10. [CrossRef]
180. Han, Y.A.; Singh, M.; Saxena, B.B. Development of vaginal rings for sustained release of nonhormonal contraceptives and anti-HIV agents. *Contraception* **2007**, *76*, 132–138. [CrossRef]
181. Malcolm, R.K.; Veazey, R.S.; Geer, L.; Lowry, D.; Fetherston, S.M.; Murphy, D.J.; Boyd, P.; Major, I.; Shattock, R.J.; Klasse, P.J.; et al. Sustained Release of the CCR5 Inhibitors CMPD167 and Maraviroc from Vaginal Rings in Rhesus Macaques. *Antimicrob. Agents Chemother.* **2012**, *56*, 2251. [CrossRef]
182. Johnson, T.J.; Gupta, K.M.; Fabian, J.; Albright, T.H.; Kiser, P.F. Segmented polyurethane intravaginal rings for the sustained combined delivery of antiretroviral agents dapivirine and tenofovir. *Eur. J. Pharm. Sci.* **2010**, *39*, 203–212. [CrossRef] [PubMed]
183. Woolfson, A.D.; Toner, C.F.; Malcolm, R.K.; Morrow, R.J.; McCullagh, S.D. Long-term, controlled release of the HIV microbicide TMC120 from silicone elastomer vaginal rings. *J. Antimicrob. Chemother.* **2005**, *56*, 954–956.
184. Baum, M.M.; Butkyavichene, I.; Gilman, J.; Kennedy, S.; Kopin, E.; Malone, A.M.; Nguyen, C.; Smith, T.J.; Friend, D.R.; Clark, M.R.; et al. An Intravaginal Ring for the Simultaneous Delivery of Multiple Drugs. *J. Pharm. Sci.* **2012**, *101*, 2833–2843. [CrossRef]

185. Johnson, T.J.; Clark, M.R.; Albright, T.H.; Nebeker, J.S.; Tuitupou, A.L.; Clark, J.T.; Fabian, J.; McCabe, R.T.; Chandra, N.; Doncel, G.F.; et al. A 90-Day Tenofovir Reservoir Intravaginal Ring for Mucosal HIV Prophylaxis. *Antimicrob. Agents Chemother.* **2012**, *56*, 6272–6283. [CrossRef]
186. Blakney, A.K.; Little, A.B.; Jiang, Y.; Woodrow, K.A. In vitro–ex vivo correlations between a cell-laden hydrogel and mucosal tissue for screening composite delivery systems. *Drug Deliv.* **2017**, *24*, 582–590. [CrossRef]
187. Rohan, L.C.; Moncla, B.J.; Ayudhya, R.P.K.N.; Cost, M.; Huang, Y.; Gai, F.; Billitto, N.; Lynam, J.; Pryke, K.; Graebing, P. In vitro and ex vivo testing of tenofovir shows it is effective as an HIV-1 microbicide. *PLoS ONE* **2010**, *5*, e9310. [CrossRef]
188. Patton, D.; Sweeney, Y.C.; Balkus, J.; Rohan, L.; Moncla, B.; Parniak, M.; Hillier, S. Preclinical safety assessments of UC781 anti-human immunodeficiency virus topical microbicide formulations. *Antimicrob. Agents Chemother.* **2007**, *51*, 1608–1615. [CrossRef]
189. Robinson, J.A.; Marzinke, M.A.; Fuchs, E.J.; Bakshi, R.P.; Spiegel, H.M.L.; Coleman, J.S.; Rohan, L.C.; Hendrix, C.W. Comparison of the Pharmacokinetics and Pharmacodynamics of Single-Dose Tenofovir Vaginal Film and Gel Formulation (FAME 05). *J. Acquir. Immune Defic. Syndr.* **2018**, *77*, 175–182. [CrossRef]
190. Hu, M.; Zhou, T.; Dezzutti, C.S.; Rohan, L.C. The effect of commonly used excipients on the epithelial integrity of human cervicovaginal tissue. *Aids Res. Hum. Retrovir.* **2016**, *32*, 992–1004. [CrossRef]
191. Merbah, M.; Introini, A.; Fitzgerald, W.; Grivel, J.C.; Lisco, A.; Vanpouille, C.; Margolis, L. Cervico-vaginal tissue ex vivo as a model to study early events in HIV-1 infection. *Am. J. Reprod. Immunol.* **2011**, *65*, 268–278. [CrossRef] [PubMed]
192. Ayehunie, S.; Cannon, C.; Lamore, S.; Kubilus, J.; Anderson, D.J.; Pudney, J.; Klausner, M. Organotypic human vaginal-ectocervical tissue model for irritation studies of spermicides, microbicides, and feminine-care products. *Toxicol. Vitr.* **2006**, *20*, 689–698. [CrossRef] [PubMed]
193. Ayehunie, S.; Cannon, C.; LaRosa, K.; Pudney, J.; Anderson, D.J.; Klausner, M. Development of an in vitro alternative assay method for vaginal irritation. *Toxicology* **2011**, *279*, 130–138. [CrossRef]
194. aniewski, P.; Gomez, A.; Hire, G.; So, M.; Herbst-Kralovetz, M.M. Human three-dimensional endometrial epithelial cell model to study host interactions with vaginal bacteria and Neisseria gonorrhoeae. *Infect. Immun.* **2017**, *85*, e01049-16. [CrossRef] [PubMed]
195. Doncel, G.F.; Clark, M.R. Preclinical evaluation of anti-HIV microbicide products: New models and biomarkers. *Antivir. Res.* **2010**, *88* (Suppl. 1), S10–S18. [CrossRef]
196. Huang, C.; Soenen, S.J.; van Gulck, E.; Vanham, G.; Rejman, J.; van Calenbergh, S.; Vervaet, C.; Coenye, T.; Verstraelen, H.; Temmerman, M.; et al. Electrospun cellulose acetate phthalate fibers for semen induced anti-HIV vaginal drug delivery. *Biomaterials* **2012**, *33*, 962–969. [CrossRef]
197. Ball, C.; Krogstad, E.; Chaowanachan, T.; Woodrow, K.A. Drug-eluting fibers for HIV-1 inhibition and contraception. *PLoS ONE* **2012**, *7*, e49792. [CrossRef]
198. Krogstad, E.A.; Woodrow, K.A. Manufacturing scale-up of electrospun poly(vinyl alcohol) fibers containing tenofovir for vaginal drug delivery. *Int. J. Pharm.* **2014**, *475*, 282–291. [CrossRef]
199. Jiang, J.; Xie, J.; Ma, B.; Bartlett, D.E.; Xu, A.; Wang, C.H. Mussel-inspired protein-mediated surface functionalization of electrospun nanofibers for pH-responsive drug delivery. *Acta Biomater.* **2014**, *10*, 1324–1332. [CrossRef] [PubMed]
200. Sun, X.-Z.; Williams, G.R.; Hou, X.-X.; Zhu, L.-M. Electrospun curcumin-loaded fibers with potential biomedical applications. *Carbohydr. Polym.* **2013**, *94*, 147–153. [CrossRef] [PubMed]
201. Berg, M.C.; Zhai, L.; Cohen, R.E.; Rubner, M.F. Controlled drug release from porous polyelectrolyte multilayers. *Biomacromolecules* **2006**, *7*, 357–364. [CrossRef] [PubMed]

7

Pterostilbene Suppresses both Cancer Cells and Cancer Stem-Like Cells in Cervical Cancer with Superior Bioavailability to Resveratrol

Hee Jeong Shin [1], Jang Mi Han [1], Ye Seul Choi [1] and Hye Jin Jung [1,2,3,*]

1 Department of Life Science and Biochemical Engineering, Sun Moon University, Asan 31460, Korea; gmlwjd903@naver.com (H.J.S.); gkswkdal200@naver.com (J.M.H.); yesll96@naver.com (Y.S.C.)
2 Genome-based BioIT Convergence Institute, Asan 31460, Korea
3 Department of Pharmaceutical Engineering and Biotechnology, Sun Moon University, Asan 31460, Korea
* Correspondence: poka96@sunmoon.ac.kr

Academic Editor: Kyoko Nakagawa-Goto

Abstract: Increasing studies have reported that cancer stem cells (CSCs) play critical roles in therapeutic resistance, recurrence, and metastasis of tumors, including cervical cancer. Pterostilbene, a dimethylated derivative of resveratrol, is a plant polyphenol compound with potential chemopreventive activity. However, the therapeutic effect of pterostilbene against cervical CSCs remains unclear. In this study, we compared the anticancer effects of resveratrol and pterostilbene using both HeLa cervical cancer adherent and stem-like cells. Pterostilbene more effectively inhibited the growth and clonogenic survival, as well as metastatic ability of HeLa adherent cells than those of resveratrol. Moreover, the superior inhibitory effects of pterostilbene compared to resveratrol were associated with the enhanced activation of multiple mechanisms, including cell cycle arrest at S and G2/M phases, induction of ROS-mediated caspase-dependent apoptosis, and inhibition of matrix metalloproteinase (MMP)-2/-9 expression. Notably, pterostilbene exhibited a greater inhibitory effect on the tumorsphere-forming and migration abilities of HeLa cancer stem-like cells compared to resveratrol. This greater effect was achieved through more potent inhibition of the expression levels of stemness markers, such as CD133, Oct4, Sox2, and Nanog, as well as signal transducer and activator of transcription 3 signaling. These results suggest that pterostilbene might be a potential anticancer agent targeting both cancer cells and cancer stem-like cells of cervical cancer via the superior bioavailability to resveratrol.

Keywords: cancer stem cell; cervical cancer; pterostilbene; resveratrol

---

1. Introduction

Cervical cancer is one of the most common types of female malignant tumor, with worldwide incidence of more than 500,000 cases and mortality rate of 9% per year [1]. High-risk human papillomavirus (HPV) types such as HPV-16 and -18 are known to cause cervical cancer through the overexpression of viral oncoproteins E6 and E7 [2]. Although the worldwide death rate from cervical cancer has declined due to the current treatment modalities, including HPV vaccines, surgery, radiation therapy, and chemotherapy, the cancer recurrence, metastasis, and the adverse drug effects remain major problems [3]. Therefore, safer and more effective therapeutic options are needed to improve the treatment of cervical cancer.

Accumulating evidence has demonstrated that cancer stem cells (CSCs), a small subpopulation of tumor cells with self-renewal and multi-lineage differentiation capacities, crucially drive the development, metastasis, relapse, and chemo/radio-resistance of cervical cancer [4,5]. In addition,

HPV oncoprotein E6 has been found to be involved in self-renewal and maintenance of stemness in cervical CSCs by upregulating Hes1, a downstream gene of Notch1 [6]. HPV16 E7 also upregulates the expression of stemness-related genes such as Oct3/4, Sox2, Nanog, and fibroblast growth factor 4 to maintain the self-renewal capacity of cervical CSCs [7]. Accordingly, targeting the cervical CSCs is a promising therapeutic strategy for the high-risk HPV-positive cervical cancer.

Various scientific studies have suggested the potential of natural active compounds isolated from plants or herbs for prevention and treatment of cancer [8,9]. Stilbenes are a class of polyphenolic compounds and naturally found in various dietary sources, such as grapes, blueberries, red wine, peanuts, and some medicinal plants [10]. Recently, stilbenes such as resveratrol (3,4′,5-trihydroxy-trans-stilbene) and its dimethylated analog, pterostilbene (trans-3,5-dimethoxy-4′-hydroxystilbene), have received considerable attention due to their potent antioxidant, anti-inflammatory, antidiabetic, and anticarcinogenic properties (Figure 1) [11,12]. Resveratrol and pterostilbene have been considered as excellent anticancer agents because of their low toxicity and abilities to regulate multiple molecular signaling pathways involved in cancer progression [13,14]. However, resveratrol has a low bioavailability that may lower its biological efficacy, while pterostilbene is more lipophilic, and thus, it exhibits better bioavailability [15]. Pterostilbene shows stronger antiproliferative and apoptotic effects than those shown by resveratrol in the human colon and cervical cancer cells [16,17]. However, the therapeutic effect and anticancer mechanism of pterostilbene against cervical CSCs compared to resveratrol have not been studied.

Here, anticancer effects of resveratrol and pterostilbene were compared using both HeLa cervical cancer adherent and stem-like cells. The abilities of the two compounds to suppress growth, migration, and stemness of HeLa cells were evaluated and the underlying molecular mechanisms were further explored. The results revealed that pterostilbene more effectively inhibited the stem-like properties of HeLa cells than resveratrol through stronger downregulation of specific CSC markers and signal transducer and activator of transcription 3 (STAT3) signaling. This is the first study to demonstrate the potential inhibitory activity of pterostilbene against cervical cancer cell stemness.

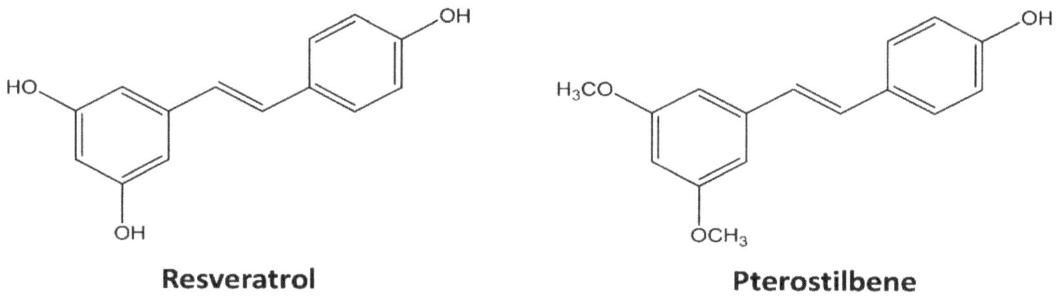

Figure 1. Chemical structures of resveratrol and pterostilbene.

2. Results

2.1. Pterostilbene Inhibited the Growth of Cervical Cancer Cells with Higher Potency Compared to Resveratrol

First, we compared the inhibitory effects of resveratrol and pterostilbene on the growth of HeLa, CaSki, and SiHa cervical cancer adherent cells using the 3-(4,5-dimethylthiazol-2-yl)-2,5-diphenyltetrazolium bromide (MTT) assay at various concentrations (0–200 μM). Resveratrol and pterostilbene suppressed the growth of HeLa, CaSki, and SiHa cells in a concentration-dependent manner (Figure 2A). The results showed that pterostilbene (IC_{50} = 32.67 μM for HeLa; 14.83 μM for CaSki; 34.17 μM for SiHa) exhibited stronger growth inhibitory effect than resveratrol (IC_{50} = 108.7 μM for HeLa; 44.45 μM for CaSki; 91.15 μM for SiHa). Next, we evaluated the effects of pterostilbene and resveratrol on the colony formation of HeLa, CaSki, and SiHa adherent cells. The colony forming ability of the cells was more effectively inhibited by pterostilbene than resveratrol (Figure 2B). These data demonstrate that pterostilbene is more potent in suppressing the growth and clonogenicity of cervical cancer adherent cells compared with resveratrol.

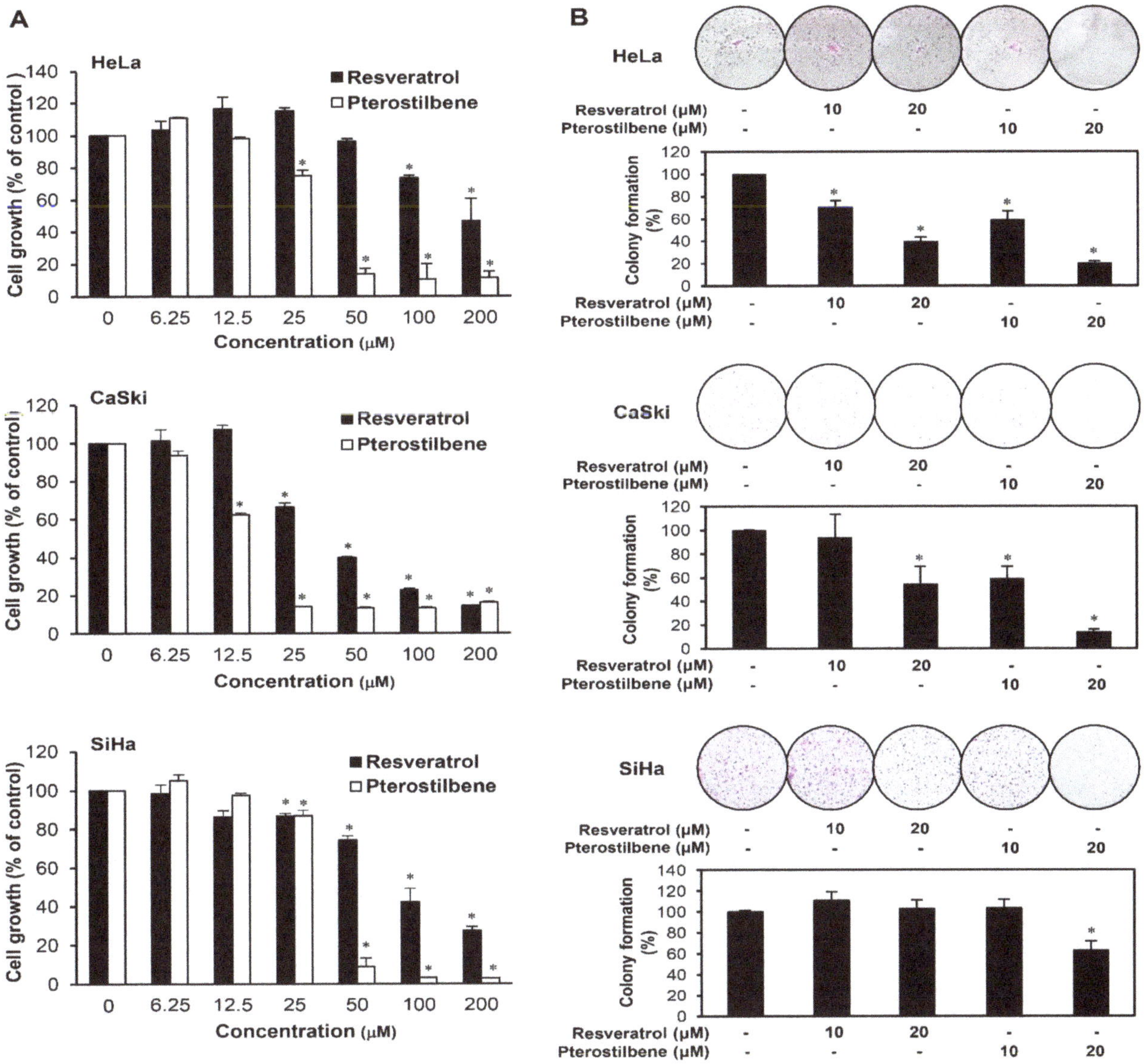

Figure 2. Growth inhibitory effects of resveratrol and pterostilbene on HeLa, CaSki, and SiHa cells. (**A**) The effects of resveratrol and pterostilbene on the growth of HeLa, CaSki, and SiHa adherent cells. The cells were treated with increasing concentrations of the two compounds (0–200 μM) for 72 h, and cell growth was measured by 3-(4,5-dimethylthiazol-2-yl)-2,5-diphenyltetrazolium bromide (MTT) assay. (**B**) The effects of resveratrol and pterostilbene on the colony forming ability of HeLa, CaSki, and SiHa adherent cells. The cells were incubated in the absence or presence of the two compounds (10 and 20 μM) for seven days. The cell colonies were detected by crystal violet staining. * $p < 0.05$ versus the control.

2.2. Pterostilbene Exhibited Stronger Migration Inhibitory Effect than Resveratrol in Cervical Cancer Cells

To compare the effects of resveratrol and pterostilbene on the metastatic ability of cervical cancer cells, we examined whether the two compounds inhibit the migration and invasion of HeLa adherent cells. A monolayer wound healing assay was performed to evaluate their effects on cell migration. Pterostilbene more markedly decreased the migration of HeLa cells at both 24 and 48 h after treatment when compared to resveratrol (Figure 3A). The effects of the two compounds on cell invasion were assessed using a Matrigel-coated Transwell chamber system. Both resveratrol and pterostilbene resulted in a significant reduction in the invasiveness of HeLa cells (Figure 3B). In particular, the invasion inhibitory effect of pterostilbene was more potent than that of resveratrol.

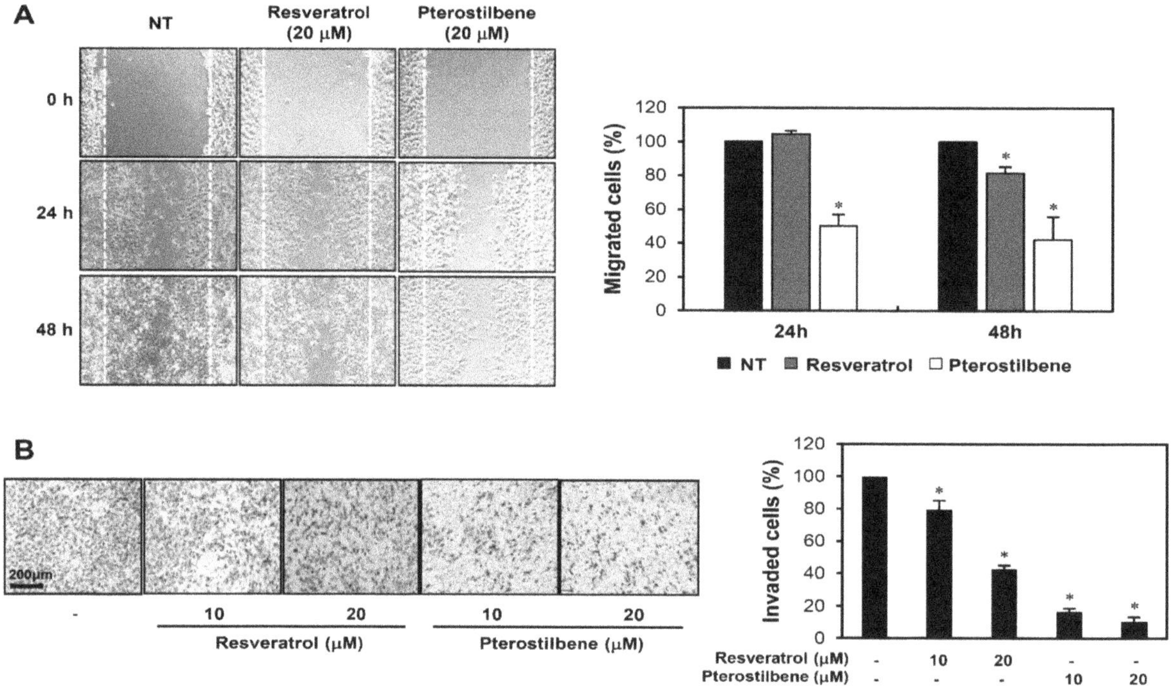

Figure 3. Effects of resveratrol and pterostilbene on the metastatic ability of HeLa cells. (**A**) The effects of resveratrol and pterostilbene on the migration of HeLa adherent cells. The migratory potential of HeLa cells was analyzed using a wound healing assay. The cells were incubated in the absence or presence of the two compounds (20 μM) for 48 h. The cells that migrated into the gap were counted using an optical microscope. Dotted white lines indicate the edge of the gap at 0 h. (**B**) The effects of resveratrol and pterostilbene on the invasion of HeLa adherent cells. The invasiveness of HeLa cells was analyzed using Matrigel-coated polycarbonate filters. The cells were incubated in the absence or presence of the two compounds (10 and 20 μM) for 48 h. The cells penetrating the filters were stained and counted using an optical microscope. * $p < 0.05$ versus the control.

2.3. Comparison of the Cell Cycle Arrest and Apoptosis-Inducing Effects of Resveratrol and Pterostilbene in Cervical Cancer Cells

To determine whether the growth inhibitory effects of resveratrol and pterostilbene on HeLa adherent cells were caused by cell cycle arrest, the effects of the two compounds on the cellular cell cycle distribution were quantified using flow cytometry analysis. Both resveratrol and pterostilbene induced cell cycle arrest at the S and G2/M phases along with a decrease in G0/G1 phase duration when compared with the control cells (Figure 4A). Notably, pterostilbene was more potent than resveratrol in blocking cell cycle progression. The induction of tumor suppressor protein p53 and its downstream target p21 can trigger cell cycle arrest by inhibiting the activity of cyclin-dependent kinase (CDK)–cyclin complexes [18]. Therefore, the effects of resveratrol and pterostilbene on the expression of these cell cycle regulators were assessed. Results revealed that the cell cycle arrest at the S and G2/M phases of HeLa adherent cells by resveratrol and pterostilbene was associated with the promotion of p53 and p21 expression and subsequent downregulation of cyclin E1 and cyclin B1 that are active in the S and G2 phases, respectively (Figure 5B). Furthermore, pterostilbene not only more significantly increased the expression levels of p53 and p21, but also decreased those of cyclin E1 and cyclin B1 compared to resveratrol.

To further elucidate the mechanisms underlying the anticancer effects of the two compounds in cervical cancer cells, cellular apoptosis was quantitatively measured using flow cytometry analysis following annexinV-FITC/propidium iodide (PI) double staining. Annexin V is a marker of early apoptosis and PI is a marker of late apoptosis and necrosis. The total amount of early and late apoptotic cells was markedly increased after resveratrol and pterostilbene treatment in comparison with the control (Figure 4B). Moreover, the apoptosis-inducing effect of pterostilbene was stronger than that of resveratrol in HeLa adherent cells (from 4.67% to 30.58% and 50.46% by resveratrol and pterostilbene, respectively). The elevation of intracellular reactive oxygen species (ROS) plays an important role in mediating apoptotic processes [19]. Thus, to determine whether ROS are involved in the regulation of resveratrol- and pterostilbene-induced apoptosis, the levels of intracellular ROS in HeLa adherent cells were measured using the fluorescent 2′,7′-dichlorofluorescein diacetate (DCFH-DA) product. Pterostilbene more prominently elevated the production of ROS in comparison with resveratrol at the indicated doses (Figure 5A). In addition, the cell apoptosis induced by resveratrol and pterostilbene was involved in the activation of caspase-3 and caspase-9, as well as the downregulation of antiapoptotic proteins such as Bcl-2 and Bcl-XL (Figure 5B) [20]. These data also showed that pterostilbene was more effective in regulating the expression of these apoptosis-related proteins than resveratrol.

Matrix metalloproteinases (MMPs) play a critical role in the degradation of the extracellular matrix (ECM) during cancer metastasis [21]. To further define the mechanism through which resveratrol and pterostilbene reduce cervical cancer cell migration and invasion, the protein expression levels of MMP-2 and MMP-9 in HeLa adherent cells were investigated. Pterostilbene more strongly suppressed the expression of MMP-2 and MMP-9 compared with resveratrol (Figure 5B). These findings suggest that pterostilbene may possess enhanced activity in inhibiting the metastasis of cervical cancer cells than resveratrol, through more effective downregulation of MMP-2 and MMP-9 expression.

Therefore, the superior growth and migration inhibitory effects of pterostilbene compared to resveratrol in HeLa adherent cells were mediated through the enhanced activation of multiple mechanisms, including cell cycle arrest at S and G2/M phases, induction of ROS-mediated caspase-dependent apoptosis, and inhibition of MMP-2/-9 expression.

A

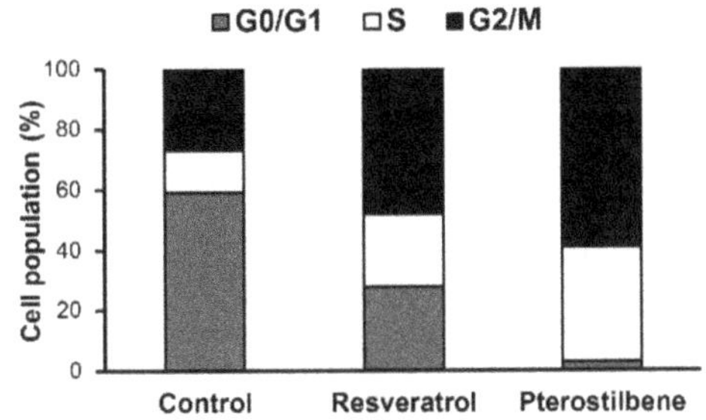

Compound	Cell cycle phase (%)		
	G0/G1	S	G2/M
Control	56.7	13.2	26.1
Resveratrol	25.7	22.1	44.6
Pterostilbene	2.6	34.2	53.5

B

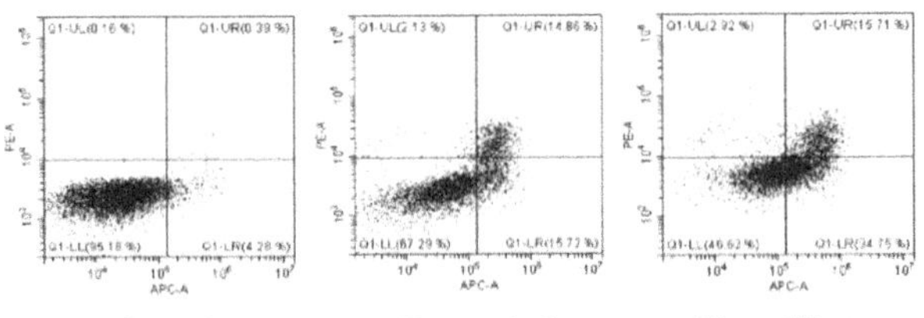

Compound	Annexin V+ /PI − (%)	Annexin V+ /PI + (%)	Apoptotic cells (%)
Control	4.28	0.39	4.67
Resveratrol	15.72	14.86	30.58
Pterostilbene	34.75	15.71	50.46

Figure 4. Effects of resveratrol and pterostilbene on the cell cycle and apoptotic cell death of HeLa cells. (**A**) The cell cycle distribution of HeLa adherent cells was evaluated by flow cytometry after the treatment of the two compounds (40 μM) for 48 h. (**B**) HeLa adherent cells were treated with resveratrol and pterostilbene (40 μM) for 48 h. Apoptotic cells were determined by flow cytometry analysis following annexin V-FITC and propidium iodide (PI) dual labeling.

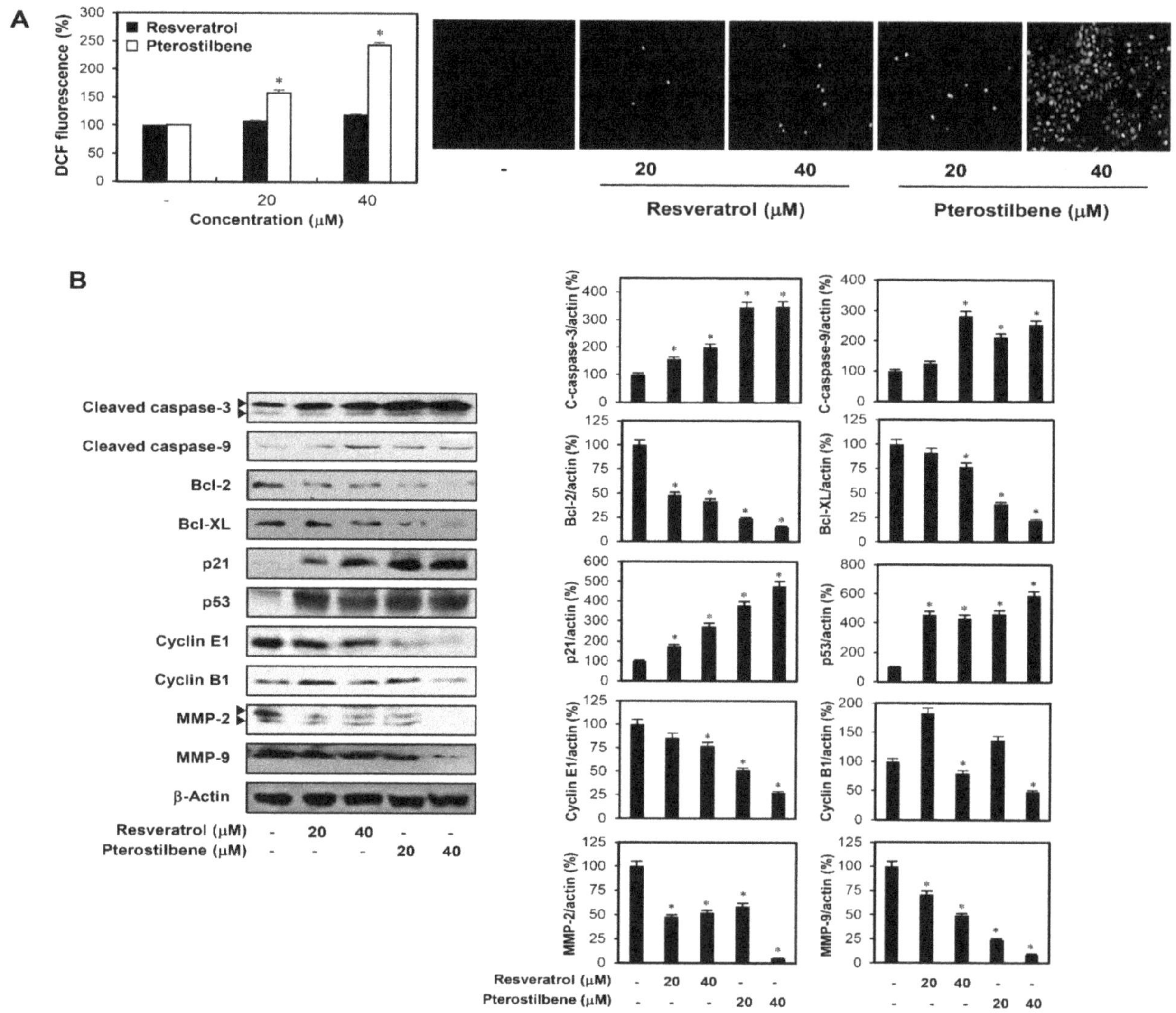

Figure 5. Identification of molecular mechanisms underlying the growth and migration inhibitory effects of resveratrol and pterostilbene in HeLa cells. (**A**) The effects of resveratrol and pterostilbene on reactive oxygen species (ROS) generation in HeLa adherent cells. The cells were treated with resveratrol and pterostilbene (20 and 40 μM) for 48 h. Intracellular ROS levels were detected with 2′,7′-dichlorofluorescein diacetate (DCFH-DA). (**B**) The effects of resveratrol and pterostilbene on the expression of cleaved caspase-3, cleaved caspase-9, Bcl-2, Bcl-XL, p21, p53, cyclin E1, cyclin B1, MMP-2, and MMP-9 in HeLa adherent cells. The cells were treated with the two compounds (20 and 40 μM) for 48 h, and the protein levels were detected by Western blot analysis using specific antibodies. The levels of β-actin were used as an internal control. Arrowheads indicate true bands for the molecular markers. * $p < 0.05$ versus the control.

2.4. Potent Inhibitory Activity of Pterostilbene against the Growth and Migration of Cervical CSCs

CSCs, which play critical roles in therapeutic resistance, recurrence, and metastasis of tumors, have been identified in various solid tumors and hematological cancers including cervical cancer [22,23]. Therefore, anticancer agents with the potential to eliminate cervical CSCs may provide novel therapeutic opportunities for more effective treatment of cervical carcinoma.

To assess the effects of resveratrol and pterostilbene against stem-like properties of cervical cancer cells, the CSC population from HeLa cells was enriched in serum-free suspended spheroid culture condition [24,25]. First, we examined whether the two compounds affect the clonogenic growth as tumorspheres of cancer stem-like cells derived from HeLa cells. The tumorsphere forming ability of HeLa cancer stem-like cells was significantly suppressed by treatment with resveratrol and pterostilbene (Figure 6A). They decreased both the number and size of HeLa cancer stem-like cells. Particularly, pterostilbene was much stronger in inhibiting the tumorsphere formation of HeLa cancer stem-like cells compared with resveratrol.

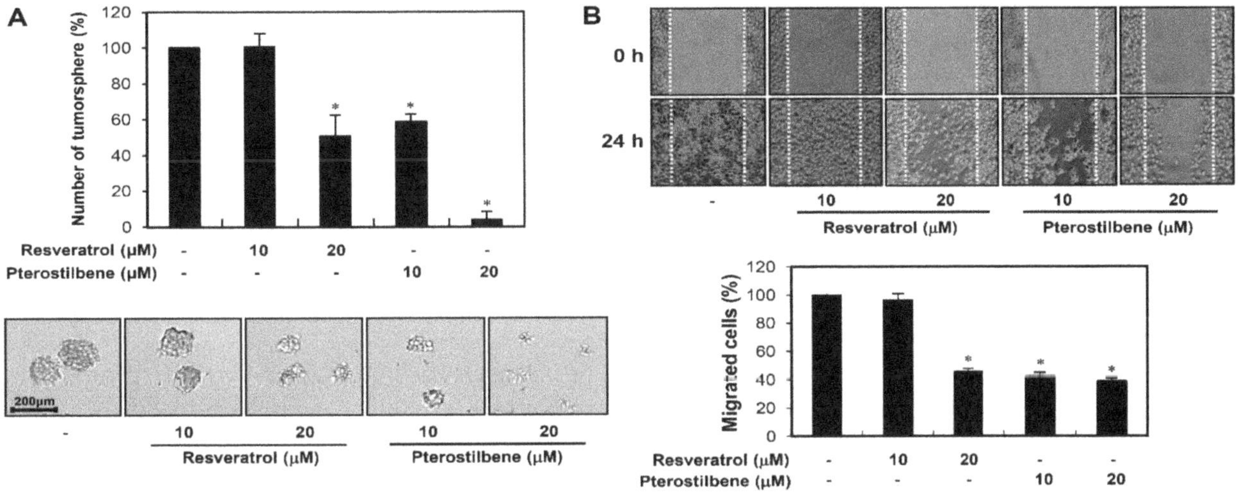

Figure 6. Effects of resveratrol and pterostilbene on the tumorsphere-forming ability and migration of cervical cancer stem cells (CSCs). (**A**) HeLa cancer stem-like cells were treated with the two compounds (10 and 20 μM) and incubated with the CSC culture media for eight days. The number of formed tumorspheres in each well was counted under a microscope. (**B**) HeLa cancer stem-like cells were seeded into laminin-coated culture plate and incubated with the CSC culture media in the absence or presence of resveratrol and pterostilbene (10 and 20 μM) for 24 h. The cells that migrated into the gap were counted under an optical microscope. White lines indicate the edge of the gap at 0 h. * $p < 0.05$ versus the control.

Next, we investigated the effects of resveratrol and pterostilbene on the migration of HeLa cancer stem-like cells. The wound healing assay showed that the two compounds reduced the migration of HeLa cancer stem-like cells when compared to the control conditions (Figure 6B). In addition, the migration inhibition activity of pterostilbene was much more potent than that of resveratrol. These findings underscore the superior therapeutic potential of pterostilbene to eliminate cervical CSCs.

2.5. Pterostilbene Exhibited Better Capacity for Inducing Cell Cycle Arrest and Apoptosis of Cervical CSCs Compared to Resveratrol

To further elucidate the inhibitory effects of resveratrol and pterostilbene on the growth of cervical CSCs, the cell cycle progression and cellular apoptosis of HeLa cancer stem-like cells were measured by flow cytometry analysis. As shown in Figure 7A, both resveratrol and pterostilbene induced S phase arrest (increase in the proportion of arrested cells from 19.87% to 23.83% and 36.93% by treatment with resveratrol and pterostilbene, respectively) when compared with the control cells. Moreover, pterostilbene more strongly induced cell cycle arrest than resveratrol in HeLa cancer stem-like cells. Our data also showed that the number of early and late apoptotic cells was markedly increased after resveratrol and pterostilbene treatment in comparison with the control (Figure 7B). The apoptosis promoting effect of pterostilbene was more potent compared to resveratrol in HeLa cancer stem-like cells (increase in the proportion of total apoptotic cells, from 15.72% to 58.65% and 83.46% by resveratrol and pterostilbene, respectively). These results indicate that pterostilbene has a better capacity for inducing cell cycle arrest and apoptosis of cervical CSCs than resveratrol, thereby causing a stronger inhibition in the tumorsphere-forming ability of cervical CSCs in comparison with resveratrol.

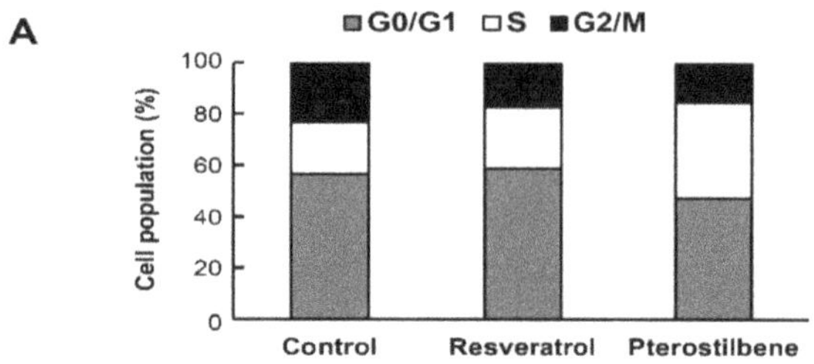

Compound	Cell cycle phase (%)		
	G0/G1	S	G2/M
Control	56.47	19.87	23.39
Resveratrol	58.10	23.83	17.17
Pterostilbene	47.01	36.93	15.30

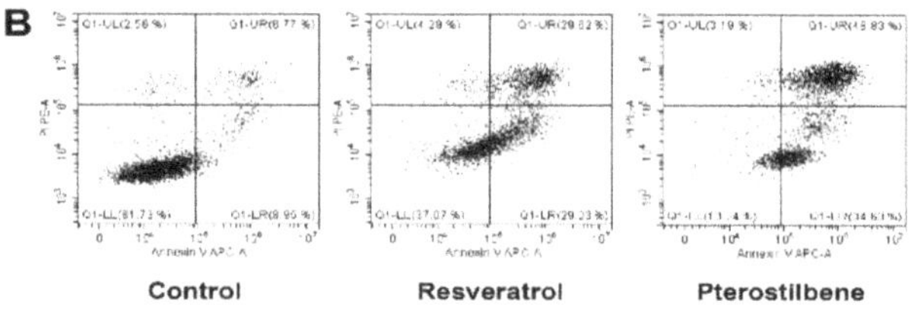

Compound	Annexin V+ /PI − (%)	Annexin V+ /PI + (%)	Apoptotic cells (%)
Control	8.95	6.77	15.72
Resveratrol	29.03	29.62	58.65
Pterostilbene	34.63	48.83	83.46

Figure 7. Effects of resveratrol and pterostilbene on the cell cycle and apoptotic cell death of cervical CSCs. (**A**) The cell cycle progression and (**B**) cellular apoptosis of HeLa cancer stem-like cells were measured by flow cytometry analysis after the treatment of resveratrol and pterostilbene (40 μM) for 48 h.

2.6. *Effect of Pterostilbene on the Expression of Stemness Markers in Cervical CSCs*

To explore the mechanism by which resveratrol and pterostilbene inhibit the growth and migration of cervical CSCs, their effects on the expression of transcription factors, Sox2, Oct4, and Nanog, were investigated. These transcription factors have been reported to induce stem-like properties, in HeLa cancer stem-like cells [26–28]. The two compounds effectively reduced the expression levels of the key stemness-related transcription factors as well as CD133, a cell surface marker for CSCs, suggesting that the inhibitory effects of resveratrol and pterostilbene against cervical CSCs may be associated with the downregulation of these stemness regulators (Figure 8A). Pterostilbene treatment more noticeably decreased the expression levels of stemness markers compared with resveratrol treatment.

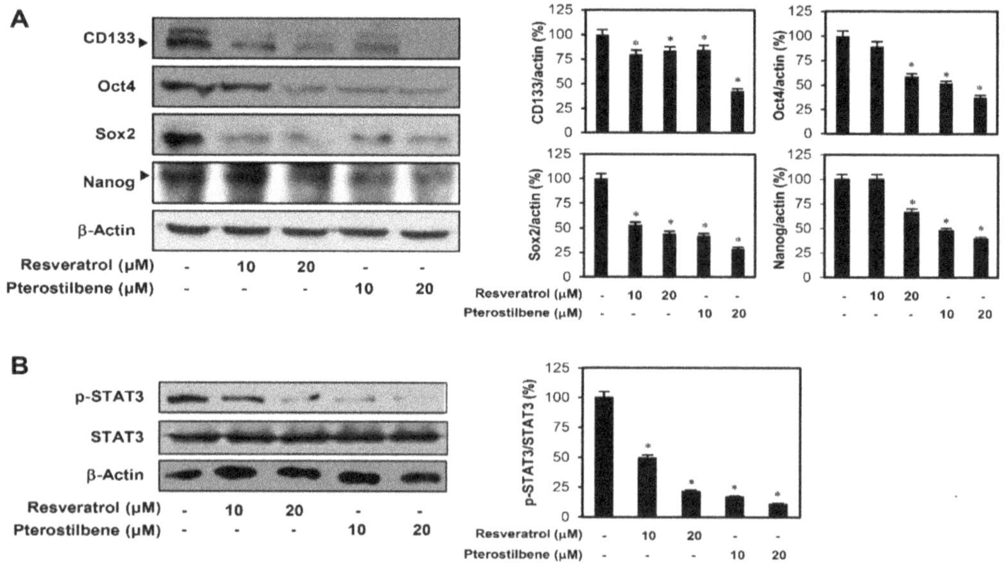

Figure 8. Effects of resveratrol and pterostilbene on stemness markers and signal transducer and activator of transcription 3 (STAT3) signaling in cervical CSCs. (**A**,**B**) HeLa cancer stem-like cells were treated with resveratrol and pterostilbene (10 and 20 μM) for 48 h, and the protein levels were detected by Western blot analysis using specific antibodies. The levels of β-actin were used as an internal control. Arrowheads indicate true bands for the molecular markers. * $p < 0.05$ versus the control.

The STAT3 pathway is involved in the maintenance of cervical CSCs by regulating the expression of stem cell-related transcription factors [29,30]. To further understand the molecular mechanism underlying the anticancer effects of resveratrol and pterostilbene against cervical CSCs, we investigated whether the two compounds affect STAT3 signaling. Our results confirmed that the compounds significantly decreased the expression levels of phosphorylated STAT3, without inhibiting the total protein levels of STAT3 in HeLa cancer stem-like cells (Figure 8B). Furthermore, pterostilbene more profoundly inhibited the phosphorylation of STAT3 than resveratrol. These results demonstrate that pterostilbene is more effective in suppressing the stem-like properties of cervical cancer cells than resveratrol through stronger downregulation of specific CSC markers and STAT3 signaling.

3. Discussion

The health beneficial effects of stilbene, a class of natural polyphenolic compounds, have been extensively studied in the past several decades [10,11]. Resveratrol and pterostilbene, the most widely known stilbenes, have gained increasing attention due to their roles in the potential prevention of major non-infectious chronic diseases such as cancer, cardiovascular disease, diabetes, and neurological degeneration [12–14]. Although both resveratrol and pterostilbene possess the therapeutic activities to inhibit various mechanisms for these human diseases, the bioavailability of pterostilbene with two methoxy groups is higher than resveratrol with two hydroxyl groups [12]. According to several studies, resveratrol and pterostilbene exhibit bioavailability at approximately 20% and 80% in vivo, respectively [31,32]. Such structural differences between the two compounds are expected to make pterostilbene more easily absorbed by oral ingestion through the promotion of lipophilicity and membrane permeability, compared with resveratrol.

The superior anticancer effects of pterostilbene have been reported in various tumors including lung, colon, breast, and cervical cancers [13]. Pterostilbene effectively suppressed cancer progression and metastasis by regulating apoptosis-dependent and apoptosis-independent signaling pathways. Accumulating evidence has shown that the anticancer effects of pterostilbene against cervical cancer are associated with the induction of apoptosis by activating the endoplasmic reticulum (ER)/nuclear factor erythroid 2-related factor 2 (Nrf2) pathway and downregulating the HPV oncoprotein E6 that causes the degradation of tumor suppressor protein p53 [17,33].

In the current study, we thoroughly investigated the cellular mechanisms responsible for the improved anticancer effects of pterostilbene compared to resveratrol in cervical cancer. Our results revealed that the superior growth and migration inhibitory effects of pterostilbene than resveratrol in HeLa cervical cancer cells could be attributed to the following reasons: the enhanced activation of multiple mechanisms, including cell cycle arrest at S and G2/M phases through the reduction of cyclin E1 and cyclin B1 expression following the induction of p53 and its downstream target p21; apoptosis through the activation of caspase-3 and caspase-9 mediated by ROS, as well as the downregulation of antiapoptotic proteins such as Bcl-2 and Bcl-XL; and the inhibition of MMP-2 and MMP-9 expression.

In addition, this is the first study to investigate the suppressive activities of pterostilbene and resveratrol against cervical cancer stemness. The critical role of CSCs in cancer progression and metastasis has already been identified and validated in many studies [4,5,22,23]. Notably, CSCs display resistance to many types of therapies, which results in cancer recurrence. Thus, it is important to suppress the self-renewal, proliferation, and metastasis abilities of CSCs for more reliable cancer treatment. In several cancers, the therapeutic effects of pterostilbene to eradicate CSCs have been confirmed. Pterostilbene inhibits the tumorsphere formation, migration, and stemness-related gene expression of CD133+ CSCs by downregulating multifaceted oncoprotein (MUC1), NF-κB, and Wnt/β-catenin-dependent signaling pathways in lung, breast, brain, and liver tumors [34–38]. However, the inhibitory effect of pterostilbene against cervical CSCs has not been studied previously.

In this study, pterostilbene significantly suppressed both the tumorsphere-forming ability and migration of HeLa cancer stem-like cells. Particularly, the therapeutic potential of pterostilbene to suppress cervical CSCs was markedly stronger than resveratrol. A tumorsphere is a solid, spherical structure developed from the proliferation of the cancer stem/progenitor cells. In these results, pterostilbene showed a better capacity for inducing cell cycle arrest and apoptosis of cervical CSCs in comparison with resveratrol. Therefore, the cell cycle arrest and apoptosis promoting effect of pterostilbene compared to resveratrol led to a stronger inhibition in the tumorsphere formation of HeLa cancer stem-like cells.

The stemness supporting transcription factors, such as Sox2, Klf4, c-Myc, Oct4, and Nanog, are upregulated in various types of CSCs [22,23,26–28]. Our results demonstrated that pterostilbene effectively decreased the expression levels of the major stemness transcription factors, including Sox2, Oct4, and Nanog, as well as a cell surface marker for CSCs, CD133, suggesting that the inhibitory effect of pterostilbene against cervical CSCs may be associated with the downregulation of these stemness regulators. In addition, pterostilbene more markedly suppressed the expression of stemness markers than resveratrol.

STAT3 is a transcription factor that is activated in many cancer types and can regulate pathways involving cell proliferation, cell survival, angiogenesis, and tumorigenesis [39]. Recent studies have revealed that STAT3 is an important regulator for self-renewal and survival of CSCs in various tumors [40]. In cervical carcinoma, STAT3 upregulates the stem-like characteristics of cervical cancer cells by increasing the expression of the stemness supporting markers such as Sox2, Oct4, and Nanog [29,30]. Therefore, targeting STAT3 signaling may be a promising approach to combat the survival of cervical CSCs. In the present study, pterostilbene resulted in a reduction in the expression levels of phosphorylated STAT3, without affecting the total protein levels of STAT3 in HeLa cancer stem-like cells. Furthermore, pterostilbene was more effective in suppressing the phosphorylation of STAT3 than resveratrol.

Our results collectively demonstrate that pterostilbene can suppress the stem-like properties of cervical cancer cells by downregulating specific CSC markers and STAT3 signaling. Thus, pterostilbene might serve as a potential anticancer agent for more effectively eradicating cervical cancer by targeting both cancer cells and CSCs, with superior bioavailability compared to resveratrol. However, the precise mechanism underlying how pterostilbene modulates the phosphorylation of STAT3 remains unclear. It is well known that STAT3 is phosphorylated by various protein kinases, including epidermal growth factor receptor (EGFR), Janus kinases (JAK), and Src family kinases (SFKs) [41]. Accumulating evidence has revealed that pterostilbene and resveratrol can induce cell cycle arrest and apoptosis by inhibiting the upstream kinase activities of STAT3 signaling in several cancers such as breast, pancreatic, prostate, and bone tumors [42–45]. Further studies to understand the mechanism of action of pterostilbene against cervical CSCs will help the discovery of the upstream cellular mediators of STAT3 activity regulated by pterostilbene. Moreover, further in vivo experiments using tumor xenograft animal models will be required to better verify the therapeutic potential of pterostilbene for cervical cancer compared to resveratrol.

4. Materials and Methods

4.1. Materials

Resveratrol and pterostilbene were purchased from Sigma-Aldrich (Saint Louis, MO, USA) and dissolved in dimethyl sulfoxide (DMSO) at a concentration of 100 mM to prepare a stock solution. Matrigel and gelatin were obtained from BD Biosciences (San Jose, CA, USA). Laminin and the Transwell chamber system were obtained from Koma Biotech (Seoul, Korea) and Corning Costar (Acton, MA, USA), respectively. Antibodies against p21, p53, MMP-2, MMP-9, Bcl-2, Bcl-XL, cleaved caspase-3, cleaved caspase-9, cyclin E1, cyclin B1, STAT3, phospho-STAT3, Sox2, Oct4, Nanog, β-actin, rabbit IgG, and mouse IgG were purchased from Cell Signaling Technology (Danvers, MA, USA). Anti-CD133 antibody was obtained from MiltenyiBiotec GmbH (BergischGladbach, Germany).

4.2. Cell Culture

Human cervical cancer HeLa, CaSki, and SiHa cell lines were obtained from the Korean Cell Line Bank (KCLB). The cells were cultured in Dulbecco's modified Eagle medium (DMEM; Gibco, Grand Island, NY, USA) supplemented with 10% fetal bovine serum (FBS; Gibco) and 1% penicillin–streptomycin–amphotericin B (Lonza, Walkersville, MD, USA) and then maintained at 37 °C in a 5% CO_2 humidified incubator.

4.3. Cell Growth Assay

HeLa, CaSki, and SiHa cells (3×10^3 cells/well) were seeded in a 96-well culture plate and then treated with various concentrations of resveratrol and pterostilbene (0–200 μM) for 72 h. Cell growth was measured with the 3-(4,5-dimethylthiazol-2-yl)-2,5-diphenyltetrazolium bromide (MTT) colorimetric assay (Sigma-Aldrich). The absorbance of each well was determined at a wavelength of 540 nm using a microplate reader (Thermo Fisher Scientific, Vantaa, Finland). The IC_{50} values from obtained data were analyzed using the curve-fitting program GraphPad Prism 5 (GraphPad Software, La Jolla, CA, USA).

4.4. Colony Formation Assay

To evaluate the colony forming inhibitory effects of resveratrol and pterostilbene, HeLa, CaSki, and SiHa cells (2.5×10^2 cells/well) were seeded in a six-well culture plate. After 24 h incubation, the cells were treated with resveratrol and pterostilbene (10 and 20 μM) and incubated for 7 days until colonies were formed. Following this, the colonies were fixed with 4% formaldehyde and stained with 0.5% crystal violet solution for 10 min and washed with double-distilled water. The number of colonies on each well was counted and the percentage of compound-treated colonies relative to DMSO-treated control colonies was calculated.

4.5. Wound Healing Assay

HeLa cells (2.5×10^5 cells/well) were seeded in a 24-well culture plate. The confluent monolayer cells were scratched using a tip and each well was washed with PBS to remove non-adherent cells. The cells were treated with resveratrol and pterostilbene (20 μM) and then incubated for up to 48 h. The perimeter of the central cell-free zone was observed under an optical microscope (Olympus, Center Valley, PA, USA).

4.6. Invasion Assay

The invasiveness of cells was examined using Transwell chamber inserts with a pore size of 8.0 μm. The lower surface of the polycarbonate filter was coated with 10 μL of gelatin (1 mg/mL), while the upper surface was coated with 10 μL of Matrigel (3 mg/mL). HeLa cells (5×10^4 cells/well) were seeded in the upper chamber of the filter; resveratrol and pterostilbene (10 and 20 μM) were added to the lower chamber filled with medium. The chamber was incubated at 37 °C for 48 h, and then the cells were fixed with 70% methanol and stained with hematoxylin and eosin (H and E). The total number of cells that invaded the lower chamber of the filter was counted using an optical microscope (Olympus).

4.7. Cell Cycle Analysis

The cell cycle distribution was analyzed using the Muse Cell Cycle Assay Kit (Millipore, Hayward, CA, USA) according to the manufacturer's instructions. To this end, HeLa cells (5×10^5 cells/dish) were seeded in a 60-mm culture dish and treated with resveratrol and pterostilbene for 48 h. The cells were collected by centrifugation and washed using PBS and fixed in ice cold 70% ethanol at −20 °C for more than 3 h. The cells were then incubated with the Muse Cell Cycle reagent for 30 min at room temperature in the dark. The cell cycle analysis was carried out using the Muse Cell Analyzer (Millipore).

4.8. Apoptosis Analysis

The apoptotic cell distribution was determined using the Muse Annexin V and Dead Cell Kit (Millipore) according to the manufacturer's instructions. Briefly, after treatment with resveratrol and pterostilbene, HeLa cells were collected and diluted with PBS containing 1% bovine serum albumin (BSA) as a dilution buffer to a concentration of 5×10^5 cells/mL. The single cell suspension was mixed with the Muse Annexin V/Dead Cell reagent at a 1:1 ratio and incubated in the dark for 20 min at room temperature. The cells were then analyzed using the Muse Cell Analyzer (Millipore).

4.9. Reactive Oxygen Species (ROS) Measurement

Intracellular ROS levels were measured using a ROS-sensitive fluorescence indicator, 2′,7′-dichlorofluorescein diacetate (DCFH-DA; Sigma-Aldrich). HeLa cells (1×10^5 cells/well) were seeded in a 96-black well culture plate and treated with resveratrol and pterostilbene (20 and 40 μM) for 48 h. The cells were then incubated with 10 μM of DCFH-DA for 20 min and washed with PBS. The fluorescence intensity of DCF was detected using a multimode microplate reader (Biotek, Inc., Winooski, VT, USA) at the excitation and emission wavelengths of 495 and 529 nm, respectively. The fluorescent images were also acquired using an Optinity KI-2000F fluorescence microscope (Korea Lab Tech, Seong Nam, Korea).

4.10. Western Blot Analysis

Cells were lysed using RIPA buffer (Sigma-Aldrich) supplemented with a protease inhibitor cocktail (Roche Diagnostics, Mannheim, Germany) on ice. Protein concentrations of the extracts were determined using a BCA Protein Assay kit (Pierce; Thermo Fisher Scientific, Inc., Waltham, MA, USA). Equal amounts of cell lysate were separated by 10% sodium dodecyl sulfate-polyacrylamide gel electrophoresis (SDS-PAGE), and the separated proteins were transferred to polyvinylidene difluoride (PVDF) membranes (EMD Millipore) using standard electroblotting procedures. The blots were blocked in Tris-buffered saline with Tween-20 (TBST) containing 5% skim milk at room temperature for 1 h and immunolabeled with primary antibodies against p21, p53, MMP-2, MMP-9, Bcl-2, Bcl-XL, cleaved caspase-3, cleaved caspase-9, cyclin E1, cyclin B1, STAT3, phospho-STAT3, Sox2, Oct4, Nanog, CD133 (dilution 1:2000), and β-actin (dilution 1:10000) overnight at 4 °C. After washing with TBST three times, the membranes were incubated with horseradish peroxidase-conjugated anti-rabbit or anti-mouse (dilution 1:3000) secondary antibody for 1 h at room temperature. Immunolabeling was detected with an enhanced chemiluminescence (ECL) kit (Bio-Rad Laboratories, Inc., Hercules, CA, USA) according to the manufacturer's instructions. The band density was analyzed using ImageJ software (version 1.5; NIH).

4.11. CSC Culture

CSCs were cultured using a non-adhesive culture method [24,25]. To propagate cervical cancer stem-like cells, HeLa cells grown in the serum-based media were cultured in Dulbecco's modified Eagle medium/nutrient mixture F-12 (DMEM/F12; Gibco) containing 1× B-27 serum-free supplement (Gibco), 5 μg/mL heparin (Sigma-Aldrich), 2 mM L-glutamine (Gibco), 20 ng/mL epidermal growth factor (EGF; Gibco), 20 ng/mL basic fibroblast growth factor (bFGF; Gibco), and 1% penicillin/streptomycin (Gibco). Tumorspheres grown in the serum-free media were subcultured every 7 days by dissociating with Accutase (Millipore) and maintained at 37 °C in a 5% CO_2 humidified incubator.

4.12. CSC Tumorsphere Formation Assay

HeLa cancer stem-like cells were seeded in a 96-well culture plate at a density of 500 cells/well using the serum-free media with EGF and bFGF. After 8 days of resveratrol and pterostilbene treatment (10 and 20 μM), the number of tumorspheres formed in each well was counted under an optical microscope (Olympus).

4.13. CSC Migration Assay

For the CSC migration assay, the ibidi culture inserts (IBIDI GmbH, Martinsried, Germany) were placed in a laminin-coated 24-well culture plate. HeLa cancer stem-like cells were prepared at a density of 5×10^5 cells/mL, of which 70 μL was transferred to each chamber. After cell attachment for 24 h, the culture inserts were removed, and the attached cells were incubated with the serum-free media containing EGF and bFGF, in the absence or presence of resveratrol and pterostilbene (10 and 20 μM) for 24 h. The perimeter of the central cell-free zone was confirmed under an optical microscope (Olympus).

4.14. Statistical Analysis

The data were presented as the mean ± standard error (SE) of three independent experiments. Student's *t*-test was used to determine statistical significance between the control and the test groups. A *p*-value of <0.05 was considered to indicate a statistically significant difference.

5. Conclusions

The present study focused on the therapeutic effect and mechanism underlying the anticancer effects of pterostilbene against both cancer cells and cancer stem-like cells in cervical cancer compared to resveratrol. Our results demonstrated that the superior inhibitory effects of pterostilbene compared to resveratrol were associated with the enhanced activation of multiple mechanisms, including cell cycle arrest at S and G2/M phases through the induction of p53 and p21 and subsequent reduction of cyclin E1 and cyclin B1; apoptosis through the activation of caspase-3 and -9 mediated by ROS and the downregulation of Bcl-2 and Bcl-XL antiapoptotic proteins; and the inhibition of MMP-2 and -9 expression. Notably, pterostilbene exhibited a greater inhibitory effect against HeLa cancer stem-like cells than resveratrol through more potent inhibition of the expression levels of stemness markers, such as CD133, Oct4, Sox2, and Nanog, as well as STAT3 signaling. Based on these findings, we conclude that pterostilbene is a better potential candidate than resveratrol for more effectively treating cervical carcinoma.

Author Contributions: H.J.J. conceived and designed the experiments; H.J.S., J.M.H. and Y.S.C. performed the experiments and analyzed the data; H.J.S. and H.J.J. wrote the paper. All authors have read and agreed to the published version of the manuscript.

References

1. Torre, L.A.; Bray, F.; Siegel, R.L.; Ferlay, J.; Lortet-Tieulent, J.; Jemal, A. Global cancer statistics, 2012. *CA Cancer J. Clin.* **2015**, *65*, 87–108. [CrossRef]
2. Schiffman, M.; Castle, P.E.; Jeronimo, J.; Rodriguez, A.C.; Wacholder, S. Human papillomavirus and cervical cancer. *Lancet* **2007**, *370*, 890–907. [CrossRef]
3. Liontos, M.; Kyriazoglou, A.; Dimitriadis, I.; Dimopoulos, M.A.; Bamias, A. Systemic therapy in cervical cancer: 30 years in review. *Crit. Rev. Oncol. Hematol.* **2019**, *137*, 9–17. [CrossRef]
4. Ortiz-Sánchez, E.; Santiago-López, L.; Cruz-Domínguez, V.B.; Toledo-Guzmán, M.E.; Hernández-Cueto, D.; Muñiz-Hernández, S.; Garrido, E.; Cantú De León, D.; García-Carrancá, A. Characterization of cervical cancer stem cell-like cells: Phenotyping, stemness, and human papilloma virus co-receptor expression. *Oncotarget* **2016**, *7*, 31943–31954. [CrossRef]
5. Huang, R.; Rofstad, E.K. Cancer stem cells (CSCs), cervical CSCs and targeted therapies. *Oncotarget* **2017**, *8*, 35351–35367. [CrossRef]
6. Tyagi, A.; Vishnoi, K.; Mahata, S.; Verma, G.; Srivastava, Y.; Masaldan, S.; Roy, B.G.; Bharti, A.C.; Das, B.C. Cervical cancer stem cells selectively overexpress HPV oncoprotein E6 that controls stemness and self-renewal through upregulation of HES1. *Clin. Cancer Res.* **2016**, *22*, 4170–4184. [CrossRef] [PubMed]
7. Organista-Nava, J.; Gómez-Gómez, Y.; Ocadiz-Delgado, R.; García-Villa, E.; Bonilla-Delgado, J.; Lagunas-Martínez, A.; Tapia, J.S.; Lambert, P.F.; García-Carrancá, A.; Gariglio, P. The HPV16 E7 oncoprotein increases the expression of Oct3/4 and stemness-related genes and augments cell self-renewal. *Virology* **2016**, *499*, 230–242. [CrossRef]
8. Cragg, G.M.; Newman, D.J. Plants as a source of anti-cancer agents. *J. Ethnopharmacol.* **2005**, *100*, 72–79. [CrossRef] [PubMed]
9. Yin, S.Y.; Wei, W.C.; Jian, F.Y.; Yang, N.S. Therapeutic applications of herbal medicines for cancer patients. *Evid. Based Complement. Alternat. Med.* **2013**, *2013*, 302426. [CrossRef] [PubMed]

10. Chong, J.; Poutaraud, A.; Hugueney, P. Metabolism and roles of stilbenes in plants. *Plant Sci.* **2009**, *177*, 143–155. [CrossRef]
11. Akinwumi, B.C.; Bordun, K.M.; Anderson, H.D. Biological activities of stilbenoids. *Int. J. Mol. Sci.* **2018**, *19*, 792. [CrossRef]
12. Tsai, H.Y.; Ho, C.T.; Chen, Y.K. Biological actions and molecular effects of resveratrol, pterostilbene, and 3′-hydroxypterostilbene. *J. Food Drug Anal.* **2017**, *25*, 134–147. [CrossRef]
13. Chen, R.J.; Kuo, H.C.; Cheng, L.H.; Lee, Y.H.; Chang, W.T.; Wang, B.J.; Wang, Y.J.; Cheng, H.C. Apoptotic and nonapoptotic activities of pterostilbene against cancer. *Int. J. Mol. Sci.* **2018**, *19*, 287. [CrossRef]
14. Xiao, Q.; Zhu, W.; Feng, W.; Lee, S.S.; Leung, A.W.; Shen, J.; Gao, L.; Xu, C. A review of resveratrol as a potent chemoprotective and synergistic agent in cancer chemotherapy. *Front. Pharmacol.* **2019**, *9*, 1534. [CrossRef] [PubMed]
15. Asensi, M.; Medina, I.; Ortega, A.; Carretero, J.; Baño, M.C.; Obrador, E.; Estrela, J.M. Inhibition of cancer growth by resveratrol is related to its low bioavailability. *Free Radic. Biol. Med.* **2002**, *33*, 387–398. [CrossRef]
16. Nutakul, W.; Sobers, H.S.; Qiu, P.; Dong, P.; Decker, E.A.; McClements, D.J.; Xiao, H. Inhibitory effects of resveratrol and pterostilbene on human colon cancer cells: A side-by-side comparison. *J. Agric. Food Chem.* **2011**, *59*, 10964–10970. [CrossRef] [PubMed]
17. Chatterjee, K.; AlSharif, D.; Mazza, C.; Syar, P.; Al Sharif, M.; Fata, J.E. Resveratrol and pterostilbene exhibit anticancer properties involving the downregulation of HPV oncoprotein E6 in cervical cancer cells. *Nutrients* **2018**, *10*, 243. [CrossRef] [PubMed]
18. Libra, M.; Scalisi, A.; Vella, N.; Clementi, S.; Sorio, R.; Stivala, F.; Spandidos, D.A.; Mazzarino, C. Uterine cervical carcinoma: Role of matrix metalloproteinases (review). *Int. J. Oncol.* **2009**, *34*, 897–903. [CrossRef]
19. Wu, G.; Lin, N.; Xu, L.; Liu, B.; Feitelson, M.A. UCN-01 induces S and G2/M cell cycle arrest through the p53/p21(waf1) or CHK2/CDC25C pathways and can suppress invasion in human hepatoma cell lines. *BMC Cancer* **2013**, *13*, 167. [CrossRef]
20. Redza-Dutordoir, M.; Averill-Bates, D.A. Activation of apoptosis signalling pathways by reactive oxygen species. *Biochim. Biophys. Acta* **2016**, *1863*, 2977–2992. [CrossRef]
21. Wu, P.P.; Chung, H.W.; Liu, K.C.; Wu, R.S.; Yang, J.S.; Tang, N.Y.; Lo, C.; Hsia, T.C.; Yu, C.C.; Chueh, F.S.; et al. Diallyl sulfide induces cell cycle arrest and apoptosis in HeLa human cervical cancer cells through the p53, caspase- and mitochondria-dependent pathways. *Int. J. Oncol.* **2011**, *38*, 1605–1613. [PubMed]
22. Reya, T.; Morrison, S.J.; Clarke, M.F.; Weissman, I.L. Stem cells, cancer, and cancer stem cells. *Nature* **2001**, *414*, 105–111. [CrossRef]
23. Jordan, C.T.; Guzman, M.L.; Noble, M. Cancer stem cells. *N. Engl. J. Med.* **2006**, *355*, 1253–1261. [CrossRef]
24. Cao, H.Z.; Liu, X.F.; Yang, W.T.; Chen, Q.; Zheng, P.S. LGR5 promotes cancer stem cell traits and chemoresistance in cervical cancer. *Cell Death Dis.* **2017**, *8*, e3039. [CrossRef]
25. Kim, B.; Jung, N.; Lee, S.; Sohng, J.K.; Jung, H.J. Apigenin inhibits cancer stem cell-like phenotypes in human glioblastoma cells via suppression of c-Met signaling. *Phytother. Res.* **2016**, *30*, 1833–1840. [CrossRef] [PubMed]
26. Yao, T.; Lu, R.; Zhang, Y.; Zhang, Y.; Zhao, C.; Lin, R.; Lin, Z. Cervical cancer stem cells. *Cell Prolif.* **2015**, *48*, 611–625. [CrossRef] [PubMed]
27. Li, Z. CD133: A stem cell biomarker and beyond. *Exp. Hematol. Oncol.* **2013**, *2*, 17. [CrossRef]
28. Bigoni-Ordóñez, G.D.; Ortiz-Sánchez, E.; Rosendo-Chalma, P.; Valencia-González, H.A.; Aceves, C.; García-Carrancá, A. Molecular iodine inhibits the expression of stemness markers on cancer stem-like cells of established cell lines derived from cervical cancer. *BMC Cancer* **2018**, *18*, 928. [CrossRef]
29. Wang, H.; Cai, H.B.; Chen, L.L.; Zhao, W.J.; Li, P.; Wang, Z.Q.; Li, Z. STAT3 correlates with stem cell-related transcription factors in cervical cancer. *J. Huazhong Univ. Sci. Technol.* **2015**, *35*, 891–897. [CrossRef]
30. Wang, H.; Deng, J.; Ren, H.Y.; Jia, P.; Zhang, W.; Li, M.Q.; Li, S.W.; Zhou, Q.H. STAT3 influences the characteristics of stem cells in cervical carcinoma. *Oncol. Lett.* **2017**, *14*, 2131–2136. [CrossRef]
31. Kapetanovic, I.M.; Muzzio, M.; Huang, Z.; Thompson, T.N.; McCormick, D.L. Pharmacokinetics, oral bioavailability, and metabolic profile of resveratrol and its dimethylether analog, pterostilbene, in rats. *Cancer Chemother. Pharmacol.* **2011**, *68*, 593–601. [CrossRef]
32. Francioso, A.; Mastromarino, P.; Masci, A.; d'Erme, M.; Mosca, L. Chemistry, stability and bioavailability of resveratrol. *Med. Chem.* **2014**, *10*, 237–245. [CrossRef] [PubMed]
33. Zhang, B.; Wang, X.Q.; Chen, H.Y.; Liu, B.H. Involvement of the Nrf2 pathway in the regulation of pterostilbene-induced apoptosis in HeLa cells via ER stress. *J. Pharmacol. Sci.* **2014**, *126*, 216–229. [CrossRef]

34. Mak, K.K.; Wu, A.T.; Lee, W.H.; Chang, T.C.; Chiou, J.F.; Wang, L.S.; Wu, C.H.; Huang, C.Y.; Shieh, Y.S.; Chao, T.Y.; et al. Pterostilbene, a bioactive component of blueberries, suppresses the generation of breast cancer stem cells within tumor microenvironment and metastasis via modulating NF-κB/microRNA 448 circuit. *Mol. Nutr. Food Res.* **2013**, *57*, 1123–1134. [CrossRef]
35. Huang, W.C.; Chan, M.L.; Chen, M.J.; Tsai, T.H.; Chen, Y.J. Modulation of macrophage polarization and lung cancer cell stemness by MUC1 and development of a related small-molecule inhibitor pterostilbene. *Oncotarget* **2016**, *7*, 39363–39375. [CrossRef] [PubMed]
36. Huynh, T.T.; Lin, C.M.; Lee, W.H.; Wu, A.T.; Lin, Y.K.; Lin, Y.F.; Yeh, C.T.; Wang, L.S. Pterostilbene suppressed irradiation-resistant glioma stem cells by modulating GRP78/miR-205 axis. *J. Nutr. Biochem.* **2015**, *26*, 466–475. [CrossRef] [PubMed]
37. Lee, C.M.; Su, Y.H.; Huynh, T.T.; Lee, W.H.; Chiou, J.F.; Lin, Y.K.; Hsiao, M.; Wu, C.H.; Lin, Y.F.; Wu, A.T.; et al. Blueberry isolate, pterostilbene, functions as a potential anticancer stem cell agent in suppressing irradiation-mediated enrichment of hepatoma stem cells. *Evid. Based Complement. Alternat. Med.* **2013**, *2013*, 258425. [CrossRef] [PubMed]
38. Paul, S.; DeCastro, A.J.; Lee, H.J.; Smolarek, A.K.; So, J.Y.; Simi, B.; Wang, C.X.; Zhou, R.; Rimando, A.M.; Suh, N. Dietary intake of pterostilbene, a constituent of blueberries, inhibits the beta-catenin/p65 downstream signaling pathway and colon carcinogenesis in rats. *Carcinogenesis* **2010**, *31*, 1272–1278. [CrossRef]
39. Chai, E.Z.; Shanmugam, M.K.; Arfuso, F.; Dharmarajan, A.; Wang, C.; Kumar, A.P.; Samy, R.P.; Lim, L.H.; Wang, L.; Goh, B.C.; et al. Targeting transcription factor STAT3 for cancer prevention and therapy. *Pharmacol. Ther.* **2016**, *162*, 86–97. [CrossRef]
40. Galoczova, M.; Coates, P.; Vojtesek, B. STAT3, stem cells, cancer stem cells and p63. *Cell. Mol. Biol. Lett.* **2018**, *23*, 12. [CrossRef]
41. Bromberg, J., Jr.; Darnell, J.E. The role of STATs in transcriptional control and their impact on cellular function. *Oncogene* **2000**, *19*, 2468–2473. [CrossRef]
42. Kotha, A.; Sekharam, M.; Cilenti, L.; Siddiquee, K.; Khaled, A.; Zervos, A.S.; Carter, B.; Turkson, J.; Jove, R. Resveratrol inhibits Src and Stat3 signaling and induces the apoptosis of malignant cells containing activated Stat3 protein. *Mol. Cancer Ther.* **2006**, *5*, 621–629. [CrossRef] [PubMed]
43. McCormack, D.; Schneider, J.; McDonald, D.; McFadden, D. The antiproliferative effects of pterostilbene on breast cancer in vitro are via inhibition of constitutive and leptin-induced Janus kinase/signal transducer and activator of transcription activation. *Am. J. Surg.* **2011**, *202*, 541–544. [CrossRef]
44. Liu, Y.; Wang, L.; Wu, Y.; Lv, C.; Li, X.; Cao, X.; Yang, M.; Feng, D.; Luo, Z. Pterostilbene exerts antitumor activity against human osteosarcoma cells by inhibiting the JAK2/STAT3 signaling pathway. *Toxicology* **2013**, *304*, 120–131. [CrossRef] [PubMed]
45. Chen, R.J.; Tsai, S.J.; Ho, C.T.; Pan, M.H.; Ho, Y.S.; Wu, C.H.; Wang, Y.J. Chemopreventive effects of pterostilbene on urethane-induced lung carcinogenesis in mice via the inhibition of EGFR-mediated pathways and the induction of apoptosis and autophagy. *J. Agric. Food Chem.* **2012**, *60*, 11533–11541. [CrossRef] [PubMed]

8

Characterization of a Reservoir-Style Implant for Sustained Release of Tenofovir Alafenamide (TAF) for HIV Pre-Exposure Prophylaxis (PrEP)

Leah M. Johnson [1,*], Sai Archana Krovi [1], Linying Li [1], Natalie Girouard [1], Zach R. Demkovich [2], Daniel Myers [3], Ben Creelman [3] and Ariane van der Straten [2]

[1] Engineered Systems, RTI International, 3040 E. Cornwallis Road, Research Triangle Park, NC 27709, USA
[2] Women's Global Health Imperative, RTI International, 351 California Street, Suite 500, San Francisco, CA 94104, USA
[3] PATH, 2201 Westlake Ave, Suite 200, Seattle, WA 98121, USA
[*] Correspondence: leahjohnson@rti.org

Abstract: Long-acting (LA) HIV pre-exposure prophylaxis (PrEP) offers the potential to improve adherence by lowering the burden of daily or on-demand regimens of antiretroviral (ARV) drugs. This paper details the fabrication and in vitro performance of a subcutaneous and trocar-compatible implant for the LA delivery of tenofovir alafenamide (TAF). The reservoir-style implant comprises an extruded tube of a biodegradable polymer, poly(ε-caprolactone) (PCL), filled with a formulation of TAF and castor oil excipient. Parameters that affect the daily release rates of TAF are described, including the surface area of the implant, the thickness of the PCL tube walls (between 45 and 200 μm), and the properties of the PCL (e.g., crystallinity). In vitro studies show a linear relationship between daily release rates and surface area, demonstrating a membrane-controlled release mechanism from extruded PCL tubes. Release rates of TAF from the implant are inversely proportional to the wall thickness, with release rates between approximately 0.91 and 0.15 mg/day for 45 and 200 μm, respectively. The sustained release of TAF at 0.28 ± 0.06 mg/day over the course of 180 days in vitro was achieved. Progress in the development of this implant platform addresses the need for new biomedical approaches to the LA delivery of ARV drugs.

Keywords: poly(ε-caprolactone) (PCL); tenofovir alafenamide (TAF); pre-exposure prophylaxis (PrEP); long-acting drug delivery systems; implant

1. Introduction

HIV pre-exposure prophylaxis (PrEP) with antiretroviral (ARV) drugs is promising among the biomedical strategies to address the global HIV epidemic. Tenofovir-based PrEP has demonstrated landmark successes with daily [1–4] and on-demand dosing [3,5] in men who have sex with men (MSM) and transgender women (TGW). Despite these advancements, adherence to time- or event-driven regimens for PrEP remains an incessant struggle [6–11]. The long-acting (LA) delivery of ARV drugs simplifies traditional dosing regimens for PrEP by alleviating the emotional and logistical burden of user-dependent methods. For example, a LA-injectable formulation of the integrase inhibitor, cabotegravir (CAB), is currently under investigation in a pair of phase two and three HIV PrEP trials [12,13]. Although injectable methods are acceptable to many users [14,15], and offer key advantages such as a bi-monthly dosing regimen and discretion, drawbacks do exist. Injectable formulations cannot be removed in the event of an adverse drug-related event and the potential exists for a long plasma "tail" of sub-therapeutic drug levels [16,17]. An alternative injectable formulation in preclinical development involves an in situ forming polymer depot for LA delivery of dolutegravir for HIV PrEP, which shows the capacity for removal within the period of drug delivery, if needed [18].

A promising biomedical approach for LA-PrEP involves implants that reside under the skin to continuously release the drug, which supports adherence over longer time periods, enables discretion of use, lowers the burden of the regimen, and remains reversible during the therapeutic duration. Polymeric implants can comprise different architectures that each have advantages for drug delivery [19–21]. Matrix-style implants contain a drug dispersed within a polymer that controls the rate of the drug exiting the implant. For example, an FDA-approved matrix-style implant for the six-month maintenance treatment of opioid addiction (Probuphine®) contains buprenorphine distributed through four individual poly(ethylene-vinyl acetate) (EVA) rods [22]. Reservoir-style implants involve a formulated drug core encapsulated by a polymeric barrier that control drug release rates. Notable examples of implants with a core-sheath configuration include the collection of subdermal contraceptive implants: Norplant and Jadelle [23,24] for the delivery of levonorgestrel (LNG) using a rod of silicone-based polymer, as well as Implanon [25] and Nexplanon [26] for the delivery of etonogestrel (ENG) using a rod of EVA-based polymer. The low dosages required for the subcutaneous delivery of hormonal contraceptives enable these implants to last multiple years. Implants also show utility for indications in ophthalmology, including intraocular implants for the delivery of ganciclovir for the treatment of cytomegalovirus retinitis (Vitrasert) [27], dexamethasone for the treatment of macular edema (Ozurdex) [28,29] and fluocinolone acetonide for the treatment of noninfectious posterior uveitis (Retisert) [30].

Several implants are currently under development for HIV PrEP, with each implant system holding unique configurations and features. A subdermal, silicone implant that delivers tenofovir alafenamide (TAF) from orthogonal channels coated with polyvinyl alcohol (PVA) showed 40-days of drug delivery in beagle dogs without observed adverse events [31]. A non-polymeric, refillable implant designed to deliver TAF and emtricitabine (FTC) from separate devices showed sustained levels of tenofovir diphosphate (TFV-DP) in peripheral blood mononuclear cells (PBMCs) over 83 days in rhesus macaques, but only 28 days for FTC-triphosphate (FTC-TP) due to the large dosing required and short plasma half-life [32]. Intarcia is developing a titanium osmotic pump system, called the Medici Drug Delivery System™, for PrEP and for type-2 diabetes [33]. A matrix-style PrEP implant for delivery of 4′-ethylnyl-2-fluoro-2′-dexoyadenosine (EFdA) has shown promising efficacy for HIV treatment and prevention, as demonstrated in animal models [34].

Concurrently with these other innovative technologies, RTI is developing a subcutaneous biodegradable implant for HIV PrEP as a single indication and as a multipurpose prevention technology (MPT) for HIV and pregnancy prevention [35,36]. The implant uses a semi-crystalline aliphatic polyester, poly(ε-caprolactone) (PCL), pioneered by Pitt et al. at RTI International in the 1980s [37] and largely neglected for nearly 20 years [38]. Renewed appeal for PCL has surfaced in light of biomedical applications, including tissue engineering [39,40] and drug delivery [41,42], that demand materials with long-term functionality, mechanical integrity, biocompatibility, and capacity for biodegradation and bioresorption. PCL is currently used in FDA-approved products for root canal fillings (Resilon) [43] and sutures (Monocryl) [44] and was previously explored for use as a 1-year contraceptive implant (Capronor) [45]. In terms of HIV PrEP, PCL implants can advantageously offer LA delivery of ARVs, while also enabling bioresorption at the end of the implant drug delivery period. An implant that is biodegradable could benefit health care systems by eliminating the need for a clinic visit to remove a depleted implant, whereby a minor surgical procedure would be required to remove the implant when discontinuing PrEP. In the case of the implant described in this paper, reversibility and retrievability can be maintained, potentially throughout the duration of treatment.

Herein, we report advancements to the fabrication and performance of a reservoir-style subcutaneous PCL implant for sustained release of TAF. We detail parameters that control release rates of TAF from the implant, including wall thickness and surface area, and further describe the effects of crystallinity on the performance of the implant. We demonstrate the fabrication and processing steps that align the implant with future manufacturing requirements, while keeping preferences of the end user in mind.

2. Materials and Methods

2.1. Implant Fabrication

PCL pellets were purchased in research-grade from Sigma Aldrich, referred to as "Sigma-PCL" throughout this paper (number average molecular weight (M_n) = 103 kDa, Cat# 440744, St. Louis, MO, USA) and in medical-grade from Corbion, referred to as "PC-12" throughout this paper (M_n = 51 kDa, PURASORB PC 12, Amsterdam, The Netherlands). PCL tubes were fabricated via a hot-melt, single screw extrusion process using solid PCL pellets at GenX Medical (Chattanooga, TN, USA). All tubes were 2.5 mm in outer diameter (OD) and had wall thicknesses of 45, 70, 100, 150 or 200 μm, as measured with a 3-axis laser measurement system and light microscopy at GenX Medical.

PCL tubes were first sealed at one end using two different approaches: impulse heat sealing and injection sealing. Implants fabricated with the impulse heat sealing were used for certain in vitro studies, such as the implants used in the surface area studies that comprised different lengths (e.g., 70 mm length), because they were too long to fit the injection sealing apparatus. Importantly, no significant differences in release rates were observed for TAF implants sealed with either approach. For the first approach, an impulse heat sealer (AIE-110T, American International Electric Sealer Supply, South El Monte, CA, USA) was used to clamp the tube flat and then apply a pulse of heat for a few seconds. The tubing was then allowed to cool for about 10 s. Thicker tubes were sealed with longer heat pulses. The sealing step fused the PCL tube wall together through melting and created a flat-shaped seal. The seal was trimmed with scissors to remove excess PCL. For the injection sealing, the PCL tube was marked and trimmed to the correct length to achieve an implant with a 40-mm paste length with 3 mm of headspace at both ends for sealing. The initial seal was then created on one end of the implant by placing the tube over a stainless steel rod that filled all the tube except for a 3 mm headspace at one end, placing a Teflon collar around the headspace to support the tube wall and injecting molten PCL into the cavity of the headspace. After the injected PCL was solidified, excess PCL was trimmed, and the collar was removed to form a cylindrical seal approximately 2 mm long that is compatible with commercial contraceptive trocars.

TAF was graciously provided by Gilead Sciences (Foster City, CA, USA). TAF was mixed with pharmaceutical grade, Super Refined™ Castor Oil (Croda, Cat# SR40890, Snaith, UK) at 2:1 mass ratio immediately prior to loading into the implant. The mixture was first ground with a mortar and pestle to create a smooth paste, and then back loaded into a 1 mL syringe fitted with a 14-gauge blunt tip needle. The TAF and castor oil paste was then extruded through the needle into the empty tube. Otherwise, the TAF formulation was loaded into the PCL tube using a modified spatula. After the filled formulation reached the 40-mm mark, the interior tube wall was cleaned with a rod and sealed in a similar manner to the first seal. After fabrication, all devices were weighed to determine the total payload and photographed with a ruler to record the final dimensions. Paste area was measured with ImageJ (Version 1.50e, NIH, Bethesda, MD, USA) and release rates were normalized to the surface area of a full-sized implant (2.5 mm OD, 40 mm in length), 314 mm^2. The end of the implants (i.e., end-seals) were not included in calculations of the implant surface area.

2.2. Device Sterilization

All implants were fabricated and handled under aseptic conditions using a biosafety cabinet. Certain devices were exposed to gamma irradiation, as indicated in the text. Devices exposed to gamma irradiation were first packed in amber glass vials and then irradiated with a dose range of 18–24 kGy at room temperature, using a Cobalt-60 gamma-ray source (Nordion Inc., Ottawa, Canada) at Steris (Mentor, OH, USA). Samples were exposed to the source on a continuous path for a period of 8 h.

2.3. *In Vitro Release Studies*

In vitro release characterization involved incubation of the implants in 40 mL 1X phosphate buffered saline (PBS) (pH 7.4) at 37 °C and placed on an orbital shaker. TAF species in the release media was measured by ultraviolet-visible (UV) spectroscopy at 260 nm using the Synergy MX multi-mode plate reader (BioTek Instruments, Inc, Winooski, VT, USA). The release buffer was sampled three times per week during which the devices were transferred to 40 mL of fresh buffer to maintain sink conditions. TAF quantity released in each PBS buffer during the time interval was calculated and cumulative mass of drug release as a function of time was determined.

2.4. *Stability Analysis of TAF Formulation*

The purity of TAF formulations inside the device reservoir was evaluated by opening a device, extracting the entire reservoir contents into an organic solution, and measuring TAF chromatographic purity using ultra performance liquid chromatography coupled with UV spectroscopy (UPLC/UV). The analysis was performed using a Waters BEH C18 column (2.1 mm × 50 mm, 1.7 µm) under gradient, reversed phase conditions with detection at 260 nm. For each device, one single aliquot was prepared and quantitated by linear regression analysis against a five-point calibration curve. TAF purity was calculated as % peak area associated with TAF relative to total peak area of TAF related degradation products (detected above the limit of detection (LOD) ≥ 0.05%). The TAF formulations within the implant were analyzed after exposure of the implant to a simulated physiological condition (i.e., 1X PBS, pH 7.4 at 37 °C) for up to 180 days.

2.5. *Characterization of PCL Extruded Tubes*

2.5.1. Differential Scanning Calorimetry (DSC)

The melting behavior of PCL samples was assessed with modulated differential scanning calorimetry (MDSC) (TA Instruments Q200, RCS90 cooling system, New Castle, DE, USA). Approximately 8 mg of extruded polymer tubing was placed in a Tzero™ Pan and sealed with a Tzero™ Lid and a dome-shaped die, resulting in a crimped seal. Samples were then placed in a nitrogen-purged DSC cell, cooled to 0 °C, then heated to 120 °C at a rate of 1 °C/min with an underlying heat-only modulation temperature scan of ± 0.13 °C every 60 s. The melting temperature (T_m) of the polymer was determined by the peak temperature of the melting endotherm, and the enthalpy associated with melting was determined by integrating linearly the area of the melt peak (between 25 and 65 °C) using the TA Universal Analysis software (version 4.5A, TA Instruments, New Castle, DE, USA). PCL samples did not exhibit exothermic peaks in the non-reversing heat flow signal indicating that PCL did not experience cold-crystallization during the melting process; therefore, the total heat flow curve was used to assess the mass % crystallinity. The mass % crystallinity was calculated using Equation (1), where X_c represents the mass fraction of crystalline domains in PCL, ΔH_m represents the enthalpy of melting measured by the DSC, and ΔH_{fus} represents the theoretical enthalpy of melting for 100% crystalline PCL, reported as 139.5 J/g [46,47].

$$X_C = \frac{\Delta H_m}{\Delta H_{fus}} \times 100 \tag{1}$$

The peak melting temperatures of polymers were used calculate crystallite sizes within the sample using the Thompson–Gibbs equation (Equation (2)) [48,49]:

$$L = \frac{2\sigma_e T_m^o}{\Delta H_m^o (T_m^o - T_m)} \tag{2}$$

where L is the crystallite size in nm, σ_e is the free energy of chain folds in mJ/m^2, T_m^o is the equilibrium melting temperature in K, T_m is the melting temperature measured by DSC in K, and ΔH_m^o is the enthalpy of fusion for 100% crystalline polymer in J/g. T_m^o and ΔH_m^o were taken from the ATHAS data bank as 342.2 K and 139.5 J/g, respectively. The free energy associated with chain folding was taken as 60 mJ/m^2 [50].

2.5.2. X-ray Diffraction (XRD)

The extruded PCL tubes at wall thickness of 100 μm were cryo-grinded in a freezer mill using liquid nitrogen. The material was ground for 1.5 min after cooling for three minutes before initiating the grinding cycle. The X-ray diffraction (XRD) patterns were acquired using a Bruker AXS, Inc D8 Advance model utilizing standard Bragg-Brentano geometry and a LynxEye XE-T high resolution detector (Bruker, Billerica, MA, USA). Samples were packed into a zero background sample holder and scanned at 40 kV and 40 mA power settings (1600 Watts) for a scan covering 5° to 70°, with a step size of 0.02° and a dwell time of 2 s per step. The MDI Jade version 9.6 software (MDI, Livermore, CA, USA) was used to analyze results and the 2019 International Center for Diffraction Data (ICDD) PDF 4+ database was used to search match crystalline phases present in the materials. The crystallite size was determined via the Scherrer equation (Equation (3)):

$$L = \frac{K\lambda}{\beta cos\theta} \tag{3}$$

where L = crystallite size, K = Scherrer constant (0.94 from literature [51,52]), λ = X-ray wavelength, β = full-width at half maximum of a crystallographic peak, and θ = Bragg angle.

2.5.3. Gel Permeation Chromatography (GPC)

The molecular weight of PCL was analyzed via GPC by first dissolving samples in tetrahydrofuran (THF) to 10 mg/mL injecting 40 μL of sample using an Agilent 1100/1200 HPLC-UV instrument (Santa Clara, CA, USA, flow rate of 1.0 mL/min). Polystyrene polymer standards (MWs of 2460 to 0.545 kDa) were used to calibrate the MW of samples.

2.5.4. Statistical Analysis

Where indicated, significance testing was performed with GraphPad Prism 7.00 (GraphPad Software, San Diego, CA, USA) using an unpaired, parametric, two tailed, t-test with a confidence level of 95%. Probability (p)-values ≤ 0.05 were considered statistically significant.

3. Results and Discussion

3.1. Tuning TAF Release Rates: Surface Area and Wall Thickness

These studies involve a reservoir-style PCL implant (Figure 1), that can deliver TAF at sustained, zero-order release kinetics. Once inserted subcutaneously, biological fluid from the surrounding environment transports through the PCL membrane into the reservoir and can solubilize TAF. TAF can partition into the PCL and transport passively through the PCL membrane to exit the implant. Transport of a drug through the PCL material is dictated by many parameters, such as the diffusion coefficient and partition coefficient, as described elsewhere [53]. As an aliphatic polyester, PCL undergoes bulk hydrolysis through random chain scission as water permeates through the polymer [37,54]. However, biodegradation of PCL is slow and can require years (e.g., 1–2 years) for complete bioresorption [37], depending on the starting MW. Because bulk erosion of PCL is slow, the faster process of drug delivery is decoupled from biodegradation, enabling zero-order release profiles of drug from the implant. At this zero-order release profile, the daily drug delivery rates are controlled by various parameters: surface area of the device, thickness of the device wall, polymer properties, and drug formulation. A digital camera image of RTI's trocar-compatible reservoir-style implant is shown in Figure 1.

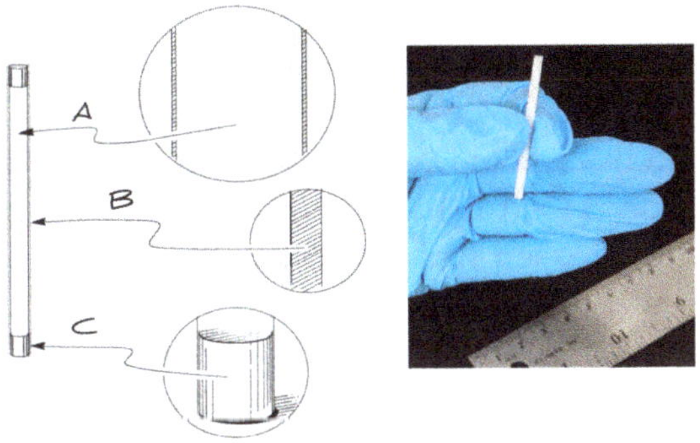

Figure 1. (Left) A schematic of a PCL reservoir-style device for delivery of TAF, which comprises a formulated drug core (A) encapsulated by a rate-controlling PCL membrane (B). The device is end-sealed using PCL material (C) for trocar compatibility. (Right) A digital camera image of the biodegradable implant.

To evaluate the relationship between release rates and the surface area of the extruded PCL tubes, implants were fabricated with three different surface areas, as generated by varying the implant length: 82 ± 1 mm^2, 311 ± 4 mm^2, and 543 ± 5 mm^2, with an average of 31, 124, and 216 mg of TAF loaded into the implant, respectively. All devices comprised Sigma-PCL with a wall thickness of 100 μm, an OD of 2.5 mm, and a formulation of 2:1 TAF:castor oil. The cumulative release of TAF from the implants were monitored for approximately 30 days, as shown in Figure 2a. As expected for a membrane-controlled system, the higher surface area results in a higher release rate of TAF from the implant. Furthermore, the linear relationship between daily release rates and surface area supports the mechanism of membrane-controlled release from these implants (Figure 2b). These results align with a previous report using reservoir-style devices with thinner walls of PCL (8.5 μm) fabricated via solvent film-casting [55]. In the current study, devices were fabricated using PCL tubes prepared via melt extrusion, which produced thicker walled tubes (between 45–200 μm). Despite the thicker PCL wall and different fabrication approach, these devices also maintained membrane-controlled release in this range of wall thickness, demonstrating the robustness of the PCL-based drug delivery platform. For the remainder of this paper, the cylindrical geometry was fixed at 2.5 mm OD and 40 mm length to accommodate commercially available trocars utilized for contraceptive implants [56,57], and the release rates were normalized to the surface area of 314 mm^2.

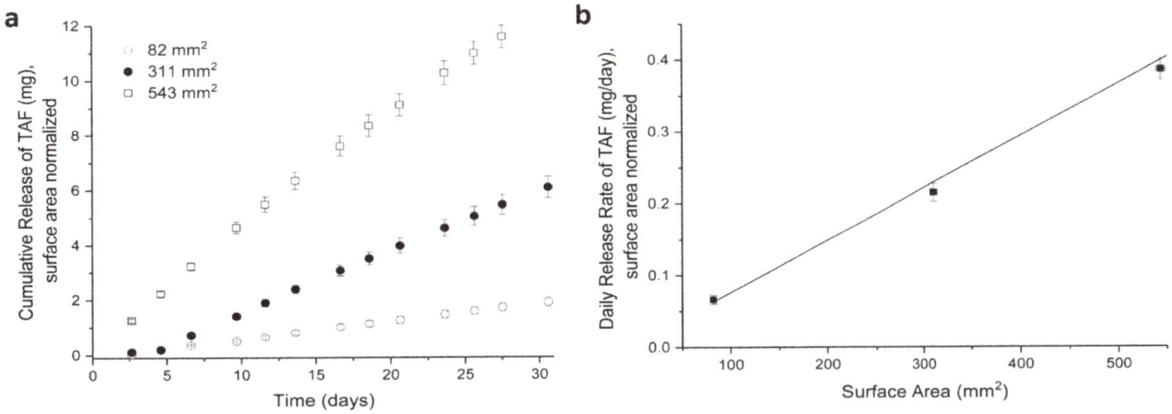

Figure 2. In vitro release studies showing (**a**) cumulative release of TAF from implants of differing surface areas and (**b**) daily release rates of TAF at day = 24 for implants with different surface areas. All implants were fabricated with Sigma-PCL, 100 μm wall thickness and a formulation of 2:1, TAF:castor oil. Surface areas were normalized according to the theoretical surface area for implant of 10, 40, 70 mm in length. Three implants were tested per condition.

The thickness of the implant walls was another attribute that affected release rates of drug. Figure 3 shows the daily release rates of TAF from implants comprising PCL of different wall thicknesses and containing a formulation of 2:1 TAF:castor oil excipient. The release rates of TAF inversely correlated with thickness of the PCL walls: 0.91 ± 0.23 mg/day (45 μm), 0.61 ± 0.09 mg/day (70 μm), 0.29 ± 0.05 mg/day (100 μm), 0.19 ± 0.04 mg/day (150 μm), and 0.15 ± 0.03 mg/day (200 μm). As the wall thickness increased from 45 to 200 μm, the release rates approach a plateau wherein the release rates of TAF show minimal change. Importantly, the daily release rates were calculated over the first 35 days of TAF release from the implants, which included a burst release that is more pronounced in thinner walled implants that results in a higher standard deviation (e.g., 45 μm walled implant). We speculate the burst release may arise from transport of drug into the PCL. This inverse relationship between the thickness of the PCL walls and the release rates of TAF was also demonstrated for thin-walled PCL implants fabricated by a solvent casting approach despite considerable differences in the device processing technique [55]. To reserve adequate volume in the reservoir for drug load, this study only investigated wall thickness up to 200 μm. Overall, these experiments demonstrate the ability to employ two parameters, surface area or wall thickness, to tailor the release rates of TAF from a reservoir-style implant fabricated with extruded PCL tubes.

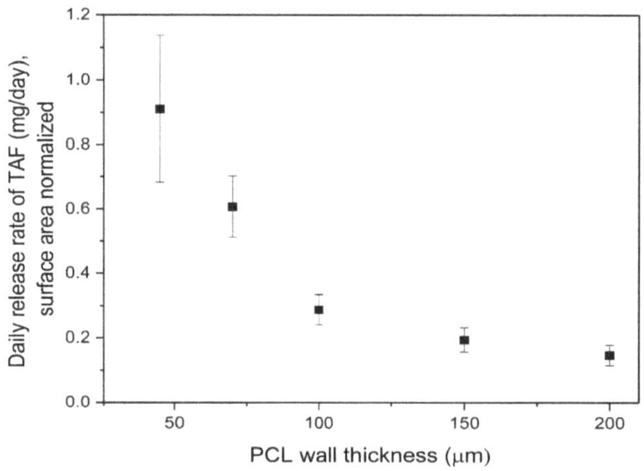

Figure 3. Daily release of TAF (mg/day) from implants with different wall thicknesses as calculated over 35 consecutive days within an in vitro assay. Implants comprised a 2:1 TAF-castor oil formulation (dimensions: 2.5 mm outer diameter (OD) by 40 mm length) fabricated with Sigma-Grade PCL. Three implants were tested per condition.

3.2. *Effects of PCL Properties on Implant Performance*

PCL is a semi-crystalline, hydrophobic polymer with biodegradation kinetics that depend on the initial MW, typically occurring in the order of 1–2 years [38], which supports a LA PrEP implant. In these studies, PCL starting material with two different MWs were selected to potentially support an implant with target duration of 6–12 months: Sigma-PCL (M_n of 103 kDa) and PC-12 PCL (M_n of 51 kDa). PCL tubes of different wall thicknesses (70, 100, 200 μm) were extruded with either Sigma-PCL or PC-12 and subsequently filled with a formulation of 2:1 TAF:castor oil. Evaluation of these implants using in-vitro release assays revealed two important concepts (Figure 4). First, the release rates of drug from the implant depended on the selection of PCL; TAF releases at a higher rate from implants comprising Sigma-PCL as compared to implants comprising PC-12. Interestingly, the influence of PCL type on TAF release rates is minimal in tubes with thicker walls (e.g., 200 μm) versus thinner walls (e.g., 70 μm). Second, Figure 4 also shows that irrespective of the PCL type used to fabricate the implant, the release rates of TAF still scales inversely with wall thickness, as also shown in Figure 3.

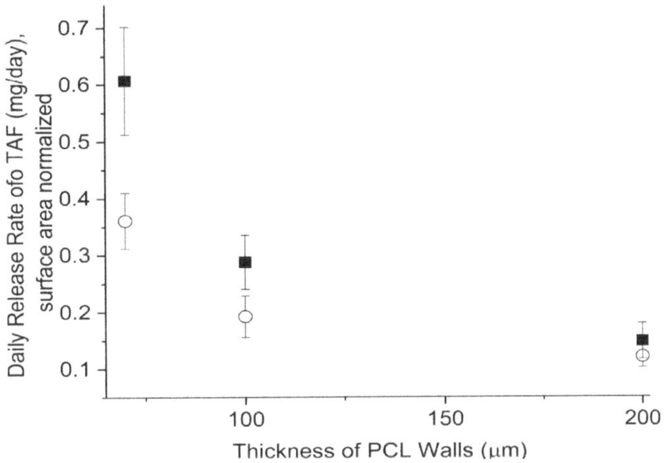

Figure 4. Effect of PCL type on daily release rates of TAF (mg/day) from implants with different wall thicknesses and fabricated with (■) Sigma -PCL or (○) PC-12. Implants contained a formulation of 2:1 TAF-castor Oil. Daily release rates were calculated from release over at 35 days and three implants were tested per condition.

It is possible that differences in crystallinity between the two types of PCL starting materials could affect the release rates of TAF from the implant. Therefore, to further understand the effect of polymer properties on release rates of drug, extruded tubes comprising PC-12 or Sigma-PCL were evaluated with DSC and XRD. Analysis by DSC showed that all PCL tubes exhibit a melting endotherm with a peak near 60 °C (Figure 5A, Figure S1), the characteristic melting temperature (T_m) of PCL [58,59]. However, notable differences in the melting endotherms were also evident, such as a narrower melt transition of PC-12 compared to Sigma-PCL and the presence of a small shoulder peak around 50 °C in Sigma-PCL which was absent in PC-12. Quantitatively, the specific T_m values also differed; Sigma-PCL showed a slightly higher T_m compared to PC-12 for all thicknesses of the tube walls (Table 1 and Figure S1). For each sample, Equation (1) was used to calculate the mass % crystallinity and Equation (2) (Thompson–Gibbs equation) was used to calculate the crystallite sizes. Results in Table 1 show that irrespective of the wall thickness, the crystallite size of PC-12 was slightly lower than the crystallite size of Sigma-PCL. Moreover, the crystallite size of Sigma-PCL slightly varied with different tube thicknesses, whereas PC-12 remained consistent. The % crystallinity was slightly higher in certain cases for PC-12 compared to Sigma-PCL, showing statistically significant differences for extruded tubes with 70 and 200 μm wall thicknesses.

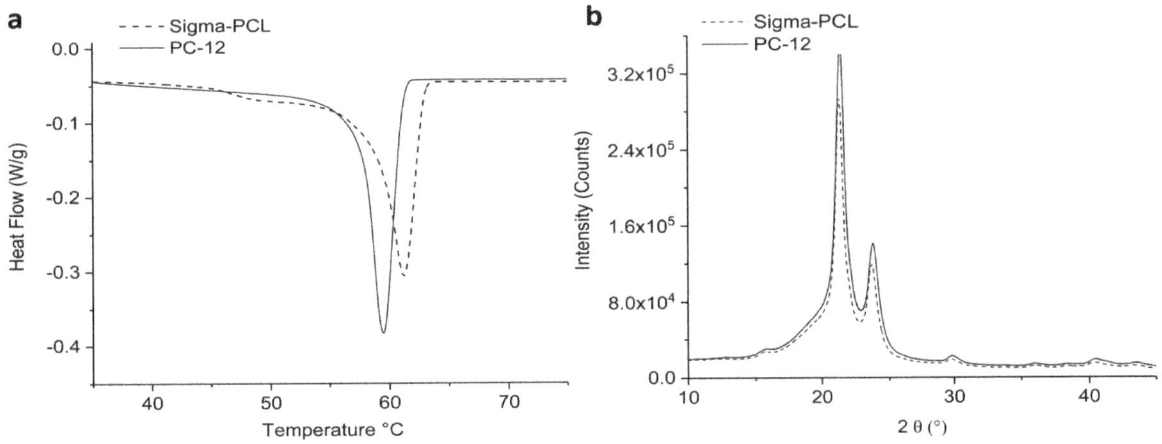

Figure 5. Exemplary graphs of (**a**) DSC heat flow curves and (**b**) XRD profiles of PCL tubes with 100 μm wall thickness.

Table 1. Thermal properties of PCL extruded tubes from DSC analysis.

PCL Type	Wall Thickness (μm)	T_m (°C)	% Crystallinity	Crystallite Size (nm)
PC-12	70	59.4 ± 0.1	56 ± 1.0	27 ± 0.2
	100	59.4 ± 0.1	53 ± 2.0	27 ± 0.4
	200	59.7 ± 0.4	56 ± 1.0	27 ± 1.2
Sigma-PCL	70	60.7 ± 0.1	53 ± 0.3	31 ± 0.2
	100	61.1 ± 0.2	52 ± 1.2	32 ± 0.6
	200	61.3 ± 0.1	53 ± 0.1	33 ± 0.3

XRD analysis was also performed to further examine the crystallite size of PCL extruded tubes using the Scherrer equation (Equation (3)). Extruded tubes (100 μm wall thickness) fabricated from Sigma-PCL and PC-12 showed similar diffraction patterns that include intense Bragg peaks at 2θ near 21.3° and 23.7°, correlating to diffraction of the (110) and (200) planes of the PCL crystallite, respectively (Figure 5B) [60,61]. Results from XRD analysis (Table 2) show that the crystallite sizes of PC-12 were slightly smaller than Sigma-PCL, where Sigma-PCL total crystallite sizes was 25 nm (14.2 + 10.8) and PCL-12 was 23.4 nm (13.2 + 10.2), which also agrees with DSC data. Both techniques used to measure crystallite size indicate a similar order of magnitude from the two PCL types, therefore it is unlikely that crystal size alone was responsible for the differences in drug diffusion kinetics from the materials considered in this study, however the observation that crystallite size increased with tube thickness for Sigma-PCL (as measured by DSC) may play a role in release kinetics.

Table 2. Thermal properties of PCL tubes * from XRD analysis.

PCL Type	Crystallite Size (nm)	
	L_{110}	L_{200}
PC-12	13.2	10.2
Sigma-PCL	14.2	10.8

* Extruded tubes comprised 100 μm wall thickness.

Taken together, these data highlight the importance in considering properties of drug transport in products comprising semi-crystalline polymers, which contain both amorphous regions amenable to drug transport when above the polymer glass transition temperature (T_g), and crystalline regions which pose a diffusive mass transport barrier. These data indicate that PCL is an ideal polymer suited for membrane-controlled drug diffusion applications given its material properties and semi-crystalline nature. For example, PCL has a T_g of −60 °C which allows for drug transport at physiological conditions (37 °C) where the amorphous regions exhibit adequate free volume for passive diffusion of small molecules and fluid driven by concentration gradients. Concurrently, PCL crystals impart structural integrity to the implant and act as a transport barrier which modulate drug diffusion and allow for sustained release of TAF. The DSC and XRD results presented here suggest that crystallite size, quantity of crystallinity, and ultimately polymer free volume within PCL will impact transport properties of TAF through the polymer, as also supported by studies with other systems [62]. Our results show that extruded tubes with lower MW (PC-12) contain smaller sizes of crystals and slightly higher % crystallinity (statistically significant for 70 and 200 μm tubes, $p = 0.008$ and $p = 0.007$, respectively) as compared to PCL with higher MW (Sigma-PCL). This suggests that higher degree of crystallinity and smaller crystallites could create a more tortuous path for diffusion of the drug, leading to a lower release rate from the implant. At 37 °C, TAF likely diffuses through the amorphous regions of PCL, where the polymer exhibits greater segmental mobility to facilitate passage of small molecules. The size and quantity of the crystal regions would affect the spatial arrangement and quantity of these amorphous regions, ultimately affecting transport kinetics. These findings are supported by the mathematical relationship between membrane flux through a given area which is inversely proportional to distance traveled (wall thickness) by the constant of mass diffusivity, i.e., Fick's first law of diffusion. The diffusion constant is a function of temperature, molecular size, and viscosity. For polymers, the viscosity term describes polymer free volume, which is impacted by crystallinity, hence the differences in material properties and resultant release rates were observed here.

In addition to the quantitative differences in polymer physicochemical properties observed in this study, three important qualitative findings are also of note. First, Sigma-PCL exhibited irregularities in the melting endotherm as evidenced by a small but apparent shoulder peak prior to the melt whereas PC-12 did not. It was likely a result of thermal history incurred in Sigma-PCL processing from the manufacturer. Given this consideration, the shoulder peak likely did not represent the PCL crystalline phase and may have contributed to an over-estimation of the crystalline content of the Sigma-PCL. A second difference was noted when comparing the width of the melt transition where PC-12 exhibited a narrower melt endotherm compared to Sigma-PCL, suggesting a tighter distribution of polymer molecular weight comprising the crystalline phase. Finally, another difference between these two grades of material was the crystallite size as a function of tube thicknesses. While PC-12 demonstrated more consistency in crystallite size, Sigma-PCL crystallite size increased with tube thickness, indicating a lack of control on the final properties during processing and perhaps explaining the large variability in release rates at low thicknesses and more consistent release rates at higher thicknesses. Sigma grade PCL also exhibited a steeper decline in release rate with respect to wall thickness, while PC-12 demonstrated a more gradual decline in release rate as a function of thickness. It was hypothesized that the concomitant increase in wall thickness and crystallite size observed with Sigma PCL was responsible for the attenuation in release rate values for the two grades of PCL at the higher wall thicknesses studied here. Taken together, these observations highlight the importance of material choices in the design of drug delivery devices from an engineering and quality control perspective.

3.3. Performance and Fabrication of a LA PCL Implant for Delivery of TAF

The duration of this reservoir-style implant for TAF is dictated by two parameters: the drug quantity within the reservoir and the rate of drug release from the implant. Using selected implant dimensions (2.5 mm OD, 40 mm length), TAF payload within the reservoir for the 2:1 TAF:castor oil formulation was approximately 115 mg for an implant with wall thicknesses of 100 μm. Within these constraints of drug payload, the duration of a single TAF implant for PrEP ultimately depends on the daily drug release required for protection as administered via the subcutaneous route, which is currently unknown. In this manuscript, in-vitro release rates from prototype implants were tailored to the range between approximately 0.2 and 0.8 mg/day from a single device, as suggested from previous animal studies and in-silico modelling set with TFV-DP target concentrations of >48 fmol/10^6 cells among 500 virtual healthly women [31,63].

Using these dimensional parameters, a batchwise process was developed to fabricate TAF implants from extruded PCL tubes, which entails loading the drug formulation into the cavity of a PCL tube and sealing the ends. Given the low melting temperature of PCL (60 °C), the implant was readily end-sealed by controllably heating PCL into the desired geometry using an in-house customized polymer extruder. Care was given to avoid contamination of the interior walls of the tube near the sealing points, which could hinder the formation of end seals during the melt sealing. This fabrication process was used to generate implants for a six-month in-vitro study to assess the release of TAF. As shown in Figure 6, implants released TAF at a rate of 0.28 ± 0.06 mg/day over the course of 180 days. After 180 days, approximately 68 mg of TAF remained within the implant, with a chromatographic purity of 89.2 ± 0.8% (Table S1). The trend of decreased TAF stability over time results from ingress of water into the implant as drug depletes, which, in turn, facilitates hydrolytic degradation of TAF [64]. We are currently evaluating other formulations of TAF that help optimize stability. The implant maintained structural integrity throughout the 180-day release period in simulated physiological conditions.

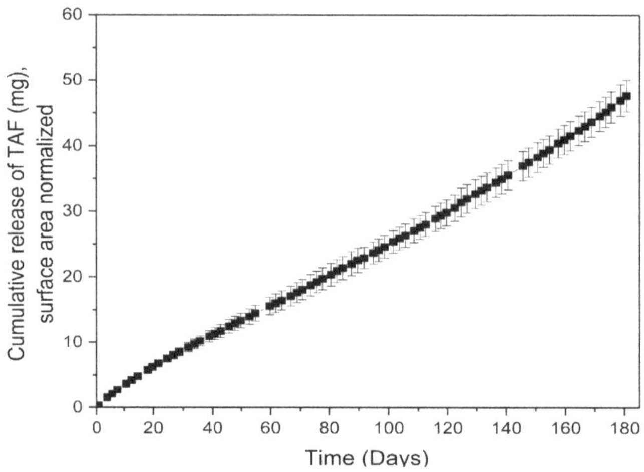

Figure 6. Cumulative release of TAF (mg) from an implant comprising Sigma-PCL of 100 μm wall thickness at 2.5 mm outer diameter and 40 mm length. Implants contained a 2:1 TAF-castor oil formulation. Three implants were tested per condition.

To support in vivo use of the implant, gamma irradiation was used to sterilize the implant after fabrication. Since gamma irradiation has been shown to affect the chemical and physical properties of PCL [65,66], studies were performed to evaluate its potential effects on the implant performance. Table S2 shows the GPC analysis of PCL, including samples of PCL raw material used for the extrusion process and extruded PCL tubes before and after gamma irradiation. Both PCL types (Sigma-PCL and PC-12) showed a slight decrease in M_n after gamma irradiation, as expected, but the extrusion process minimally affected the M_n of PCL. To further ascertain release rates of TAF from the implant after gamma irradiation, in vitro release assays were performed on implants with and without gamma irradiation at dosages between 18–24 kGy. As shown in Table 3, the release rates were comparable irrespective of treatment with gamma irradiation and the difference in release rates were not statistically significant when comparing non-irradiated and gamma irradiated release rates ($p = 0.27$ and $p = 0.42$ for Sigma-PCL at 70 and 100 μm, respectively; $p = 0.11$ and $p > 0.99$ for PC-12 at 70 and 100 μm, respectively).

Table 3. Daily TAF release rates from implants pre- and post-gamma irradiation.

PCL Type	Wall Thickness (μm)	Release Rates of TAF (mg/Day)	
		Non-Irradiated	Gamma Irradiated
Sigma-PCL	70	0.62 ± 0.09	0.54 ± 0.06
	100	0.29 ± 0.05	0.32 ± 0.03
PC-12	70	0.37 ± 0.05	0.30 ± 0.03
	100	0.20 ± 0.03	0.20 ± 0.02

Formulation of 2:1, TAF:castor oil; Daily release rates calculated from 30 days of consecutive release.

In summary, the in vitro studies presented in this manuscript demonstrate a new fabrication method to produce reservoir-style PCL implants using a batchwise process of polymer tube extrusion, formulation filling, and implant sealing via melt procedures. Although this fabrication process is not currently conducive to high-throughput manufacture, incremental steps detailed here support future production and implementation efforts. For instance, use of melt extrusion to produce PCL tubes presents an improvement over previously reported thin-film casting techniques, in terms of throughput of tube manufacturing and ultimate robustness of the implant. By increasing the implant wall thickness (e.g., from 70 to 200 μm) using an extrusion method, the implants were more aesthetically pleasing, exhibited greater mechanical sturdiness during handling and therapeutic use, while simultaneously retaining sustained release kinetics of drug. Moreover, the injection end-sealing method presented here produces an implant suitable for commercially available trocars, and is loaded with enough of the drug to last longer than six months; all considerations that were deemed preferable by end-users [67,68]. With an eye towards product development needs for clinical implementation, compatibility with applicators already clinically employed offers options to adopt existing procedures to support LA-PrEP rollout.

4. Conclusions

As the field of HIV PrEP rapidly progresses, new LA drug delivery systems must respond to evolving clinical and socio-behavioral insights in terms of effective ARV dosing, desired duration, and product acceptability. This paper describes a reservoir-style implant with the flexibility to adapt to needs of this advancing field by readily tailoring properties of the implant, including surface area, wall thickness, and properties of PCL. The first section of this manuscript describes the ability to control release rates of TAF via dimensions of extruded PCL tubes (i.e., surface area, wall thickness). We report an inverse correlation between wall thickness and drug release rates and this feature was further used to tune TAF dosing between 0.91 ± 0.23 mg/day (45 μm wall thickness) and 0.15 ± 0.03 mg/day (200 μm wall thickness). Our studies further show that the release rates of TAF scale proportionally with the surface area of the implant, demonstrating the membrane-controlled release from extruded PCL tubes. These results build from previous work using implants made of thin-films of PCL, which reported similar trends with the ability to tune release rates from reservoir-style devices between 8 and 15 μm thick [55]. However, the replacement of solvent-cast thin films with extruded tubes, as described here, supports the development of future manufacturing processes and ultimately provides robust implants with thicker walls for greater ease of handling. Although outside the scope of this manuscript, additional strategies to further increase drug stability, dosing and duration from a single implant, while simultaneously maintaining compatibility with market-available trocars, include modifications to the formulations such as selection and quantity of excipient. Although in vivo studies were not reported in this paper, the in vitro assay conditions used here have shown good in vitro/in vivo correlations previously [57]. Future in vivo studies will further advance this implant technology.

We also described a batchwise fabrication of implants using two types of PCL starting materials, either PC-12 or Sigma-PCL. In these studies, the selection of PCL starting material affects the release rates of TAF from the implant; TAF releases faster from implants fabricated with Sigma-PCL as compared to PC-12. Analysis via DSC and XRD were used to probe the reason for these differences. Analysis by DSC revealed slight differences in the mass percent of crystallinity from both PCL types (70 and 200 μm wall thickness) and showed slight differences in the crystalline sizes. Although additional studies are needed to further characterize these differences, our results do suggest that a smaller crystalline size and higher mass % crystallinity within the polymeric material retard the diffusion of TAF through PCL. Interestingly, when using these thicker walled tubes (e.g., 200 μm walls), the effect of PCL type on release rate is less pronounced. Using down-selected parameters, we demonstrate delivery of TAF in vitro for 180 days at a dose of 0.28 ± 0.06 mg/day and the TAF within the implant maintains stability at 89.2% ± 0.8% at the end of this duration. This is the first report of a six-month in vitro study showing sustained release of TAF from a biodegradable trocar-compatible implant. This manuscript also shows that the use of gamma irradiation (dosages 18–24 kGy) as a sterilization technique minimally affects the release rates of TAF, which benefits future in vivo studies. Overall, this implantable drug delivery system holds various parameters that can be tuned to achieve a targeted dose of TAF. Although the final design of this drug delivery system for TAF awaits feedback from dosing requirements, these promising results help to highlight the path towards the goal of developing LA delivery of TAF for HIV PrEP.

Author Contributions: Conceptualization and Design, L.M.J., S.A.K., L.L., N.G., A.v.d.S.; Methodology, L.M.J., S.A.K., L.L., N.G., D.M., B.C.; Formal Analysis: L.M.J., S.A.K., L.L., N.G.; Writing: L.M.J., L.L., N.G., Z.R.D., A.v.d.S.; Review & Editing, L.M.J., S.A.K., L.L., Z.R.D., D.M., B.C., A.v.d.S.; Project Administration, Z.R.D.; Funding Acquisition, A.v.d.S.

Acknowledgments: This research was made possible by the generous support of the American people through the U.S. President's Emergency Plan for AIDS Relief. The contents are the responsibility of the authors and do not necessarily reflect the views of USAID, PEPFAR, or the United States Government. We thank The Bill and Melinda Gates Foundation for support of this work (OPP1149227). We thank Gilead Sciences, Inc. for graciously providing TAF. We thank RTI team members: Christine Areson, Marza Hill, Pafio Johnson, Todd Ennis, and Teresa Jester for data collection, Ellen Luecke for program management, and Dayle Johnson for Figure 1 drawing and the TOC graphic.

References

1. Grant, R.M.; Lama, J.R.; Anderson, P.L.; McMahan, V.; Liu, A.Y.; Vargas, L.; Goicochea, P.; Casapía, M.; Guanira-Carranza, J.V.; Ramirez-Cardich, M.E.; et al. Preexposure Chemoprophylaxis for HIV prevention in men who have sex with men. *N. Engl. J. Med.* **2010**, *363*, 2587–2599. [CrossRef] [PubMed]
2. Baeten, J.M.; Donnell, D.; Ndase, P.; Mugo, N.R.; Campbell, J.D.; Wangisi, J.; Tappero, J.W.; Bukusi, E.A.; Cohen, C.R.; Katabira, E.; et al. Antiretroviral prophylaxis for HIV prevention in heterosexual men and women. *N. Engl. J. Med.* **2012**, *367*, 399–410. [CrossRef] [PubMed]
3. Molina, J.-M.; Capitant, C.; Spire, B.; Pialoux, G.; Cotte, L.; Charreau, I.; Tremblay, C.; Le Gall, J.-M.; Cua, E.; Pasquet, A.; et al. On-Demand preexposure prophylaxis in men at high risk for HIV-1 infection. *N. Engl. J. Med.* **2015**, *373*, 2237–2246. [CrossRef] [PubMed]
4. McCormack, S.; Dunn, D.T.; Desai, M.; Dolling, D.I.; Gafos, M.; Gilson, R.; Sullivan, A.K.; Clarke, A.; Reeves, I.; Schembri, G.; et al. Pre-exposure prophylaxis to prevent the acquisition of HIV-1 infection (PROUD): Effectiveness results from the pilot phase of a pragmatic open-label randomised trial. *Lancet* **2016**, *387*, 53–60. [CrossRef]
5. Cranston, R.D.; Lama, J.R.; Richardson, B.A.; Carballo-Diéguez, A.; Kunjara Na Ayudhya, R.P.; Liu, K.; Patterson, K.B.; Leu, C.-S.; Galaska, B.; Jacobson, C.E.; et al. MTN-017: A Rectal Phase 2 extended safety and acceptability study of tenofovir reduced-glycerin 1% gel. *Clin. Infect. Dis.* **2016**, *64*, 614–620. [CrossRef]
6. Marrazzo, J.M.; Ramjee, G.; Richardson, B.A.; Gomez, K.; Mgodi, N.; Nair, G.; Palanee, T.; Nakabiito, C.; van der Straten, A.; Noguchi, L.; et al. Tenofovir-based preexposure prophylaxis for HIV infection among African women. *N. Engl. J. Med.* **2015**, *372*, 509–518. [CrossRef] [PubMed]
7. Hosek, S.G.; Rudy, B.; Landovitz, R.; Kapogiannis, B.; Siberry, G.; Rutledge, B.; Liu, N.; Brothers, J.; Mulligan, K.; Zimet, G.; et al. An HIV preexposure prophylaxis demonstration project and safety study for young MSM. *J. Acquir. Immune Defic. Syndr.* **2017**, *74*, 21–29. [CrossRef]
8. Hosek, S.G.; Landovitz, R.J.; Kapogiannis, B.; Siberry, G.K.; Rudy, B.; Rutledge, B.; Liu, N.; Harris, D.R.; Mulligan, K.; Zimet, G.; et al. Safety and feasibility of antiretroviral preexposure prophylaxis for adolescent men who have sex with men aged 15 to 17 years in the United States. *JAMA Pediatrics* **2017**, *171*, 1063–1071. [CrossRef]
9. Morgan, E.; Ryan, D.T.; Newcomb, M.E.; Mustanski, B. High rate of discontinuation may diminish PrEP coverage among young men who have sex with men. *AIDS Behav.* **2018**, *22*, 3645–3648. [CrossRef]
10. Deutsch, M.B.; Glidden, D.V.; Sevelius, J.; Keatley, J.; McMahan, V.; Guanira, J.; Kallas, E.G.; Chariyalertsak, S.; Grant, R.M.; For the iPrEx Study Team. HIV pre-exposure prophylaxis in transgender women: A subgroup analysis of the iPrEx trial. *Lancet* **2015**, *2*, e512–e519. [CrossRef]
11. Van Damme, L.; Corneli, A.; Ahmed, K.; Agot, K.; Lombaard, J.; Kapiga, S.; Malahleha, M.; Owino, F.; Manongi, R.; Onyango, J.; et al. Preexposure prophylaxis for HIV infection among African women. *N. Engl. J. Med.* **2012**, *367*, 411–422. [CrossRef] [PubMed]
12. HPTN. HPTN 083. A Phase 2b/3 Double Blind Safety and Efficacy Study of Injectable Cabotegravir Compared to Daily Oral Tenofovir Disoproxil Fumarate/Emtricitabine (TDF/FTC), for Pre-Exposure Prophylaxis in HIV-Uninfected Cisgender Men and Transgender Women who have Sex with Men. Available online: https://www.hptn.org/research/studies/hptn083 (accessed on 1 July 2019).
13. HPTN. HPTN 084. A Phase 3 Double Blind Safety and Efficacy Study of Long-Acting Injectable Cabotegravir Compared to Daily Oral TDF/FTC for Pre-Exposure Prophylaxis in HIV-Uninfected Women. Available online: https://www.hptn.org/research/studies/hptn084 (accessed on 1 July 2019).

14. van der Straten, A.; Agot, K.; Ahmed, K.; Weinrib, R.; Browne, E.N.; Manenzhe, K.; Owino, F.; Schwartz, J.; Minnis, A.; on behalf of the TRIO Study Team. The Tablets, Ring, Injections as Options (TRIO) study: What young African women chose and used for future HIV and pregnancy prevention. *J. Int. AIDS Soc.* **2018**, *21*, e25094. [CrossRef] [PubMed]
15. Landovitz, R.J.; Li, S.; Grinsztejn, B.; Dawood, H.; Liu, A.Y.; Magnus, M.; Hosseinipour, M.C.; Panchia, R.; Cottle, L.; Chau, G.; et al. Safety, tolerability, and pharmacokinetics of long-acting injectable cabotegravir in low-risk HIV-uninfected individuals: HPTN 077, a phase 2a randomized controlled trial. *PLoS Med.* **2018**, *15*, e1002690. [CrossRef] [PubMed]
16. Markowitz, M.; Frank, I.; Grant, R.M.; Mayer, K.H.; Elion, R.; Goldstein, D.; Fisher, C.; Sobieszczyk, M.E.; Gallant, J.E.; Van Tieu, H.; et al. Safety and tolerability of long-acting cabotegravir injections in HIV-uninfected men (ECLAIR): A multicentre, double-blind, randomised, placebo-controlled, phase 2a trial. *Lancet HIV* **2017**, *4*, e331–e340. [CrossRef]
17. Penrose, K.J.; Parikh, U.M.; Hamanishi, K.A.; Else, L.; Back, D.; Boffito, M.; Jackson, A.; Mellors, J.W. Selection of Rilpivirine-Resistant HIV-1 in a Seroconverter From the SSAT 040 Trial Who Received the 300-mg Dose of Long-Acting Rilpivirine (TMC278LA). *J. Infect. Dis.* **2016**, *213*, 1013–1017. [CrossRef] [PubMed]
18. Kovarova, M.; Benhabbour, S.R.; Massud, I.; Spagnuolo, R.A.; Skinner, B.; Baker, C.E.; Sykes, C.; Mollan, K.R.; Kashuba, A.D.M.; García-Lerma, J.G.; et al. Ultra-long-acting removable drug delivery system for HIV treatment and prevention. *Nat. Commun.* **2018**, *9*, 4156. [CrossRef] [PubMed]
19. Solorio, L.; Carlson, A.; Zhou, H.; Exner, A.A. Implantable drug delivery systems. In *Engineering Polymer Systems for Improved Drug Delivery*, 1st ed.; Bader, R.A., Putnam, D.A., Eds.; John Wiley & Sons, Inc.: Hoboken, NJ, USA, 2014. [CrossRef]
20. Yang, W.-W.; Pierstorff, E. Reservoir-based polymer drug delivery systems. *J. Lab. Autom.* **2012**, *17*, 50–58. [CrossRef] [PubMed]
21. Langer, R. Implantable controlled release systems. *Pharmacol. Ther.* **1983**, *21*, 35–51. [CrossRef]
22. Highlights of Prescribing Information, Probuphine (Buprenorphine) Implant for Subdermal Administration. Available online: https://probuphine.com/prescribing-information/ (accessed on 1 July 2019).
23. Highlights of Prescribing Information, Jadelle (Levonogestrel Implant). Available online: https://www.accessdata.fda.gov/drugsatfda_docs/label/2016/020544s010lbl.pdf (accessed on 1 July 2019).
24. "Norplant® II" Levonorgestrel Implants (Jadelle®), Supplement 003. Council, P. (Ed.) Vol. NDA 20-544. Available online: https://www.accessdata.fda.gov/drugsatfda_docs/label/2002/20544se2-003_jadelle_lbl.pdf (accessed on 1 July 2019).
25. Highlights of Prescribing Information, Implanon (Etonogestrel Implant). Available online: https://www.merck.com/product/usa/pi_circulars/i/implanon/implanon_pi.pdf (accessed on 1 July 2019).
26. Highlights of Prescribing Information, Nexplanon (etonogestrel implants). Available online: https://www.merck.com/product/usa/pi_circulars/n/nexplanon/nexplanon_pi.pdf (accessed on 1 July 2019).
27. Musch, D.C.; Martin, D.F.; Gordon, J.F.; Davis, M.D.; Kuppermann, B.D. Treatment of cytomegalovirus retinitis with a sustained-release ganciclovir implant. *N. Engl. J. Med.* **1997**, *337*, 83–90. [CrossRef]
28. The Highlights of Prescribing Information Ozurdex (Dexamethasone Intravitreal Implant). Available online: https://www.accessdata.fda.gov/drugsatfda_docs/label/2014/022315s009lbl.pdf (accessed on 1 July 2019).
29. Haller, J.A.; Bandello, F.; Belfort, R.; Blumenkranz, M.S.; Gillies, M.; Heier, J.; Loewenstein, A.; Yoon, Y.-H.; Jacques, M.-L.; Jiao, J.; et al. Randomized, sham-controlled trial of dexamethasone intravitreal implant in patients with macular edema due to retinal vein occlusion. *Ophthalmology* **2010**, *117*, 1134–1146. [CrossRef]
30. Jaffe, G.J.; Martin, D.; Callanan, D.; Pearson, P.A.; Levy, B.; Comstock, T. Fluocinolone Acetonide Implant (Retisert) for Noninfectious Posterior Uveitis: Thirty-Four–Week results of a multicenter randomized clinical study. *Ophthalmology* **2006**, *113*, 1020–1027. [CrossRef] [PubMed]
31. Gunawardana, M.; Remedios-Chan, M.; Miller, C.S.; Fanter, R.; Yang, F.; Marzinke, M.A.; Hendrix, C.W.; Beliveau, M.; Moss, J.A.; Smith, T.J.; et al. Pharmacokinetics of long-acting tenofovir alafenamide (GS-7340) subdermal implant for HIV prophylaxis. *Antimicrob. Agents Chemother.* **2015**, *59*, 3913–3919. [CrossRef] [PubMed]
32. Chua, C.Y.X.; Jain, P.; Ballerini, A.; Bruno, G.; Hood, R.L.; Gupte, M.; Gao, S.; Di Trani, N.; Susnjar, A.; Shelton, K.; et al. Transcutaneously refillable nanofluidic implant achieves sustained level of tenofovir diphosphate for HIV pre-exposure prophylaxis. *J. Control. Release* **2018**, *286*, 315–325. [CrossRef] [PubMed]

33. Pipeline and Partners. Available online: https://www.intarcia.com/pipeline-technology/itca-650.html (accessed on 1 July 2019).
34. Barrett, S.E.; Teller, R.S.; Forster, S.P.; Li, L.; Mackey, M.A.; Skomski, D.; Yang, Z.; Fillgrove, K.L.; Doto, G.J.; Wood, S.L.; et al. Extended-Duration MK-8591-Eluting Implant as a Candidate for HIV Treatment and Prevention. *Antimicrob. Agents Chemother.* **2018**, *62*, e01058-18. [CrossRef] [PubMed]
35. Gatto, G.; Girouard, N.; Brand, R.M.; Johnson, L.; Marzinke, M.A.; Rowshan, S.; Engstrom, J.C.; McGowan, I.; Demkovich, Z.; Luecke, E.; et al. Pharmacokinetics of Tenofovir Alafenamide by Subcutaneous Implatn for HIV PrEP. In Proceedings of the Conference on Retrovirusus and Opportunistic Infections (CROI) 2018, Boston, MA, USA, 7 March 2018.
36. New Multipurpose Device to Help Prevent HIV and Pregnancy—RTI International Awarded Project to Develop a Device to Help Women in Africa. Available online: https://www.rti.org/news/new-multipurpose-device-help-prevent-hiv-and-pregnancy (accessed on 1 July 2019).
37. Pitt, C.G.; Chasalow, F.I.; Hibionada, Y.M.; Klimas, D.M.; Schindler, A. Aliphatic Polyesters. I. The Degradation of Poly(ε-caprolactone) In Vivo. *J. Appl. Polym. Sci.* **1981**, *26*, 3779–3787. [CrossRef]
38. Woodruff, M.A.; Hutmacher, D.W. The return of a forgotten polymer—Polycaprolactone in the 21st century. *Prog. Polym.Sci.* **2010**, *35*, 1217–1256. [CrossRef]
39. Dong, L.; Wang, S.-J.; Zhao, X.-R.; Zhu, Y.-F.; Yu, J.-K. 3D-Printed Poly(ε-caprolactone) Scaffold Integrated with Cell-laden Chitosan Hydrogels for Bone Tissue Engineering. *Sci. Rep.* **2017**, *7*, 13412. [CrossRef]
40. Patrício, T.; Domingos, M.; Gloria, A.; Bártolo, P. Characterisation of PCL and PCL/PLA Scaffolds for Tissue Engineering. *Procedia CIRP* **2013**, *5*, 110–114. [CrossRef]
41. Grossen, P.; Witzigmann, D.; Sieber, S.; Huwyler, J. PEG-PCL-based nanomedicines: A biodegradable drug delivery system and its application. *J. Control. Release* **2017**, *260*, 46–60. [CrossRef]
42. Dash, T.K.; Konkimalla, V.B. Polymeric modification and its implication in drug delivery: Poly-epsilon-caprolactone (PCL) as a model polymer. *Mol. Pharm.* **2012**, *9*, 2365–2379. [CrossRef]
43. Shrestha, D.; Wei, X.; Wu, W.-C.; Ling, J.-Q. Resilon: A methacrylate resin-based obturation system. *J. Dental Sci.* **2010**, *5*, 47–52. [CrossRef]
44. Trott, A.T. Chapter 8—Instruments, Suture Materials, and Closure Choices. In *Wounds and Lacerations*, 4th ed.; Trott, A.T., Ed.; W.B. Saunders: Philadelphia, PA, USA, 2012; pp. 82–94. [CrossRef]
45. Ory, S.J.; Hammond, C.B.; Yancy, S.G.; Wayne Hendren, R.; Pitt, C.G. The effect of a biodegradable contraceptive capsule (Capronor) containing levonorgestrel on gonadotropin, estrogen, and progesterone levels. *Am. J. Obstet. Gynecol.* **1983**, *145*, 600–605. [CrossRef]
46. Gupta, B.; Geeta; Ray, A.R. Preparation of poly(ε-caprolactone)/poly(ε-caprolactone-*co*-lactide) (PCL/PLCL) blend filament by melt spinning. *J. Appl. Polym. Sci.* **2012**, *123*, 1944–1950. [CrossRef]
47. Obregon, N.; Agubra, V.; Pokhrel, M.; Campos, H.; Flores, D.; De la Garza, D.; Mao, Y.; Macossay, J.; Alcoutlabi, M. Effect of Polymer Concentration, Rotational Speed, and Solvent Mixture on Fiber Formation Using Forcespinning®. *Fibers* **2016**, *4*, 20. [CrossRef]
48. Su, H.-H.; Chen, H.-L.; Díaz, A.; Casas, M.T.; Puiggalí, J.; Hoskins, J.N.; Grayson, S.M.; Pérez, R.A.; Müller, A.J. New insights on the crystallization and melting of cyclic PCL chains on the basis of a modified Thomson–Gibbs equation. *Polymer* **2013**, *54*, 846–859. [CrossRef]
49. Menczel, J.D.; Judovits, L.; Prime, R.B.; Bair, H.E.; Reading, M.; Swier, S. Chapter 2-Differential Scanning Calorimetry (DSC). In *Thermal Analysis of Polymers: Fundamentals and Applications*; Menczel, J.D., Prime, R.B., Eds.; Wiley: Hoboken, NJ, USA, 2009.
50. Núñez, E. Crystallization in Constrained Polymer Structures: Approaching the Unsolved Problems in Polymer Crystallization. Ph.D. Thesis, KTH, Stockholm, Sweden, 2006.
51. Tuba, F. Towards the Understanding of the molecular weight dependence of essential work of fracture in semi-crystalline polymers: A study on poly(ε-caprolactone). *Express Polym. Lett.* **2014**, *8*, 869–879. [CrossRef]
52. Kosobrodova, E.; Kondyurin, A.; Chrzanowski, W.; Theodoropoulos, C.; Morganti, E.; Hutmacher, D.; Bilek, M.M.M. Effect of plasma immersion ion implantation on polycaprolactone with various molecular weights and crystallinity. *J. Mater. Sci. Mater. Med.* **2017**, *29*, 5. [CrossRef] [PubMed]
53. Schlesinger, E.; Ciaccio, N.; Desai, T.A. Polycaprolactone thin-film drug delivery systems: Empirical and predictive models for device design. *Mater. Sci. Eng. C Mater. Biol. Appl.* **2015**, *57*, 232–239. [CrossRef]

54. Lam, C.X.; Savalani, M.M.; Teoh, S.H.; Hutmacher, D.W. Dynamics of in vitro polymer degradation of polycaprolactone-based scaffolds: Accelerated versus simulated physiological conditions. *Biomed. Mater.* **2008**, *3*, 034108. [CrossRef]
55. Schlesinger, E.; Johengen, D.; Luecke, E.; Rothrock, G.; McGowan, I.; van der Straten, A.; Desai, T. A Tunable, Biodegradable, Thin-Film Polymer Device as a Long-Acting Implant Delivering Tenofovir Alafenamide Fumarate for HIV Pre-exposure Prophylaxis. *Pharm. Res.* **2016**, *33*, 1649–1656. [CrossRef]
56. Steiner, M.J.; Boler, T.; Obhai, G.; Hubacher, D. Assessment of a disposable trocar for insertion of contraceptive implants. *Contraception* **2010**, *81*, 140–142. [CrossRef] [PubMed]
57. Gatto, G.J.; Brand, R.M.; Girouard, N.; Li, L.A.; Johnson, L.; Marzinke, M.A.; Krogstad, E.; Siegel, A.; Helms, E.; Demkovich, Z.; et al. Development of an End-user Informed Tenofovir Alafenamide (TAF) Implant for Long-acting (LA)-HIV Pre-exposure Prophylaxis (PrEP). In Proceedings of the HIV Research for Prevention (HIVR4P) 2018, Madrid, Spain, 25 October 2018.
58. Wang, Y.; Rodriguez-Perez, M.A.; Reis, R.L.; Mano, J.F. Thermal and Thermomechanical Behaviour of Polycaprolactone and Starch/Polycaprolactone Blends for Biomedical Applications. *Macromol. Mater. Eng.* **2005**, *290*, 792–801. [CrossRef]
59. Speranza, V.; Sorrentino, A.; De Santis, F.; Pantani, R. Characterization of the Polycaprolactone Melt Crystallization: Complementary Optical Microscopy, DSC, and AFM Studies. *Sci. World J.* **2014**, *2014*, 9. [CrossRef] [PubMed]
60. Hu, H.; Dorset, D.L. Crystal structure of poly(iε-caprolactone). *Macromolecules* **1990**, *23*, 4604–4607. [CrossRef]
61. Lv, Q.; Wu, D.; Xie, H.; Peng, S.; Chen, Y.; Xu, C. Crystallization of poly(ε-caprolactone) in its immiscible blend with polylactide: Insight into the role of annealing histories. *RSC Adv.* **2016**, *6*, 37721–37730. [CrossRef]
62. Scheler, S. The polymer free volume as a controlling factor for drug release from poly(lactide-*co*-glycolide) microspheres. *J. Appl. Polym. Sci.* **2014**, *131*. [CrossRef]
63. Rajoli, R.; Demkovish, Z.; van der Straten, A.; Flexner, C.; Owen, A.; Siccardi, M. In Silico simulation of long-acting tenofovir alafenamide subcutaneous implant. In Proceedings of the CROI 2019, Seatle, WA, USA, 4–7 March 2019.
64. Golla, V.M.; Kurmi, M.; Shaik, K.; Singh, S. Stability behaviour of antiretroviral drugs and their combinations. 4: Characterization of degradation products of tenofovir alafenamide fumarate and comparison of its degradation and stability behaviour with tenofovir disoproxil fumarate. *J. Pharm. Biomed. Anal.* **2016**, *131*, 146–155. [CrossRef]
65. Navarro, R.; Burillo, G.; Adem, E.; Marcos-Fernández, A. Effect of Ionizing Radiation on the Chemical Structure and the Physical Properties of Polycaprolactones of Different Molecular Weight. *Polymers* **2018**, *10*, 397. [CrossRef]
66. Cooke, S.L.; Whittington, A.R. Influence of therapeutic radiation on polycaprolactone and polyurethane biomaterials. *Mater. Sci. Eng. C* **2016**, *60*, 78–83. [CrossRef]
67. Krogstad, E.A.; Montgomery, E.T.; Atujuna, M.; Minnis, A.M.; O'Rourke, S.; Ahmed, K.; Bekker, L.-G.; van der Straten, A. Design of an Implant for Long-Acting HIV Pre-Exposure Prophylaxis: Input from South African Health Care Providers. *AIDS Patient Care STDs* **2019**, *33*, 157–166. [CrossRef]
68. Krogstad, E.A.; Atujuna, M.; Montgomery, E.T.; Minnis, A.; Ndwayana, S.; Malapane, T.; Shapley-Quinn, M.K.; Manenzhe, K.; Bekker, L.-G.; van der Straten, A. Perspectives of South African youth in the development of an implant for HIV prevention. *J. Int. AIDS Soc.* **2018**, *21*, e25170. [CrossRef] [PubMed]

9

Tenofovir Hot-Melt Granulation using Gelucire to Develop Sustained-Release Vaginal Systems for Weekly Protection against Sexual Transmission of HIV

Fernando Notario-Pérez [1], Raúl Cazorla-Luna [1], Araceli Martín-Illana [1], Roberto Ruiz-Caro [1], Juan Peña [2] and María-Dolores Veiga [1,*]

[1] Departamento de Farmacia Galénica y Tecnología Alimentaria, Facultad de Farmacia, Universidad Complutense de Madrid, 28040 Madrid, Spain; fnotar01@ucm.es (F.N.-P.); racazorl@ucm.es (R.C.-L.); aracelimartin@ucm.es (A.M.-I.); rruizcar@ucm.es (R.R.-C.)

[2] Departamento de Química en Ciencias Farmacéuticas, Facultad de Farmacia, Universidad Complutense de Madrid, 28040 Madrid, Spain; juanpena@ima.ucm.es

* Correspondence: mdveiga@ucm.es

Abstract: Hot-melt granulation is a technique used to obtain granules by dispersing a drug in polymers at a high temperature. Tenofovir, an antiretroviral drug with proven activity as a vaginal microbicide, was dispersed in melted Gelucire® (or a mixture of different Gelucire®) to obtain drug-loaded granules. Studies performed on the granules proved that the drug is not altered in the hot-melt granulation process. The granules obtained were included in a matrix formed by the hydrophilic polymers hydroxypropylmethylcellulose and chitosan to obtain vaginal tablets that combine different mechanisms of controlled release: The Gelucire® needs to soften to allow the release of the Tenofovir, and the hydrophilic polymers must form a gel so the drug can diffuse through it. The studies performed with the tablets were swelling behavior, Tenofovir release, and ex vivo mucoadhesion. The tablets containing granules obtained with Tenofovir and Gelucire® 43/01 in a ratio of 1:2 in a matrix formed by hydroxypropylmethylcellulose and chitosan in a ratio of 1.9:1 were selected as the optimal formulation, since they release Tenofovir in a sustained manner over 216h and remain attached to the vaginal mucosa throughout. A weekly administration of these tablets would therefore offer women protection against the sexual transmission of HIV.

Keywords: controlled release; ex vivo bioadhesion; Gelucire®; Human Immunodeficiency Virus; mucoadhesive vaginal compacts; Tenofovir

---

1. Introduction

The hot-melt granulation technique consists of dissolving or dispersing an active principle in one or more melted polymers in order, after cooling, to obtain granules with a defined structure [1]. The melt entropy of the different components determines whether they will crystallize simultaneously, in turn conditioning the microstructure of the granules in the solid state [2].

The most common applications of this technique in pharmaceutical development are targeted drug release, masking the taste of active substances, and particularly improving the solubility of poorly soluble drugs [3]. In the latter case, solid dispersions of the drug are usually prepared in an inert hydrophilic matrix, causing the active principle to convert from its crystalline state to an amorphous form and improving its solubility [4]. However, this technique could also be applied in reverse to delay the dissolution of water-soluble drugs, which would aid the development of sustained-release systems capable of releasing the drug at a given rate, thereby achieving a constant concentration of the active principle at the site of action [3,4]. Some references to this possibility can be found in the literature: Mini-matrices have been developed where the drug is found in polymers as diverse as ethyl cellulose and xanthan gum [5], polyvinylpyrrolidone (PVP) [6], thermoplastic polyurethane [7] or ethylene vinyl acetate and polyethylene oxide [8]. One alternative yet to be explored would be to develop these systems using as carriers various Gelucire®, a group of amphiphilic excipients commonly used to develop sustained-release matrices [9,10]. Another advantage is that Gelucire® is commercialized with different melting points and hydrophilic-lipophilic balances (HLB), offering a wide range of options from which to select the most suitable for our purposes [11].

This last option—developing systems for the sustained release of drugs—raises the possibility of applying this technique to produce a vaginal microbicide to prevent the sexual transmission of the human immunodeficiency virus (HIV). A vaginal microbicide is any suitably formulated compound which, when applied in the vagina before intercourse, has the ability to prevent or reduce the transmission of sexually-transmitted diseases. The latest published data reflect the gender inequality in HIV protection, with an estimated 18.6 million women and girls living with the virus, and three young women infected every four minutes [12]. This explains the growing interest in recent decades in developing this type of formulations as a tool to protect women from the sexual acquisition of HIV.

Tenofovir (TFV) is an antiretroviral drug, specifically a nucleotide analogue reverse transcriptase inhibitor, approved by the Food and Drug Administration and recommended by the World Health Organization for its use as a first-line drug for the treatment of HIV [13]. It has also been extensively studied for the development of vaginal microbicides, mainly since the publication in 2010 of the results of the CAPRISA 004 trial, in which a 1% TFV gel showed a 39% effectiveness in protecting against HIV infection [14]. However, the fact that it required a daily application reduced the effectiveness of the formulation, so the current trend is to develop sustained-release formulations that require less frequent administration [15]. TFV is a hydrophilic drug that is soluble in aqueous media, such as vaginal fluid, requiring techniques to obtain sustained-release formulations that slow its dissolution rate in the vaginal environment.

The aim of this work is to prepare granules of TFV by hot-melt granulation using one or more Gelucire® containing mono-, di- and triglyceride esters of fatty acids (C8 to C18), –Gelucire® 39/01 (G39) and Gelucire® 43/01 (G43)–, which are characterized by their low HLB value (HLB = 1) and low melting point (39 °C and 43 °C respectively). However, rather than manufacturing matrices, the granules are incorporated in a hydrophilic matrix formed by a combination of hydroxypropylmethyl cellulose (HPMC) and chitosan (CH), two polymers that are capable of swelling in the presence of vaginal fluid and have proven to be an excellent choice for the development of sustained drug-delivery systems [16]. Vaginally administered tablets could then be developed in which the release of the drug would be conditioned by multiple factors. A Gelucire® with a predominantly lipophilic rather than hydrophilic character would prevent the dissolution of the granules in the vaginal medium, while their low melting point would cause Gelucire® to soften at body temperature and allow the vaginal fluid to diffuse through it and dissolve the drug; alternatively, the combination of HPMC and CH would swell with the vaginal fluid and form a gel which would initially delay the arrival of the vaginal fluid at the granules, and subsequently hinder the diffusion of the dissolved drug through the gel to reach the vaginal environment. The aim is to develop mucoadhesive systems that offer weekly protection against HIV infection and encourage greater adherence to the use of the microbicide, due to their lower frequency of administration, and consequently achieve greater protective efficacy.

2. Materials and Methods

2.1. Materials

Gelucire® 39/01 (G39, lot: 3E3701-2) and Gelurice® 43/01 (G43, lot: 1E5203-2) were a gift from Gattefossé (Saint-Priest, France). Tenofovir (TFV, lot: FT104801401) was supplied by Carbosynth Limited (Berkshire, UK). Chitosan, whose properties were characterized experimentally determining that it has a molecular weight of 32.1 kDa—being therefore a low-molecular-weight chitosan-, with an intrinsic viscosity of 24.75 dL/g and a degree of deacetylation of 54. 7% [17] (CH, lot: 0055790), was provided by Guinama (La Pobla de Vallbona, Spain). Hydroxypropylmethylcellulose—Methocel® K 100 M (HPMC; lot: SB13012N31) was kindly supplied by Colorcon Ltd. (Kent, UK). Anhydrous calcium hydrogen phosphate—Emprove®—(ACDP; lot: K93487944416) was supplied by Merck (Darmstadt, Germany). Polyvinylpyrrolidone—Kollidon® 30—(PVP; lot: 98-0820) was purchased from BASF Aktiengesellschaft (Ludwigshafen, Germany). Magnesium stearate PRS-CODEX (MgSt; lot: 85269 ALP) was acquired from Panreac (Barcelona, Spain).

All other reagents in this study were of analytical grade and used without further purification. Demineralized water was used in all cases.

2.2. Preparation of the Granules

The granules were prepared using G39, G43 and a mixture of both in equal proportions in the carrier/TFV ratios, shown in Table 1. The granules were obtained by first melting the Gelucire® in an oil bath (Selecta® Univeba-401, Barcelona, Spain), taking care to ensure the temperature never exceeded 50°C. Once completely melted, the TFV was incorporated and the mixture was stirred until the drug was homogeneously dispersed. The mixture was then spread over a smooth non-stick surface and left to stand at room temperature for a few minutes to solidify. Finally, the solidified mixture was forced through a 1 mm mesh to obtain the granules. Thus, this ensured that all granules obtained had a size of < 1mm in diameter.

Table 1. Granule composition (mg).

Granules	Tenofovir	Gelucire® 39	Gelucire® 43
TFV-1-G43-2	30		60
TFV-1-G43-1	30		30
TFV-2-G43-1	30		15
TFV-1-G41-2	30	30	30
TFV-1-G39-2	30	60	

2.3. Characterization of the Granules

2.3.1. Infrared Spectroscopy

Fourier Transform Infrared Attenuated Total Reflection Spectroscopy (FTIR-ATR) was used to characterize the pure materials and prepared granules with a Perkin-Elmer spectrophotometer equipped with a MIRacle™ accessory designed for FTIR-ATR measurements (Perkin-Elmer, Waltham, MA, USA).

2.3.2. Thermal Analysis

Hot-stage microscopy studies were performed between 30 °C and 350 °C. Approximately 1 mg of each sample was placed on a microscope slide with a cover on a Kofler stage and heated at a rate of 2 °C/min. A thermogalen microscope fitted with the Kofler stage (Leica, Wetzlar, Germany) was used for the microscopy examinations.

Thermogravimetric analysis (TGA) and differential scanning calorimetry (DSC) were done in an SDT-Q 600 TA Instruments TG/DTA analyzer (TA Instruments, New Castle, DE, USA). In this case, about 5–10 mg of samples were placed in a pinholed aluminium sample pan with a lid and heated in atmospheric air to between 30 °C and 500 °C at a rate of 10 °C/min.

2.3.3. X-ray Diffraction

An automated Philips X'Pert-MPD X-ray diffractometer with Bragg–Brentano geometry (Malvern Panalytical Ltd., Royston, UK) was used to obtain the X-ray diffraction patterns of pure materials and all granulated systems. Monochromatized Cu-Kα radiation (λ = 1.5406 Å) was irradiated over the samples at 45 kV, 40 mA and a time per step of 2 s, and analyzed between 2θ angles of 5° and 50°.

An X-ray thermodiffraction of the TFV was also performed using an X'Pert PRO MPD in theta-theta configuration with an Anton Paar HTK1200 high-temperature camera (Malvern Panalytical Ltd., Royston, UK). Monochromatized Cu-Kα radiation (λ = 1.5406 Å) was irradiated over the sample at 45 kV and 40 mA. The sample was heated to 5 °C/min and analyzed between 2θ angles of 5° and 50° at 25 °C, 150 °C, 175 °C and 225 °C. The sample was then cooled at the same rate and analyzed at 200 °C, 150 °C and 25 °C under the same conditions.

2.4. *Preparation of the Tablets*

Vaginal tablets were developed with a combination of hydrophilic polymers (HPMC and CH) containing the granules developed previously. Each granulated system was in turn included in three different combinations of HPMC and CH. HPMC, CH and ACDP were mixed, and the mixture was then wetted with a solution of PVP in ethanol to produce a mass, which was granulated using a 1 mm mesh. Three granulates were obtained (C1, with a ratio of 1:1 HPMC/CH; C2, with a ratio of 1.9:1 HPMC/CH; and C3, with a ratio of 1:1.9 HPMC/CH) and dried at room temperature for 24 h. Lastly, each granulate was mixed with the TFV granules for a final content of 30 mg of drug and 290 mg of hydrophilic polymer per tablet. All granulates were prepared by forcing them through the same mesh to ensure that all granules—polymeric and TFV-loaded granules—had the same size (<1 mm in diameter), and the blends were homogeneous. MgSt was added to the total dried granules before tableting. The final content of each batch is shown in Table 2.

Table 2. Tablet composition (mg/unit).

Batch	HPMC	CH	ACDP	PVP	TFV	G43	G39	MgSt
TFV-1-G43-2 C1	145	145	45	27	30	60		3
TFV-1-G43-2 C2	190	100	45	27	30	60		3
TFV-1-G43-2 C3	100	190	45	27	30	60		3
TFV-1-G43-1 C1	145	145	45	27	30	30		3
TFV-1-G43-1 C2	190	100	45	27	30	30		3
TFV-1-G43-1 C3	100	190	45	27	30	30		3
TFV-2-G43-1 C1	145	145	45	27	30	15		3
TFV-2-G43-1 C2	190	100	45	27	30	15		3
TFV-2-G43-1 C3	100	190	45	27	30	15		3
TFV-1-G41-2 C1	145	145	45	27	30	30	30	3
TFV-1-G41-2 C2	190	100	45	27	30	30	30	3
TFV-1-G41-2 C3	100	190	45	27	30	30	30	3
TFV-1-G39-2 C1	145	145	45	27	30		60	3
TFV-1-G39-2 C2	190	100	45	27	30		60	3
TFV-1-G39-2 C3	100	190	45	27	30		60	3

HPMC: Hydroxypropylmethylcellulose; CH: Chitosan; ACDP: Anhydrous calcium hydrogen phosphate.

The tablets were produced using a press similar to the one used for preparing solid samples for analysis by IR spectroscopy. A constant pressure of 5 tons was applied for four minutes using a punch. The resulting tablets were cylindrical in shape with a diameter of 13 mm and a height of 2.5–2.8 mm.

2.5. *Assessment of the Tablets*

2.5.1. Swelling Behavior

The method described by Ruiz-Caro et al. [18] was used to analyze the swelling behavior of each batch in simulated vaginal fluid (SVF) [19]. The test was done in triplicate in a shaking water bath (Selecta® UNITRONIC320 OR, Barcelona, Spain) at 37 °C and 15 opm. The discs were removed from the medium at predetermined times, placed on filter paper to eliminate excess liquid and weighed.

The swelling ratio (SR) was calculated following Equation (1) where T_s and T_d correspond to the swollen and dry tablet weights respectively:

$$SR = \frac{T_s - T_d}{T_d} \cdot 100. \tag{1}$$

Since the initial tablet weight varies depending on the amount of Gelucire® it contains, the *SR* of different batches was compared by determining the adjusted swelling ratio (*ASR*), where the weight increment is related to the amount of swellable polymer, as shown in Equation (2) where *SR*, T_d and *SP* correspond respectively to the swelling ratio determined by Equation (1), the dry tablet weight, and the amount of swellable polymer in the tablet:

$$ASR = \frac{SR \cdot T_d}{SP}. \tag{2}$$

2.5.2. Release Study

The release of TFV from the batches was evaluated with the method described by Sánchez-Sánchez et al. [20]. The tablets were immersed in 80 mL of SVF in a borosilicate glass bottle and placed in a shaking water bath (Selecta® UNITRONIC320 OR, Barcelona, Spain) at 37 °C and 15 opm. The test was performed in triplicate. Release tests are performed in sink conditions because the solubility of TFV in SVF, measured at room temperature, is 4 mg/mL. 5 mL samples were taken and filtered at given times, and the medium was replaced with the same volume of SVF at the same temperature. The TFV released was quantified by UV spectroscopy at a wavelength of 260 nm in a Shimadzu® UV-1700 (Kyoto, Japan).

The similarity factor (f_2) (Equation (3)) was calculated in order to statistically demonstrate the differences between the batches.

$$f_2 = 50 \times \log \left\{ \left[1 + \left(\frac{1}{n} \right) \sum_{j=1}^{n} W_j \left| R_j - T_j \right|^2 \right]^{-0.5} \times 100 \right\}. \tag{3}$$

This is a model-independent index described by Moore and Flanner [21], where n is the number of samples for each dissolution test, R_j and T_j are the drug release percentage at each time for the reference and test product respectively, and W_j is a weight factor, which in this study is equal to 1. A value of $f_2 > 65$ means similarity between the profiles of over 95%, while $f_2 < 65$ indicates that the profiles are significantly different [22].

Finally, the experimental drug-release data were fitted to different model-dependent methods (zero order, first order, Higuchi, Hixson-Crowell, Hopfenberg and Korsmeyer-Peppas models) to investigate the drug release kinetics [23].

2.5.3. Mucoadhesion Test

The method described by Notario-Pérez et al. [24] was used to evaluate ex vivo mucoadhesion time. A sample of freshly excised veal vaginal mucosa was obtained from a local slaughterhouse and attached to an 8.5 cm × 5 cm stainless steel plate with a cyanoacrylate adhesive. Each tablet was then placed over the mucosa and weight of 500 g was applied for 30 s. The system was placed at an angle of 60° in a beaker containing 150 mL of SVF and then in the shaking water bath (Selecta® UNITRONIC320 OR, Barcelona, Spain) at 37 °C and 15 opm. All batches were tested in duplicate.

3. Results and Discussion

3.1. Characterization of the Granules

3.1.1. Infrared Spectroscopy

The analysis of the granules by FTIR-ATR, and the subsequent comparison with the spectrum obtained by analyzing the raw materials used in their preparation, reveal any possible interactions that may have occurred at the molecular level during the granulation process. These interactions—if they occur—require an in-depth analysis to ensure that the therapeutic efficacy of the TFV has not been modified.

The two types of Gelucire® analyzed (G39 and G43) showed a very similar FTIR-ATR spectrum, which is to be expected given their close structural similarity (Figure 1B). These spectra are also clearly similar to those obtained by other authors with other types of Gelucire® [25]. Characteristics worth noting include a band at around 1650 cm^{-1} corresponding to the C–O bonds and another double band around 2800 cm^{-1}, due to the C=O bond [26].

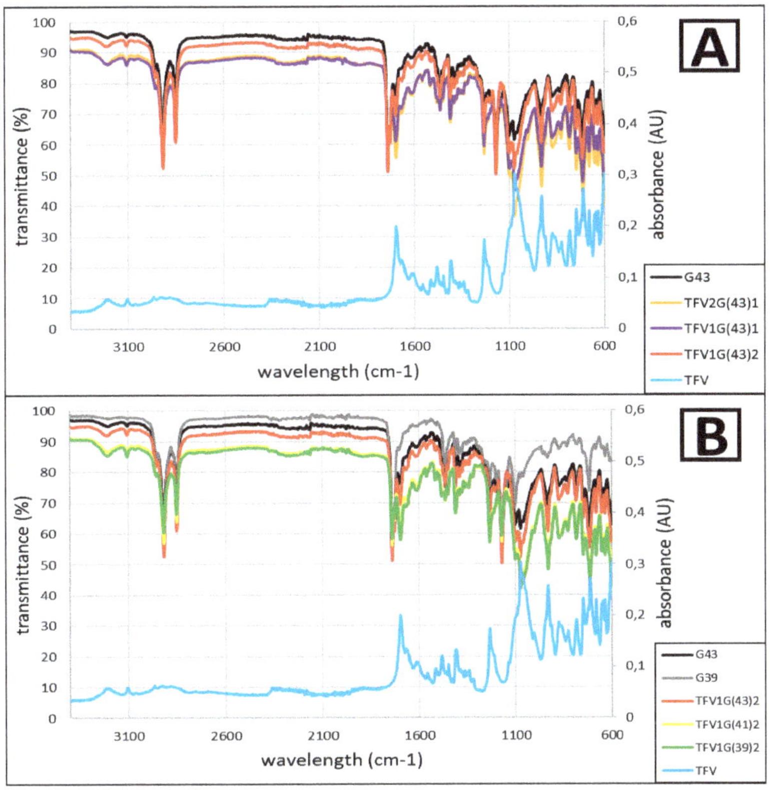

Figure 1. FTIR-ATR spectra of TFV, G43 and their combinations (**A**); and TFV, G43, G39 and their combinations in a 1:2 ratio of TFV/Gelucire® (**B**). The absorbance spectra (right axes) correspond to TFV.

TFV is notable for a band around 1700 cm^{-1}, corresponding to C=O stretching [27]. It also has bands at 3100 cm^{-1} and 3200 cm^{-1} corresponding to C–H and N–H bonds respectively [28] (Figure 1).

The results of the spectra obtained with the prepared granules are in all cases very similar, and always resemble the results that would be obtained by superimposing the spectra for the raw materials (Figure 1).

The FTIR-ATR analysis confirms that the raw materials—Gelucire® and TFV—do not interact with each other at a molecular level during the granulation process, thus maintaining the drug's properties.

3.1.2. Thermal Analysis

Thermal analysis was performed in order to determine the characteristics of the granules in greater detail. The TGA analysis (Figure 2) shows the weight lost by the granules during heating. The raw materials were also analyzed using this technique. In the case of TFV, about 5% of the weight is lost at around 90 °C (this is probably a loss of the water captured by the drug during storage), followed by a strong degradation that possibly corresponds to the drug decomposition, beginning at around 320 °C. At 500 °C, the sample maintains about 65% of its initial weight. In contrast, the Gelucire® samples show no water loss in the TGA analysis, due to the Gelucire®'s limited uptake of water at ambient humidity conditions [29], and there is no change in the TGA curves until around 240 °C. From this point until 370 °C the samples undergo a marked decomposition and lose over 80% of their weight. With further heating, Gelucire® samples continue losing weight more slowly and when the test ends at 500 °C, less than 5% of the initial weight remains. Both G43 and G39 show similar results, but should be noted that the final weight loss is lower in the G39 sample. These minor differences between the different Gelucire® products can be attributed to the slight variations in their composition [11]. Granules combining TFV and Gelucire® in all cases display an intermediate behavior between the raw materials used in their manufacture. The comparison of granules with different TFV/Gelucire® ratios show that the greater the amount of Gelucire® included in the sample, the higher the final weight loss (Figure 2A). The variations are almost negligible in granules prepared with different Gelucire®, although the inclusion of more G39 than G41 can still be seen to cause the granules to degrade more, as in the case of the raw materials. Finally, it should also be noted that no weight loss is observed in the TGA analysis of the granules at around 90 °C, as occurs in the TFV sample, which confirms that the weight loss is due to water, as the raw materials are heated and the water has already been removed during the preparation of the granules.

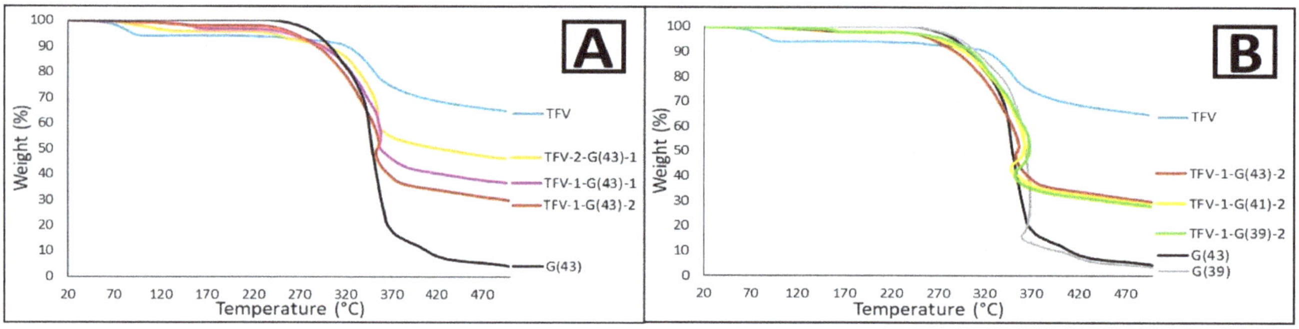

Figure 2. Thermogravimetric analysis (TGA) curves of TFV, G43 and their combinations (**A**); and TFV, G43, G39 and their combinations in a ratio of 1:2 of TFV/Gelucire® (**B**).

DSC analyses were performed to check if during the process of preparation of the solid dispersion it occurs the dissolution of the active principle in the molten vehicle, which would later be reversible by crystallization of the TFV during the cooling of the binary system, and the results are shown in Figure 3. The TFV DSC curve is characteristic, due to an endothermic peak at around 160 °C and an exothermic peak at around 220 °C, which may correspond to changes in the crystallinity of the drug. A stronger endothermic peak beginning at 295 °C corresponds to the TFV melting point [30]. Finally, drug decomposition is observed at around 315 °C.

An endothermic peak can be seen in both G43 and G39 at approximately their respective melting points. These melting points begin shortly after ambient temperature, as has already been observed by other researchers [31], and can be explained by the fact that Gelucire® are multicomponent mixtures with a semi-solid nature. Exothermic readings beginning at 230 °C are observed in both Gelucire®, and the main difference is in their decomposition, which in both cases begins after 400 °C but is much more vigorous for G43 than for G39.

When analyzing the DSC curves from the granules combining one or both Gelucire® with TFV, the main observation is an intermediate curve between the curves obtained from the raw materials. The three characteristic peaks of TFV appear in all the prepared granules, so mixing with Gelucire® apparently has no effect on the drug. Nevertheless, it should be noted that the inclusion of TFV appears to lower the melting point of Gelucire® (Figure 3).

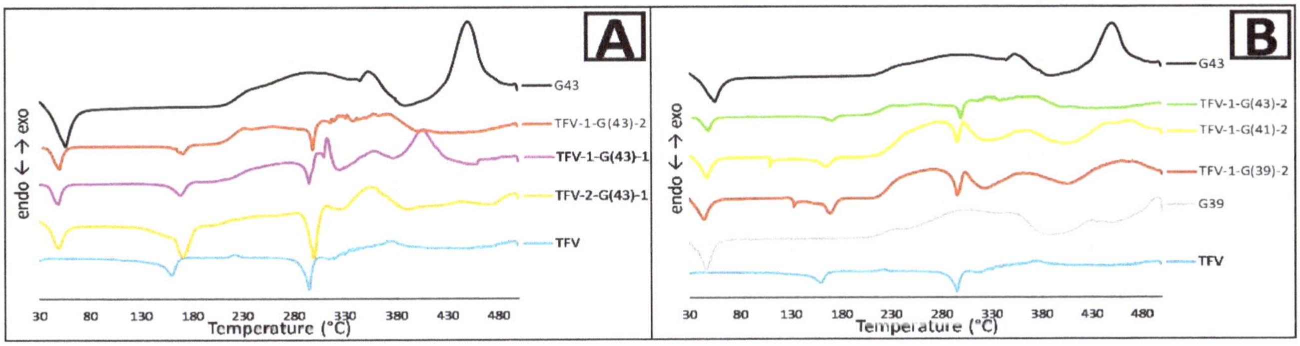

Figure 3. Differential scanning calorimetry (DSC) curves of TFV, G43 and their combinations (**A**); and TFV, G43, G39 and their combinations in a ratio of 1:2 of TFV/Gelucire® (**B**).

Finally, hot stage microscopy (HSM) was performed to complete the thermal analysis of the samples. TFV can be seen as a crystalline substance in the visualization. When heating the sample, some changes in the shape of particles are observed at 167 °C. The temperature continues rising and a similar behavior can be seen on reaching 220°C. These two changes may correspond to crystalline transitions of TFV, as was assumed to occur when analyzing the DSC curve. Finally, the sample begins to melt at around 265 °C.

Both Gelucire® appear as irregularly-shaped particles of a waxy substance with a rough surface. They are crystalline, since polarized light can pass through the samples. The start of the melting process is identified by HSM at a somewhat lower temperature than indicated by the supplier (40 °C for G43 and 36 °C for G39), as shown in the DSC analysis (Figure 3). G39 turns brown at around 310°C, as though the sample had charred, and it appears to start boiling.

Very similar results are obtained when analyzing the granules by HSM. The main changes are summarized in Figure 4. They all appear in the microscope as irregular particles that allow the partial passage of polarized light. In all the samples, the first change observed is the melting of the Gelucire®. The more G39 there is in the granules, the lower the melting point (Figure 4). When comparing samples containing only G41 and TFV, the granules with twice as much TFV as G41 have a higher melting point. However, the melting of G41 is more difficult to visual identify, due to its low proportion, so it probably occurs before it can be visually detected (when a halo of melted Gelucire® is seen around the TFV particles). Once the Gelucire® is completely melted, there are more particles that allow the passage of polarized light, corresponding to TFV crystals surrounded by melted Gelucire®. The first crystalline transition in the TFV raw material is not detected in any of the granules. However, an interesting phenomenon occurs at the temperature of the second crystalline transition of TFV. From 212 °C to 226 °C, depending on the sample, the TFV crystals that allow the passage of polarized light to disappear, probably because after the change in its crystallinity TFV is able to dissolve into the melted Gelucire®. This ability of melted Gelucire® to dissolve drugs has also been noted by other researchers [31]. However, some TFV crystals are still in evidence, so the amount of molten Gelucire® is insufficient to dissolve all the TFV present in the sample. A little later, at between 224 °C and 251°C, the sample carbonizes and turns brown, probably because the dissolved TFV has burned. Between 262–270 °C, the remaining particles that still allow the passage of polarized light disappear completely in some samples, corresponding to the melting of the undissolved TFV, which occurs at the temperature at which the TFV raw material melts. Finally, at around 290 °C, the Gelucire® can be seen to be boiling. After analyzing all the information from the thermal analysis of the granules, it can be confirmed that no interaction between Gelucire® and TFV occurs at the manufacturing temperatures; however, a more in-depth study was made using X-ray diffraction techniques to confirm the TFV transitions and some of the interactions that are assumed to occur at higher temperatures.

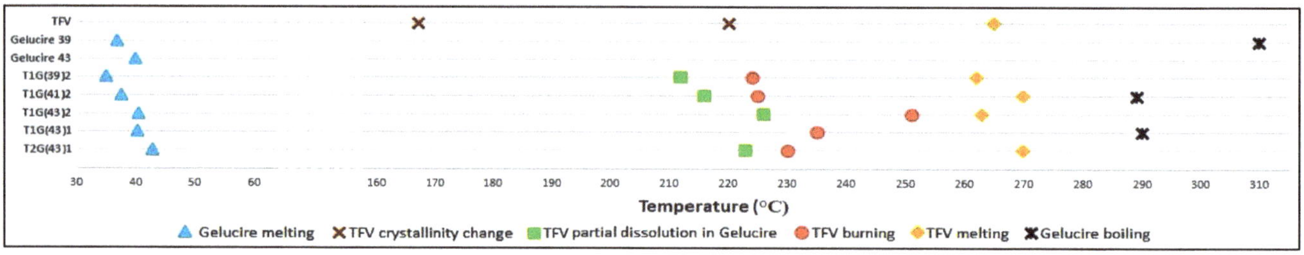

Figure 4. Diagram of the changes visualized during the observation of TFV, Gelucire® and the granules by hot stage microscopy.

3.1.3. X-ray Diffraction

X-ray spectrometry studies were performed to evaluate if these is any change in the crystalline state of the drug during the granulation process. These studies could also corroborate the hypotheses formulated after the thermal analysis of the granules. First the raw materials (TFV, G43 and G39) and the manufactured granules were analyzed to compare them and confirm that there is no interaction between the drug and the carriers during granulation.

The X-ray diffraction pattern for TFV reveals the four characteristic peaks of the drug at 7.3, 14.7, 18.3 and 23.4° 2θ [32]. This clearly confirms that TFV is a crystalline substance, as observed in HSM. There are hardly any differences between G43 and G39, and both are crystalline (as observed in HSM) with two intense peaks at 20.9 and 23.1° 2θ. This agrees with the results obtained for other Gelucire®, which also present peaks at between 20–25° 2θ [33]. A third peak of lower intensity can also be distinguished at around 6.8° 2θ, which is more clearly visible in G39 (Figure 5). The spectra observed in the granules is a mixture of the spectra obtained with their component raw materials, and the lower the proportion of each material in the composition of the granules, the lower the intensity of the characteristic peaks (Figure 5).

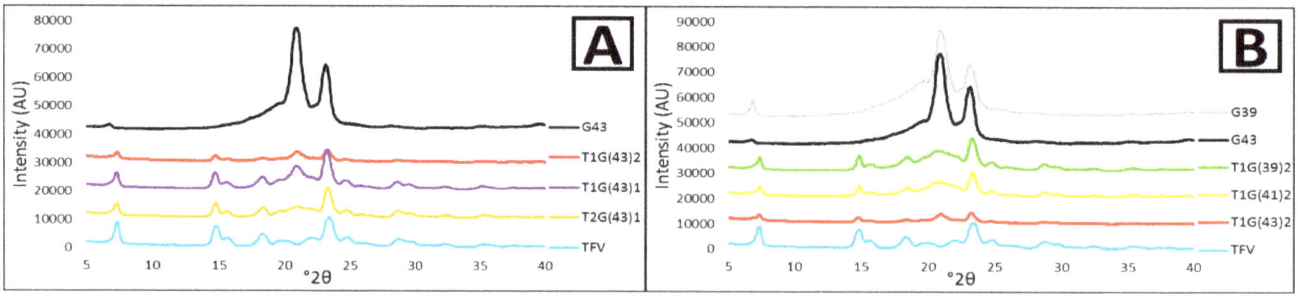

Figure 5. X-ray diffraction patterns of pure TFV, G43 and their combinations (**A**); and TFV, G43, G39 and their combinations in a ratio of 1:2 TFV/Gelucire® (**B**).

In conclusion, this analysis allows us to confirm that no drug-Gelucire® interaction occurs in the granulation process.

However, various changes were observed in TFV in DSC and HSM that have been attributed to the crystalline transition of the drug, although a further study was done to confirm this.

The X-Ray thermodiffraction technique revealed the changes in the drug's crystallinity caused by temperature. A study was done to confirm that the changes observed in DSC and HSM at 167 °C and 220 °C correspond to the crystalline transition of TFV. This consisted of measuring a sample of pure TFV by X-ray diffraction at room temperature (25 °C) and then after heating. The temperature was maintained for five minutes before and after the temperatures at which changes were observed, then a measurement was taken by X-ray diffraction. After reaching 225 °C, higher than the temperatures at which the previous change had occurred, the sample was cooled and new measurements were taken using the same procedure to determine whether the temperature-related changes are reversible.

The spectra observed when the sample was analyzed at 25 °C is exactly the same as in the previous study at room temperature (Figures 5 and 6). Although other authors have found that the crystallinity of TFV does not change with temperature, their studies reached only 80 °C [32,34]. In our study, the sample was heated to 150 °C before taking the second measurement, prior to the first change in the structure of TFV. Surprisingly, changes can be seen in TFV at this temperature. This is probably because the first transition has already begun, as the characteristic peaks have been displaced to 7.3° and 23.4° 2θ, the peak that was present at 14.7° 2θ has disappeared, and a series of peaks have appeared between 16–19° 2θ. At 175 °C, the spectrum is completely different to the one obtained at 25 °C, with a double peak between 8–9° 2θ, another two double peaks around 17–18° 2θ, and a band with multiple peaks between 19–20° 2θ that were not observed at lower temperatures. This clearly confirms that the first crystalline transition of TFV is complete (Figure 6). At 225 °C the spectrum is slightly different: The peak at 9° 2θ disappears and the intensity of the peak at 17° 2θ decreases. The second crystalline change is therefore complete at 225 °C, allowing the dissolution of TFV in its new state in the melted Gelucire®, as observed in the HSM studies. Finally, the sample was cooled and new measurements were taken, and no change was observed in X-ray diffraction, thus confirming that the crystalline changes in TFV are irreversible.

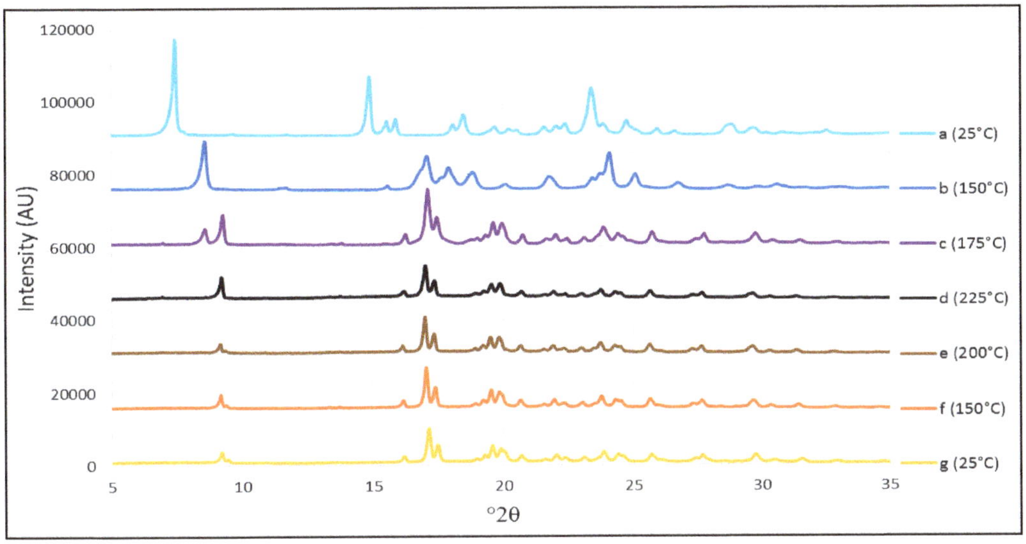

Figure 6. X-ray thermodiffraction patterns of pure TFV while heating to 25 °C (a), 150 °C (b), 175 °C (c) and 225 °C (d); and then while cooling to 200 °C (e), 150 °C (f) and 25 °C (g).

After the IR, thermal and X-ray analysis of the prepared granules, we can confirm that TFV is not altered in the hot-melt granulation process but conserves its therapeutic properties, thus enabling the use of the granules for prevention of HIV.

3.2. *Assessment of the Tablets*

3.2.1. Swelling Behavior

The evaluation of the swelling behavior of the formulations has a twofold importance: The capture of water is the main mechanism controlling the release of the drug, since it is unable to diffuse until the hydrophilic polymer swells and the water surrounds the granules [35]; and the swelling of the formulations can be seen as a way of improving adherence to prophylactic treatment, as the lower water capture would make the tablets more comfortable for women.

The inclusion of the drug granulated with G43 in the polymer matrix clearly improves the formulation in terms of swelling. As can be seen in Figure 7, the maximum swelling ratio is notably lower than in the formulations containing the drug without Gelucire® [16], and especially in the formulations in which HPMC is greater than or equal to CH, due to the predominantly hydrophobic character of Gelucire®. The formulation achieves complete erosion sooner with the addition of the granules: After 216 h instead of the 264 h for the original formulation. This behavior would imply greater adherence to prophylaxis, since the formulation would remain less time in the vaginal environment after the drug release, making it more comfortable for women. The more HPMC there is in the formulation, the higher the maximum swelling ratio. This was expected, as the swelling capacity of HPMC is higher than CH [24]. Finally, no clear differences ca be seen between the formulations containing granules with a different G43/TFV ratio (Figure 7).

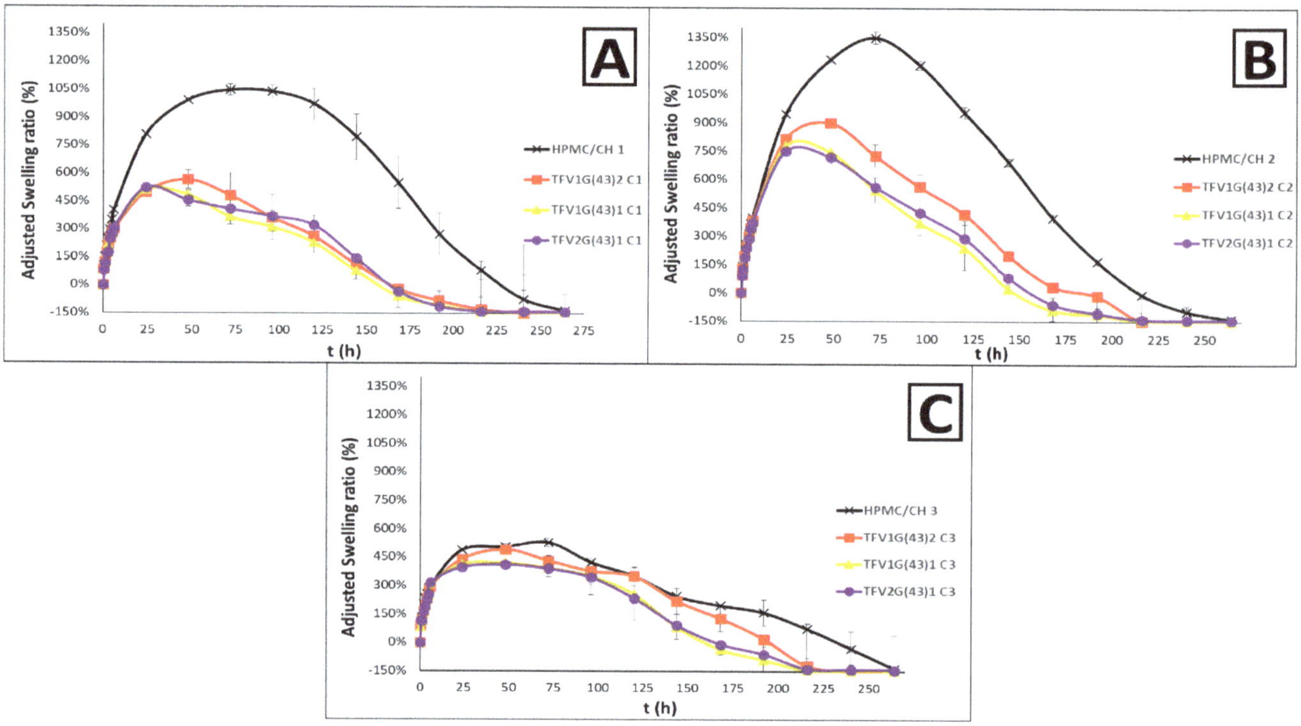

Figure 7. Adjusted swelling ratio profiles obtained from batches containing TFV/G43 drug-loaded granules in HPMC/CH matrices with equal ratios of both polymers (**A**); more HPMC than CH (**B**); and more CH than HPMC (**C**). They are all compared with standard formulations of HPMC/CH [16].

The use of different G39 or a mixture of G39 and G43 does not appear to change the swelling behavior of the formulations. This is to be expected since HPMC and CH are polymers with a capacity to capture water, and both Gelucire® act similarly as a barrier to water diffusion. Only the tablets with more HPMC than CH show a slight difference in the formulations containing G39 (or a G39/G43 mixture), which have a lower water capture than tablets with only G43. Nevertheless, an improvement is again observed compared to the formulations without Gelucire® (Figure 8).

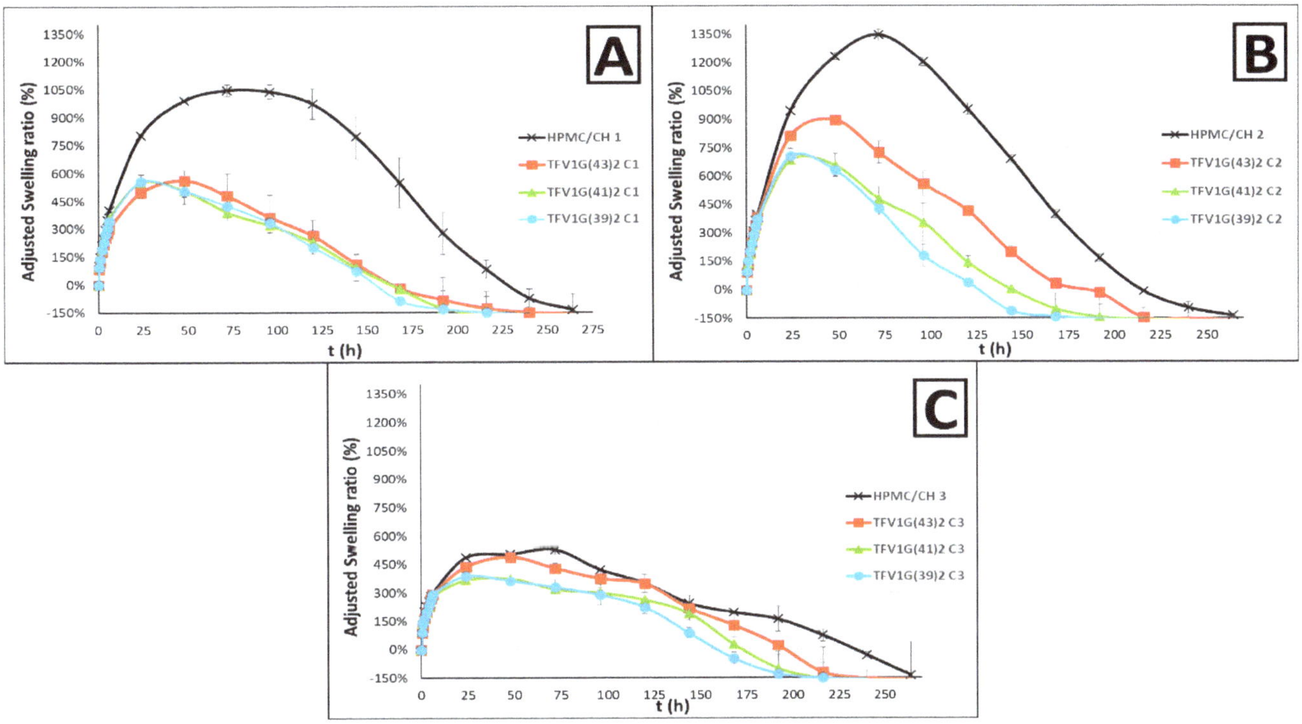

Figure 8. Adjusted swelling ratio profiles obtained from batches containing TFV/Gelucire® (in a 1:2 ratio) granules in HPMC/CH matrices with equal ratios of both polymers (**A**); more HPMC than CH (**B**); and more CH than HPMC (**C**). They are all compared with standard formulations of HPMC/CH [16].

The inclusion of the granules creates barriers within the tablet that hinder the diffusion of water and leads to lower water capture. This not only makes the tablets more comfortable, but would also probably prevent the loss of the drug, since it contains less water through which to diffuse. We can therefore formulate the hypothesis that this formulation would be more effective for the controlled release of TFV, although this must be confirmed in subsequent drug-release studies.

3.2.2. Release Study

As can be seen in Figure 9, the inclusion of mixed TFV/G43 granules in the formulations enhances the controlled release of the drug. These differences can be observed from the beginning of the drug release test, as the Gelucire® must soften as it forms granules with the drug to allow the release of the TFV. This softening is enabled by the presence of water and body temperature. Once the Gelucire® is softened and the drug diffuses through it, it is incorporated in a matrix of HPMC and CH polymers, which form a gel in the vaginal medium through which the drug must diffuse. As has been observed in the swelling test, the presence of the granules hinders the swelling of the polymers, which also causes the drug to be released from the tablet in a more sustained way.

In the samples containing granules with equal or more TFV than G43 (TFV2G(43)1 and TFV1G(43)1), the TFV drug release profiles obtained are quite similar. In these samples the main improvement is the slowdown of the release of TFV, since almost all the drug is released at 120 h (as occurred in the samples that do not use Gelucire®), although there are significant differences in the drug release behavior. In batches with TFV1G(43)2 granules, which include twice the amount of G43 as TFV, the improvement is much more marked (as an example, at 24 h approximately half the amount of drug has been released as in standard batches). This is because of the higher amount of G43 impedes softening and it takes longer for the drug to be released from the granules. Drug release is prolonged to 216–240 h, thus achieving 9−10 days of a controlled release of TFV. This is double the time taken without Gelucire® granules, and could represent a milestone in HIV transmission, since a degradable vaginal formulation capable of reaching these controlled release times has never previously been achieved.

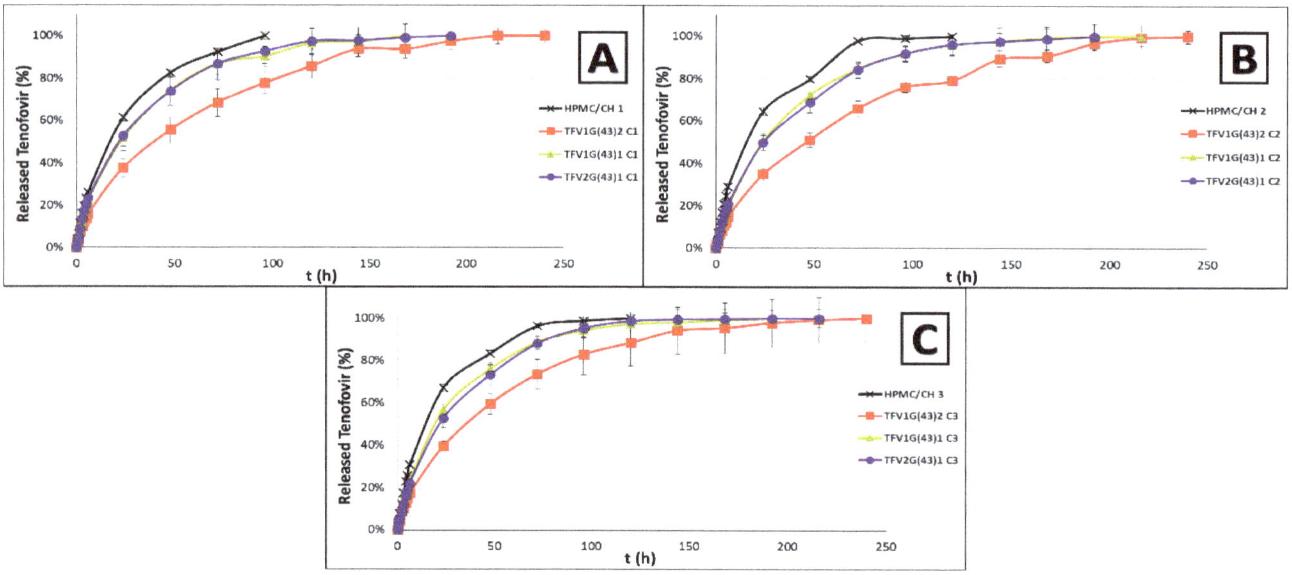

Figure 9. TFV release profiles obtained from batches including TFV/G43 drug-loaded granules in HPMC/CH matrices with equal ratios of both polymers (**A**), more HPMC than CH (**B**) and more CH than HPMC (**C**). All of them are compared with standard formulations of HPMC/CH [16].

It was also necessary to evaluate whether a Gelucire® with a melting point that was closer to body temperature would alter the release of the drug. Figure 10 shows that when G39 or a mixture of G39 and G41 is used to manufacture the granules, TFV is released faster than in tablets with TFV/G43 granules. These batches confirm that the softening of the Gelucire® is a crucial factor for controlling TFV release; this agrees with other authors, who also highlight that in the case of Gelucire® that melt above body temperature, the release of the drug depends on the composition and HLB value [36].

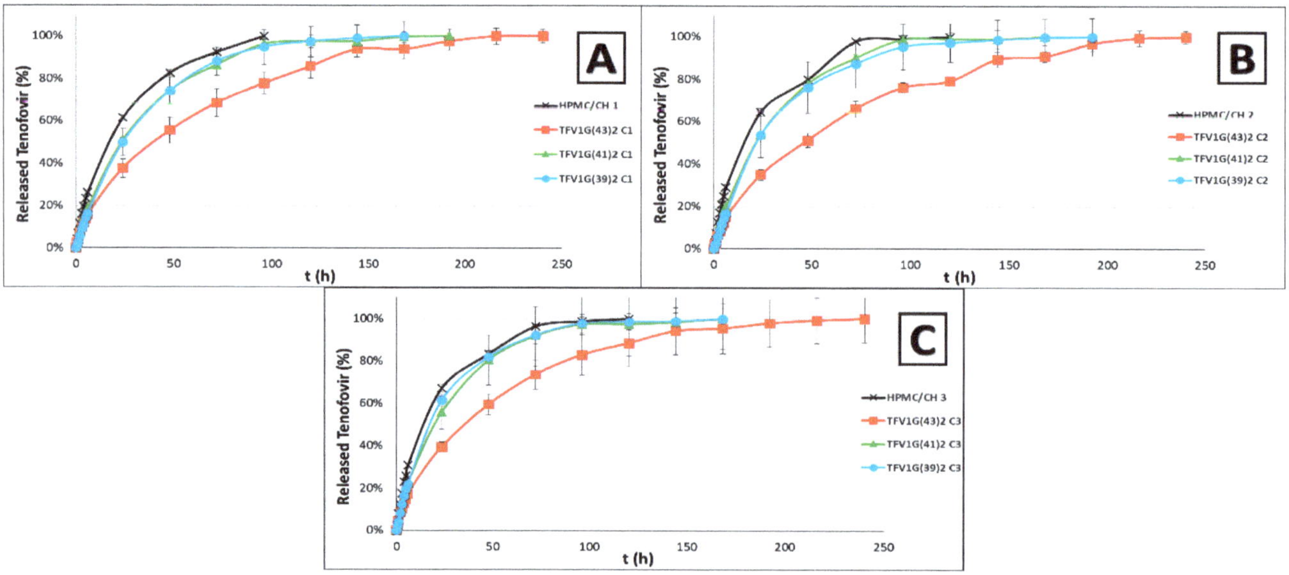

Figure 10. TFV release profiles obtained from batches containing TFV/Gelucire® (in a ratio of 1:2) granules in HPMC/CH matrices with equal ratios of both polymers (**A**); more HPMC than CH (**B**); and more CH than HPMC (**C**). All are compared with standard formulations of HPMC/CH [16].

The TFV1G(43)2 granules are therefore undoubtedly the best formulation. Finally, a comparison must be made of the formulations containing different proportions of HPMC/CH. Although the three proportions have similar TFV release profiles, the formulation with the most HPMC (TFV1G(43)2 C2) shows the greatest controlled release (Figure 10B).

Although the figures visually identify the improvements achieved with the formulations, the f_2 similarity factor was also calculated as a statistical analysis that could demonstrate these differences [37]. Table 3 shows the f_2 values for all the formulations.

Table 3. Similarity factor (f_2) values for the release profiles obtained from reference and problem formulations. Comparisons with significant difference ($f_2 < 65$) are in bold.

REFERENCE	PROBLEM	f_2	REFERENCE	PROBLEM	f_2	REFERENCE	PROBLEM	f_2
C1	T1G(43)2 C1	**44.6**	C1	C2	84.3	T1G(43)2 C1	T1G(43)2 C2	83.4
C1	T1G(43)1 C1	**64.7**	C1	C3	76.9	T1G(43)2 C1	T1G(43)2 C3	78.4
C1	T2G(43)1 C1	66.9	C2	C3	85.6	T1G(43)2 C2	T1G(43)2 C3	68.1
C1	T1G(41)2 C1	**60.4**	T1G(43)2 C1	T1G(43)1 C1	**54.5**	T1G(43)1 C1	T1G(43)1 C2	83.5
C1	T1G(39)2 C1	**60.5**	T1G(43)2 C1	T2G(43)1 C1	**53.7**	T1G(43)1 C1	T1G(43)1 C3	84.9
C2	T1G(43)2 C2	**40.9**	T1G(43)2 C1	T1G(41)2 C1	**56.3**	T1G(43)1 C2	T1G(43)1 C3	75.1
C2	T1G(43)1 C2	**55.8**	T1G(43)2 C1	T1G(39)2 C1	**57.2**	T2G(43)1 C1	T2G(43)1 C2	81.3
C2	T2G(43)1 C2	**56.7**	T1G(43)2 C2	T1G(43)1 C2	**50.0**	T2G(43)1 C1	T2G(43)1 C3	94.5
C2	T1G(41)2 C2	**60.5**	T1G(43)2 C2	T2G(43)1 C2	**51.0**	T2G(43)1 C2	T2G(43)1 C3	84.8
C2	T1G(39)2 C2	**54.7**	T1G(43)2 C2	T1G(41)2 C2	**48.4**	T1G(41)2 C1	T1G(41)2 C2	86.2
C3	T1G(43)2 C3	**43.3**	T1G(43)2 C2	T1G(39)2 C2	**50.0**	T1G(41)2 C1	T1G(41)2 C3	73.7
C3	T1G(43)1 C3	**60.5**	T1G(43)2 C3	T1G(43)1 C3	**54.6**	T1G(41)2 C2	T1G(41)2 C3	83.7
C3	T2G(43)1 C3	**56.5**	T1G(43)2 C3	T2G(43)1 C3	**59.1**	T1G(39)2 C1	T1G(39)2 C2	88.1
C3	T1G(41)2 C3	**61.9**	T1G(43)2 C3	T1G(41)2 C3	**52.4**	T1G(39)2 C1	T1G(39)2 C3	**62.7**
C3	T1G(39)2 C3	**64.1**	T1G(43)2 C3	T1G(39)2 C3	**49.3**	T1G(39)2 C2	T1G(39)2 C3	67.4

The first point to emphasize is that all the formulations developed in the present work improve those with the same proportion of HPMC/CH but without Gelucire® (except for formulation TFV2G(43)1 C1, which has a slight similarity with the formulation without Gelucire®). This highlights the role of Gelucire® in controlling the release of TFV from the tablets. However, when comparing formulations with the same granules but with a different proportion of the HPMC/CH mixture, significant differences were observed in only one case (batches TFV1G(39)2 C1 and TFV1G(39)2 C3). This reaffirms the fact that the combination of HPMC and CH forms a very robust mixed gel capable of delaying the release of TFV regardless of the proportion of polymer [16]. Although the granules' ability to control the release has been demonstrated, these results must be compared with formulations with the same proportion of HPMC/CH but different granules, in order to determine which granules are the most suitable. The comparison of these formulations confirms that the granules identified in Figure 9 as best controlling TFV release (TFV1G(43)2) always present significant differences with the other granules, regardless of the proportion of HPMC/CH in the tablets that include the granules.

The statistical analysis therefore shows that the TFV1G(43)2 granules are the best option for preparing our formulations, although it is impossible to specify the most appropriate proportion of hydrophilic polymers to include in these granules since they are all very similar.

Finally, the experimental data obtained in the drug release tests were adjusted to different mathematical models (zero order, first order, Higuchi, Hixson-Crowell, Hopfenberg and Korsmeyer-Peppas). The correlation coefficients (r^2) obtained after the adjustment are shown in Table 4.

Table 4. Correlation coefficients obtained when experimental data are fitted to different mathematical models.

Batch	Correlation Coefficients (r^2)					
	Zero Order	First Order	Higuchi	Hixson-Crowell	Hopfenberg	Korsmeyer-Peppas
TFV1G(43)2 C1	0.9557	0.7162	0.9975	0.9888	0.9824	0.9915
TFV1G(43)2 C2	0.9658	0.7139	0.9961	0.9925	0.9877	0.9876
TFV1G(43)2 C3	0.9567	0.7188	0.9971	0.9922	0.9858	0.9911
TFV1G(43)1 C1	0.9140	0.6436	0.9885	0.9749	0.9624	0.9795
TFV1G(43)1 C2	0.9298	0.6610	0.9911	0.9884	0.9771	0.9887
TFV1G(43)1 C3	0.9110	0.6514	0.9878	0.9835	0.9690	0.9896
TFV2G(43)1 C1	0.9190	0.6474	0.9920	0.9852	0.9723	0.9801
TFV2G(43)1 C2	0.9351	0.6671	0.9954	0.9911	0.9813	0.9864
TFV2G(43)1 C3	0.9306	0.6849	0.9939	0.9938	0.9834	0.9933
TFV1G(41)2 C1	0.9377	0.663	0.9930	0.9958	0.9877	0.9850
TFV1G(41)2 C2	0.9307	0.6604	0.9912	0.9963	0.9897	0.9889
TFV1G(41)2 C3	0.9148	0.6139	0.9886	0.9918	0.9775	0.9662
TFV1G(39)2 C1	0.9384	0.6522	0.9886	0.9948	0.9850	0.9862
TFV1G(39)2 C2	0.9270	0.6708	0.9854	0.9916	0.9796	0.9941
TFV1G(39)2 C3	0.9005	0.6437	0.9819	0.9879	0.9705	0.9983

As can be seen, all the formulations have a similar drug release profile and a good fit to the kinetics of Higuchi, Hixson-Crowell, Hopfenberg and Korsmeyer-Peppas (Table 4). However, there are slight differences between the batches that merit discussion. One observation is that all batches containing G43 tend to have a better fit to Higuchi kinetics. This model is often used to describe the behavior of matrix tablets, where the drug is released through a diffusion mechanism [38]. The most likely reason that these batches fit this kinetic more closely is that the G43 softens slowly, and the gelation of the outer layer of the hydrophilic polymer has already taken place when it occurs. This explains why the drug release is predominantly controlled by the diffusion mechanism (through both the softened Gelucire® and the gel formed by the HPMC/CH mixture).

The tablets containing the mixture of G43 and G39 have a better fit to the Hixson-Crowell kinetics, a mathematical model applied when the drug is released from the parallel planes of the dosage form, which maintains its shape while its size decreases [39]. In these cases the Gelucire® mixture softens a little faster than in the previous ones; one possible explanation for this drug-release mechanism is that the hydrophilic polymers gel from the outer to the inner layers, and the Gelucire® softens as the vaginal fluid reaches the granules through the gel. This explains why the drug is released in layers, first diffusing the TFV in the outer layers of the tablet, and then the drug in the innermost layers.

Finally, batches with G39 are better fitted to the Korsmeyer-Peppas kinetics (except batch TFV1G(39)2 C1, which has a better fit to the Hixson-Crowell kinetics, although it also fits the Korsmeyer-Peppas kinetics quite well) (Table 4). The Korsmeyer-Peppas model gives us the most information about the drug-release mechanism, since the drug is released in different ways depending on the value of n obtained in the adjustment [40]. Thus for cylindrical tablets, TFV release follows a pure diffusion process ($n \leq 0.45$) or an anomalous transport with simultaneous structural modification and diffusion ($0.45 < n < 0.89$). If there is a structural modification of the polymer matrix, the release is classified as transport case II ($n = 0.89$) or transport Supercase II ($n > 0.89$).

In our case, almost all the formulations can be seen to follow a simultaneous mechanism of structural modification and diffusion (Table 5), which is to be expected since it is first necessary for the hydrophilic polymer gel and the Gelucire® to soften (structural modification) and the TFV to subsequently diffuse before the drug can be released. However, there are three exceptions which present a Supercase II release and are precisely the three that include G39 in the granules (Table 5). In these cases, the melting temperature of the vehicle is so low that the G39 softens as soon as it is at body temperature, even before the vaginal fluid reaches the granules, implying that the structure of the tablet changes even before the HPMC/CH mixture begins to gel.

Table 5. TFV release kinetics from the different batches showing the kinetic constants for the models with the best fit.

Batch	Higuchi	Hixson-Crowell	Hopfenberg	Korsmeyer-Peppas	
	K_H	K_{HC}	K_{HF}	K_{KP}	n
TFV1G(43)2 C1	0.083	0.0040	0.0054	0.042	0.68
TFV1G(43)2 C2	0.080	0.0039	0.0052	0.036	0.71
TFV1G(43)2 C3	0.088	0.0045	0.0060	0.046	0.67
TFV1G(43)1 C1	0.102	0.0059	0.0075	0.045	0.82
TFV1G(43)1 C2	0.103	0.0060	0.0076	0.037	0.86
TFV1G(43)1 C3	0.106	0.0065	0.0081	0.048	0.81
TFV2G(43)1 C1	0.103	0.0061	0.0077	0.056	0.73
TFV2G(43)1 C2	0.108	0.0058	0.0074	0.047	0.78
TFV2G(43)1 C3	0.105	0.0065	0.0081	0.052	0.75
TFV1G(41)2 C1	0.107	0.0067	0.0083	0.038	0.85
TFV1G(41)2 C2	0.111	0.0076	0.0091	0.040	0.86
TFV1G(41)2 C3	0.110	0.0073	0.0089	0.043	0.88
TFV1G(39)2 C1	0.108	0.0066	0.0083	0.026	0.97
TFV1G(39)2 C2	0.109	0.0067	0.0084	0.029	0.93
TFV1G(39)2 C3	0.112	0.0075	0.0091	0.042	0.93

In addition to providing an insight into the mechanism of TFV release, this adjustment allows us to identify which formulation best controls the drug release based on the values of the release constants (K_H, K_{HC}, K_{HF} and K_{KP}). A comparison of these constants conclusively highlights the batches with the TFV1(G43)2 granules previously identified as the most suitable for controlled-release formulations. Taking the Higuchi kinetic as an example, which has the best fit for these formulations (Table 4), the batches that include these granules have a K_H value of 0.08, while the K_H value of the other batches is always greater than 0.1 (Table 5). This points to the greater control over the release of the TFV from these batches, but once again makes it impossible to select the ideal proportion of HPMC/CH, given the close similarity of the constants obtained with batches C1, C2 and C3.

3.2.3. Mucoadhesion Test

Finally, another crucial parameter to evaluate was the mucoadhesion residence time of the formulations. Mucoadhesion is important because the tablets must remain adhered to the vaginal mucosa during the time TFV is being released [41]. The detachment of the formulation would imply an incomplete prophylactic treatment and discomfort for women, leading to a decrease in the use of the formulations.

A comparison of formulations with different ratios of TFV/G43 reveals that the more G43 the formulation contains, the longer it remains adhered to the vaginal mucosa (Figure 11). As this excipient has no adhesive properties this bioadhesion cannot be directly attributed to G43, so the only possible explanation is that it acts as a structural agent that helps form a more robust gel—as observed in the swelling test (Figure 7)—and hence remains attached for longer. In terms of the influence of the type of Gelucire®, it can be seen that the lower the melting point of the Gelucire®, the shorter the mucoadhesion time. This is probably due to the easier and faster softening of G39, which again causes the tablets to erode faster. Finally, the C2 batches appear to be the most mucoadhesive, undoubtedly due to the higher mucoadhesion of HPMC than CH [24].

TFV1G(43)2 granules therefore confer the strongest adhesive properties on the tablets. Among these batches, it is worth highlighting TFV1G(43)2 C2, which remains adhered to the vaginal mucosa for almost 225 h.

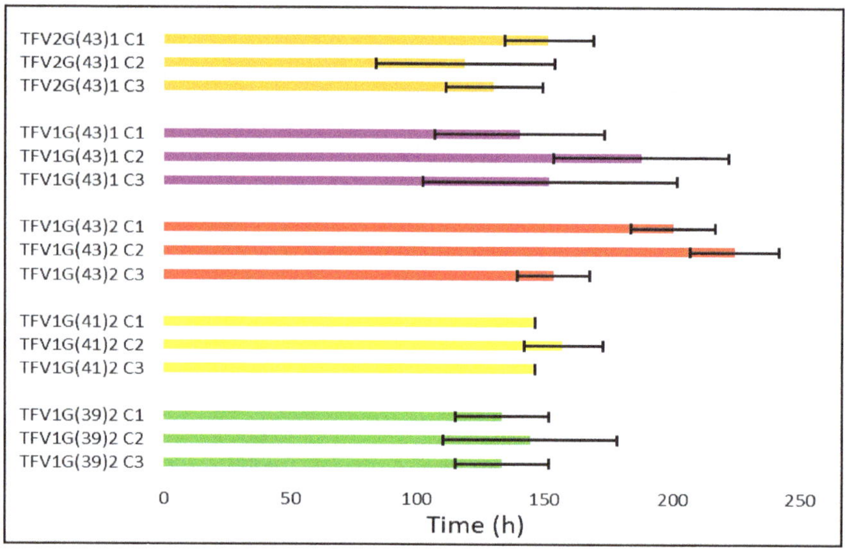

Figure 11. Mucoadhesion residence time in the simulated vaginal fluid in the batches.

The results of these studies, which are summarized in Figure 12, can be used to select the optimal formulation for preventing the sexual transmission of HIV.

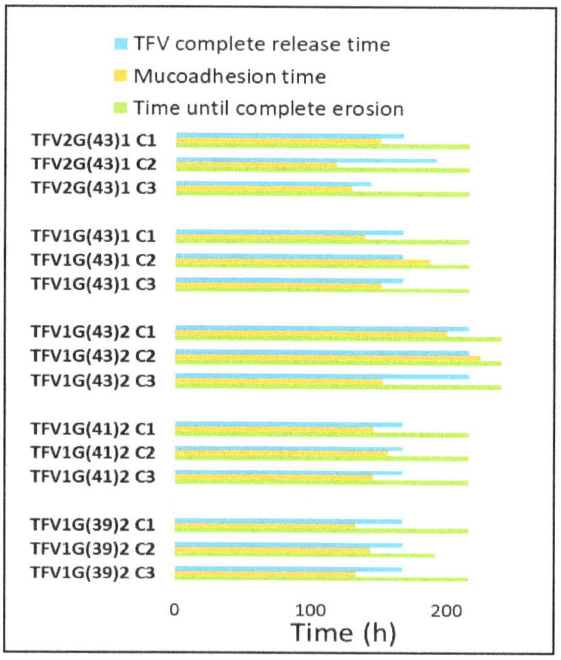

Figure 12. Summary of the data obtained from the drug release, mucoadhesion and swelling test. TFV complete release time (blue), mucoadhesion time (orange) and time until complete erosion (green) are shown for each batch.

The main parameter is undoubtedly the time taken to release the TFV from the formulation, since the aim of this work was to develop weekly sustained-release tablets whose administration could be markedly spaced in order to improve women's adherence to prophylactic treatment, which is currently the main problem with vaginal microbicides. Batches containing TFV1G(43)2 granules achieve the longest controlled release of TFV (216h), above the established target. However, the objective was not only to achieve a longer release time, but also to ensure the mucoadhesion of the formulation for as long as the drug is being released; there are only two formulations whose mucoadhesion time exceeds their complete TFV release time (batches TFV1G(43)1 C2 and TFV1G(43)2 C2). Finally, the formulation must not remain for long in the vaginal environment after the complete TFV release.

Batch TFV1G(43)2 C2 is conclusively selected as the optimal formulation for HIV prevention, since it is able to release TFV in a sustained manner for 216 h and remains attached to the vaginal mucosa throughout. Almost all the formulation has been eroded by the end of the process (with complete disintegration at 240 h), making it comfortable for women and enabling the next dose of the prophylactic treatment to be easily administered.

4. Conclusions

The combination of hydrophobic granules (prepared with Gelucire®) and hydrophilic matrices (HPMC and CH) in the development of vaginal mucoadhesive tablets allow the sustained-release of TFV.

The ratio TFV-Gelucire, as well as the proportion of HPMC and CH is critical for the development of the optimal formulation. Thus, the one with the best results contains TFV1G(43)2 granules in a mixture of HPMC and CH in a ratio of 1.9:1, which allows the sustained release of TFV for 216 h. The formulation remains adhered to the vaginal mucosa throughout this time, so a weekly administration of the tablets could protect women again the sexual transmission of HIV.

Author Contributions: Investigation, F.N.-P., R.C.-L., A.M.-I. and J.P.; Writing—original draft, F.N.-P.; Writing—review and editing, M.-D.V. and R.R.-C.

Acknowledgments: Fernando Notario-Pérez is beneficiary of a predoctoral researcher training fellowship from the Spanish Ministry of Economy and Business. Raúl Cazorla-Luna and Araceli Martín-Illana are beneficiaries of a university professor training fellowship from the Spanish Ministry of Education, Culture and Sport. We are grateful to the Carnes Barbero slaughterhouse (El Barraco, Avila, Spain) for supplying the biological samples. Acknowledgments to María Hernando, veterinarian of the Junta de Castilla y León, for verifying the suitability of the biological samples. TGA and DSC were characterized by the Escuela Politécnica de Cuenca (UCLM).

References

1. Chaudhary, R.S.; Amankwaa, E.; Kumar, S.; Hu, T.; Chan, M.; Sanghvi, P. Application of a hot-melt granulation process to enhance fenofibrate solid dose manufacturing. *Drug Develop. Ind. Pharm.* **2015**, *42*, 1137–1148. [CrossRef] [PubMed]
2. Jakson, K.A.; Hunt, J.D. Binary eutectic solidification. *Trans Met Soc AIME* **1966**, *236*, 843–852.
3. Patil, H.; Tiwari, R.V.; Repka, M.A. Hot-Melt Extrusion: From Theory to Application in Pharmaceutical Formulation. *AAPS PharmSciTech* **2015**, *17*, 20–42. [CrossRef] [PubMed]
4. Chen, Y.-C.; Ho, H.-O.; Chiou, J.-D.; Sheu, M.-T. Physical and dissolution characterization of cilostazol solid dispersions prepared by hot melt granulation (HMG) and thermal adhesion granulation (TAG) methods. *Int. J. Pharm.* **2014**, *473*, 458–468. [CrossRef] [PubMed]
5. Verhoeven, E.; De Beer, T.; Mooter, G.V.D.; Remon, J.; Vervaet, C. Influence of formulation and process parameters on the release characteristics of ethylcellulose sustained-release mini-matrices produced by hot-melt extrusion. *Eur. J. Pharm. Biopharm.* **2008**, *69*, 312–319. [CrossRef] [PubMed]
6. Özgüney, I.; Shuwisitkul, D.; Bodmeier, R. Development and characterization of extended release Kollidon® SR mini-matrices prepared by hot-melt extrusion. *Eur. J. Pharm. Biopharm.* **2009**, *73*, 140–145. [CrossRef]
7. Verstraete, G.; Mertens, P.; Grymonpré, W.; Van Bockstal, P.-J.; De Beer, T.; Boone, M.N.; Van Hoorebeke, L.; Remon, J.; Vervaet, C. A comparative study between melt granulation/compression and hot melt extrusion/injection molding for the manufacturing of oral sustained release thermoplastic polyurethane matrices. *Int. J. Pharm.* **2016**, *513*, 602–611. [CrossRef]
8. Almeida, A.; Saerens, L.; De Beer, T.; Remon, J.; Vervaet, C. Upscaling and in-line process monitoring via spectroscopic techniques of ethylene vinyl acetate hot-melt extruded formulations. *Int. J. Pharm.* **2012**, *439*, 223–229. [CrossRef]
9. El Hadri, M.; Achahbar, A.; El Khamkhami, J.; Khelifa, B.; Faivre, V.; Abbas, O.; Bresson, S. Lyotropic behavior of Gelucire 50/13 by XRD, Raman and IR spectroscopies according to hydration. *Chem. Phys. Lipids* **2016**, *200*, 11–23. [CrossRef]

10. Chambin, O.; Jannin, V. Interest of Multifunctional Lipid Excipients: Case of Gelucire® 44/14. *Drug Develop. Ind. Pharm.* **2005**, *31*, 527–534. [CrossRef]
11. Upadhyay, P.; Pandit, J.K.; Wahi, A.K. Gelucire: An alternative formulation technological tool for both sustained and fast release of drugs in treating diabetes mellitus type II disease. *J. Sci. Ind. Res.* **2013**, *72*, 776–780.
12. UNAIDS. When Women Lead Change Happens. Available online: http://www.unaids.org/sites/default/files/media_asset/when-women-lead-change-happens_en.pdf (accessed on 30 December 2017).
13. Aurpibul, L.; Puthanakit, T. Review of Tenofovir Use in HIV-infected Children. *Pediatric Infect. Dis. J.* **2015**, *34*, 383–391. [CrossRef]
14. Mertenskoetter, T.; Kaptur, P. Update on microbicide research and development-seeking new HIV prevention tools for women. *Eur. J. Med Res.* **2011**, *16*, 1–6. [CrossRef]
15. Hankins, C.A.; Dybul, M.R. The promise of pre-exposure prophylaxis with antiretroviral drugs to prevent HIV transmission: A review. *Curr. Opin. HIV AIDS* **2013**, *8*, 50–58. [CrossRef]
16. Notario-Pérez, F.; Cazorla-Luna, R.; Martín-Illana, A.; Ruiz-Caro, R.; Tamayo, A.; Rubio, J.; Veiga, M.-D. Optimization of tenofovir release from mucoadhesive vaginal tablets by polymer combination to prevent sexual transmission of HIV. *Carbohydr. Polym.* **2018**, *179*, 305–316. [CrossRef]
17. Cazorla-Luna, R.; Notario-Pérez, F.; Martín-Illana, A.; Ruiz-Caro, R.; Tamayo, A.; Rubio, J.; Veiga, M.D. Chitosan-Based Mucoadhesive Vaginal Tablets for Controlled Release of the Anti-HIV Drug Tenofovir. *Pharmaceutics* **2019**, *11*, 20. [CrossRef]
18. Ruiz-Caro, R.; Veiga-Ochoa, M.D. Characterization and Dissolution Study of Chitosan Freeze-Dried Systems for Drug Controlled Release. *Molecules* **2009**, *14*, 4370–4386. [CrossRef]
19. Owen, D.H.; Katz, D.F. A vaginal fluid simulant. *Contraception* **1999**, *59*, 91–95. [CrossRef]
20. Sánchez-Sánchez, M.-P.; Martín-Illana, A.; Ruiz-Caro, R.; Bermejo, P.; Abad, M.-J.; Carro, R.; Bedoya, L.-M.; Tamayo, A.; Rubio, J.; Fernández-Ferreiro, A.; et al. Chitosan and Kappa-Carrageenan Vaginal Acyclovir Formulations for Prevention of Genital Herpes. In Vitro and Ex Vivo Evaluation. *Mar. Drugs* **2015**, *13*, 5976–5992. [CrossRef]
21. Moore, J.W.; Flanner, H.H. Mathematical comparison of dissolution profiles. *Pharma Tec.* **1996**, *20*, 64–74.
22. Mamani, P.L.; Ruiz-Caro, R.; Veiga, M.D. Matrix Tablets: The Effect of Hydroxypropyl Methylcellulose/Anhydrous Dibasic Calcium Phosphate Ratio on the Release Rate of a Water-Soluble Drug Through the Gastrointestinal Tract I. In Vitro Tests. *AAPS PharmSciTech* **2012**, *13*, 1073–1083. [CrossRef]
23. Dash, S.; Murthy, P.N.; Nath, L.; Chowdhury, P. Kinetic modeling on drug release from controlled drug delivery systems. *Acta Pol. Pharm.* **2010**, *67*, 217–223.
24. Notario-Pérez, F.; Martín-Illana, A.; Cazorla-Luna, R.; Ruiz-Caro, R.; Bedoya, L.-M.; Tamayo, A.; Rubio, J.; Veiga, M.-D.; Harding, D.; Sashiwa, H. Influence of Chitosan Swelling Behaviour on Controlled Release of Tenofovir from Mucoadhesive Vaginal Systems for Prevention of Sexual Transmission of HIV. *Mar. Drugs* **2017**, *15*, 50. [CrossRef]
25. Ochiuz, L.; Grigoras, C.; Popa, M.; Stoleriu, I.; Munteanu, C.; Timofte, D.; Profire, L.; Grigoras, A.G. Alendronate-Loaded Modified Drug Delivery Lipid Particles Intended for Improved Oral and Topical Administration. *Molecules* **2016**, *21*, 858. [CrossRef]
26. Eloy, J.D.O.; Saraiva, J.; De Albuquerque, S.; Marchetti, J.M.; Albuquerque, S. Solid Dispersion of Ursolic Acid in Gelucire 50/13: A Strategy to Enhance Drug Release and Trypanocidal Activity. *AAPS PharmSciTech* **2012**, *13*, 1436–1445. [CrossRef]
27. Patil, S.; Kadam, C.; Pokharkar, V. QbD based approach for optimization of Tenofovir disoproxil fumarate loaded liquid crystal precursor with improved permeability. *J. Adv. Res.* **2017**, *8*, 607–616. [CrossRef]
28. Ramkumaar, G.R.; Srinivasan, S.; Bhoopathy, T.J.; Gunasekaran, S. Vibrational Spectroscopic Studies of Tenofovir Using Density Functional Theory Method. *J. Chem.* **2013**, *2013*, 1–12. [CrossRef]
29. Svensson, A.; Neves, C.; Cabane, B. Hydration of an amphiphilic excipient, Gelucire® 44/14. *Int. J. Pharm.* **2004**, *281*, 107–118. [CrossRef]
30. National Center for Biotechnology Information. PubChem Compound Database, CID=464205. Available online: https://pubchem.ncbi.nlm.nih.gov/compound/464205 (accessed on 1 July 2017).
31. Veiga, M.; Bernad, M.; Escobar, C. Thermal behaviour of drugs from binary and ternary systems. *Int. J. Pharm.* **1993**, *89*, 119–124. [CrossRef]

32. Agrahari, V.; Putty, S.; Mathes, C.; Murowchick, J.B.; Youan, B.-B.C. Evaluation of degradation kinetics and physicochemical stability of tenofovir. *Drug Test. Analysis* **2014**, *7*, 207–213. [CrossRef]
33. Albarahmieh, E.; Qi, S.; Craig, D.Q. Hot melt extruded transdermal films based on amorphous solid dispersions in Eudragit RS PO: The inclusion of hydrophilic additives to develop moisture-activated release systems. *Int. J. Pharm.* **2016**, *514*, 270–281. [CrossRef] [PubMed]
34. Zhang, T.; Zhang, C.; Agrahari, V.; Murowchick, J.B.; Oyler, N.A.; Youan, B.B.C. Spray drying tenofovir loaded mucoadhesive and pH-sensitive microspheres intended for HIV prevention. *Antivir. Res.* **2013**, *97*, 334. [CrossRef] [PubMed]
35. Yin, X.; Li, H.; Guo, Z.; Wu, L.; Chen, F.; De Matas, M.; Shao, Q.; Xiao, T.; York, P.; He, Y.; et al. Quantification of Swelling and Erosion in the Controlled Release of a Poorly Water-Soluble Drug Using Synchrotron X-ray Computed Microtomography. *AAPS J* **2013**, *15*, 1025–1034. [CrossRef] [PubMed]
36. Geeta, M.P.; Madhabhai, M.P. Design and in vitro evaluation of a novel vaginal drug delivery system based on gelucire. *Curr Drug Deliv* **2009**, *6*, 159–165. [PubMed]
37. Stevens, R.E.; Gray, V.; Dorantes, A.; Gold, L.; Pham, L. Scientific and Regulatory Standards for Assessing Product Performance Using the Similarity Factor, f2. *AAPS J* **2015**, *17*, 301–306. [CrossRef] [PubMed]
38. Paul, D. Elaborations on the Higuchi model for drug delivery. *Int. J. Pharm.* **2011**, *418*, 13–17. [CrossRef] [PubMed]
39. Hixson, A.W.; Crowell, J.H. Dependence of reaction velocity upon surface and agitation: Theoretical considerations. *Ind Eng Chem.* **1931**, *23*, 923–931. [CrossRef]
40. Korsmeyer, R.W.; Gurny, R.; Doelker, E.; Buri, P.; Peppas, N.A. Mechanisms of solute release from porous hydrophilic polymers. *Int. J. Pharm.* **1983**, *15*, 25–35. [CrossRef]
41. Caramella, C.M.; Rossi, S.; Ferrari, F.; Bonferoni, M.C.; Sandri, G. Mucoadhesive and thermogelling systems for vaginal drug delivery. *Adv. Drug Deliv. Rev.* **2015**, *92*, 39–52. [CrossRef]

10

Quercetin Inhibits Cell Survival and Metastatic Ability via the EMT-Mediated Pathway in Oral Squamous Cell Carcinoma

So Ra Kim [1,2], Eun Young Lee [1,2], Da Jeong Kim [1], Hye Jung Kim [2,*] and Hae Ryoun Park [1,2,*]

1 Department of Oral Pathology, and BK21 PLUS Project, School of Dentistry, Pusan National University, Yangsan 50612, Korea; ksr9307@pusan.ac.kr (S.R.K.); eunyeong26@pusan.ac.kr (E.Y.L.); ttakjjung@gmail.com (D.J.K.)

2 Periodontal Disease Signaling Network Research Center (MRC), School of Dentistry, Pusan National University, Yangsan 50612, Korea

* Correspondence: kimhj2850@naver.com (H.J.K.); parkhr@pusan.ac.kr (H.R.P.)

Academic Editor: Kyoko Nakagawa-Goto

Abstract: This study aimed to investigate whether quercetin exerts anticancer effects on oral squamous cell carcinoma (OSCC) cell lines and to elucidate its mechanism of action. These anticancer effects in OSCC cells were assessed using an MTT assay, flow cytometry (to assess the cell cycle), wound-healing assay, invasion assay, Western blot analysis, gelatin zymography, and immunofluorescence. To investigate whether quercetin also inhibits transforming growth factor β1 (TGF-β1)-induced epithelial–mesenchymal transition (EMT) in human keratinocyte cells, HaCaT cells were treated with TGF-β1. Overall, our results strongly suggest that quercetin suppressed the viability of OSCC cells by inducing cell cycle arrest at the G2/M phase. However, quercetin did not affect cell viability of human keratinocytes such as HaCaT (immortal keratinocyte) and nHOK (primary normal human oral keratinocyte) cells. Additionally, quercetin suppresses cell migration through EMT and matrix metalloproteinase (MMP) in OSCC cells and decreases TGF-β1-induced EMT in HaCaT cells. In conclusion, this study is the first, to our knowledge, to demonstrate that quercetin can inhibit the survival and metastatic ability of OSCC cells via the EMT-mediated pathway, specifically Slug. Quercetin may thus provide a novel pharmacological approach for the treatment of OSCCs.

Keywords: quercetin; oral squamous cell carcinoma cells; metastasis; cell cycle arrest; epithelial-to-mesenchymal transition; matrix metalloproteinase; transforming growth factor-β1

1. Introduction

Oral squamous cell carcinoma (OSCC) is the most common malignancy, accounting for about 90% of head and neck cancers, and develops at the lips, tongue, salivary glands, gums, bottom of the mouth, pharynx, and surfaces within the oral cavity [1–6]. OSCC, an aggressive human cancer with the highest mortality, has a significant impact on the quality of life of patients [6,7]. Early OSCC is treated with a combination of surgery and radiation therapy; however, this strategy does not significantly increase survival in OSCC patients. Thus, many studies have focused on compounds derived from natural products as potential candidate agents for treating or preventing OSCCs. OSCC is known to have multifactorial etiologies, including tobacco, alcohol, and viruses [6,8–10]. Several reviews suggest that periodontal disease (PD) results in a high risk of developing OSCC [8,11]. In "Cancer Facts & Figures 2018" provided by the American Cancer Society, the oral cavity is the most common site of onset of oral cancer, followed by the tongue and pharynx [12]. Therefore, we used oral squamous cell carcinoma HN22 and tongue squamous cell carcinoma such as OSC20 and SAS to confirm the effect of quercetin in oral cancer.

Cancer metastasis involves a complex process that includes primary tumor formation, angiogenesis, invasion, and metastatic colonization [8]. In the initial stages of cancer metastasis, epithelial–to–mesenchymal transition (EMT) causes a loss of adhesion and increases the motility of primary tumor cells [3,13–15]. The matrix metalloproteinase (MMP) is an important extracellular protease that breaks down the extracellular matrix (ECM) and allows cancer cells to migrate into the lymph and blood vessels [16–18]. Some studies have demonstrated that EMT and MMP support the invasion and metastasis of OSCC [19,20]. Therefore, this study investigated whether quercetin exhibits anticancer effects on OSCC cell lines and its mechanism of action.

Quercetin is a plant flavonol of the flavonoid polyphenol group found in many fruits, vegetables, leaves, and grains [21–23]. Although numerous studies have demonstrated that quercetin plays a role in the prevention of various cancers [24–26], it is still an interesting target for OSCCs. Previous studies have reported the antibacterial effects of quercetin against *Actinobacillus actinomycetemcomitans (Aa)* and *Porphyromonas gingivalis (Pg)*, which are the major pathogens in PD [27,28]. Moreover, recently, studies have reported that quercetin inhibits the cell viability, migration, and invasion of OSCC cells [29–32]. However, its potential actions in OSCCs have been poorly explored. Therefore, in this study, we sought to investigate whether quercetin exhibits anticancer effects on OSCC cell lines and to elucidate its mechanism of action.

2. Results

2.1. Quercetin Reduced Cell Viability and Arrested G2 Phase Cell Cycle in OSCC Cells

To determine the effect of quercetin on cell viability, OSCC cell lines (OSC20, SAS, and HN22 cells) were treated with various concentrations (0~160 μM) of quercetin for 24 h, and cell viability was determined using the MTT assay. The results showed that quercetin decreased cell viability in OSCC cell lines (Figure 1A). In particular, cell viability in OSC20 and SAS cells, except HN22 cells, was reduced in a quercetin dose-dependent manner. Treatment with 160 μM quercetin for 24 h reduced cell viability by approximately 50% in all cell lines ($p < 0.01$), whereas treatment with low concentrations (10–40 μM) reduced cell viability slightly (approximately 5–30%) ($p < 0.05$) compared to the control (Figure 1A). To determine the function of quercetin in the regulation of the cell cycle, OSCC cell lines were stimulated with low levels of quercetin (10–40 μM) for 24 h and analyzed the distribution of the cell cycle using flow cytometry. As shown in Figure 1B, the cell populations at the G2/M stage were increased by treatment with quercetin in the OSCC cell lines (OSC20 cell, 7.66% ± 3.92% in the control vs. 36.22% ± 4.10% in quercetin 40 μM, $p < 0.01$; SAS cell, 22.85% ± 3.04% in the control vs. 45.49% ± 1.38% in quercetin 40 μM, $p < 0.005$; and HN22 cell, 23.37% ± 4.13% in control vs. 50.40% ± 5.05% in quercetin 40 μM, $p < 0.05$). However, the cell proportion in the G0/G1 phase decreased (OSC20 cell, 35.99 ± 1.89% in the control vs. 14.06% ± 1.26% in quercetin 40 μM, $p < 0.001$; SAS cell, 33.03% ± 1.12% in the control vs. 8.14% ± 4.39% in quercetin 40 μM, $p < 0.005$; and HN22 cell, 35.05% ± 1.62% in control vs. 6.53% ± 4.34% in quercetin 40 μM, $p < 0.001$). The results indicate that quercetin suppressed the viability of OSCC cells by inducing cell cycle arrest in the G2/M phase.

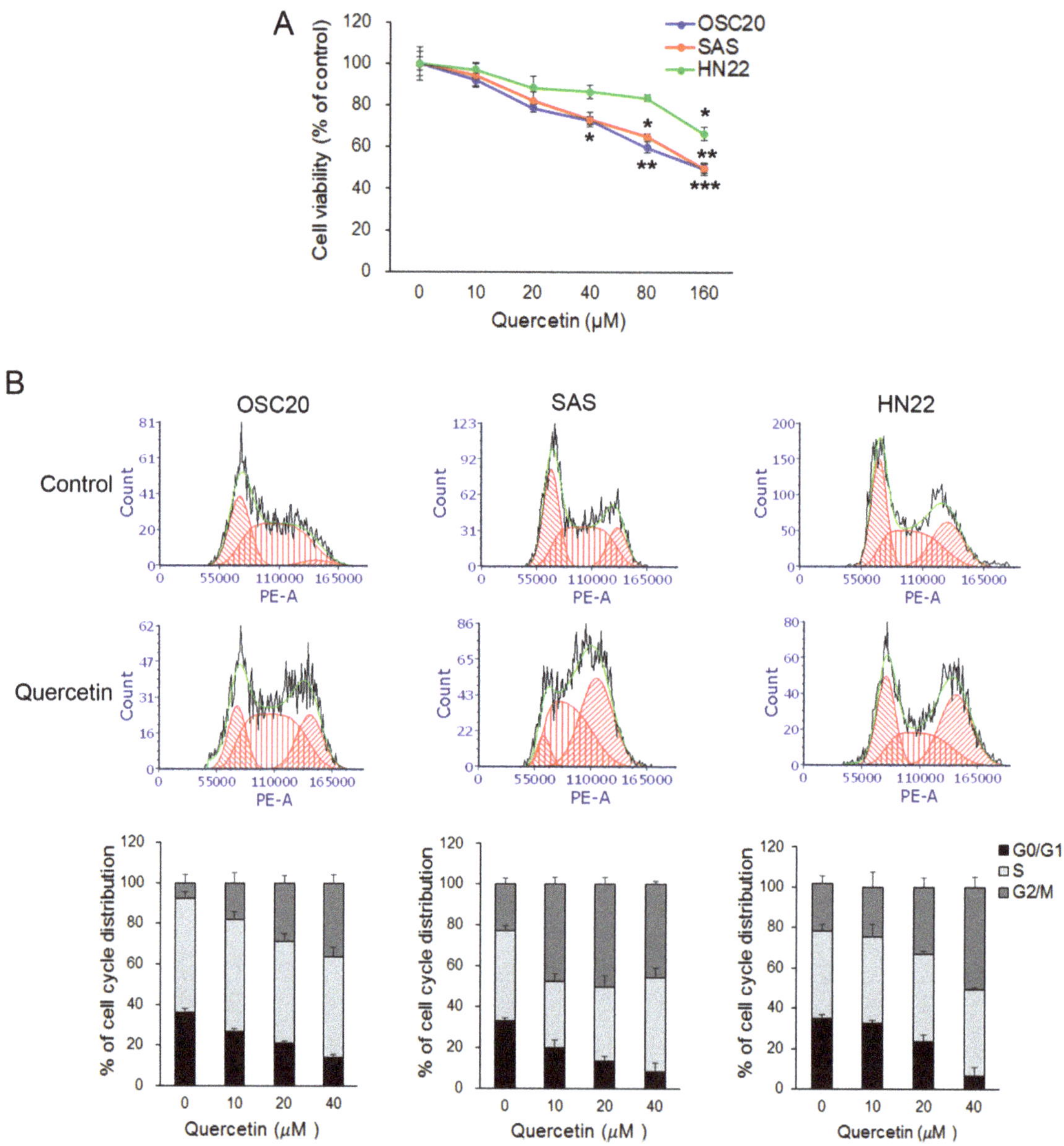

Figure 1. Quercetin reduced cell viability and arrested the G2/M phase cell cycle in oral squamous cell carcinoma (OSCC) cells. (**A**) Cell viability was investigated by an MTT assay. Oral squamous cell carcinoma cell lines (OSC20, SAS, and HN22 cells) were treated with quercetin (10, 20, 40, 80, and 160 μM). (**B**) Quercetin was shown to induce cell cycle arrest in OSC20, SAS, and HN22 cells. Data are the means ± SEM. * $p < 0.05$ and ** $p < 0.01$ vs. corresponding control (quercetin 0 μM).

2.2. *Quercetin Suppressed the Migration Potential of OSCC Cells*

We performed a wound-healing assay to evaluate the inhibitory effects of quercetin on migration. To observe the effects of quercetin on cell migration, the cell proliferation of OSC20, SAS, and HN22 cells was inhibited by treatment with thymidine (1 mM) for 2 h prior to treatment with quercetin (40 μM). After 24 h, the wound area of the control was almost completely reduced compared to the initial area; however, the quercetin-treated cells did not show any decrease (Figure 2A,B). The migration of quercetin-treated cells was significantly decreased in a dose-dependent manner (not shown). This result suggests that the migratory properties were completely lost upon quercetin treatment for 24 h in the OSCC cell lines.

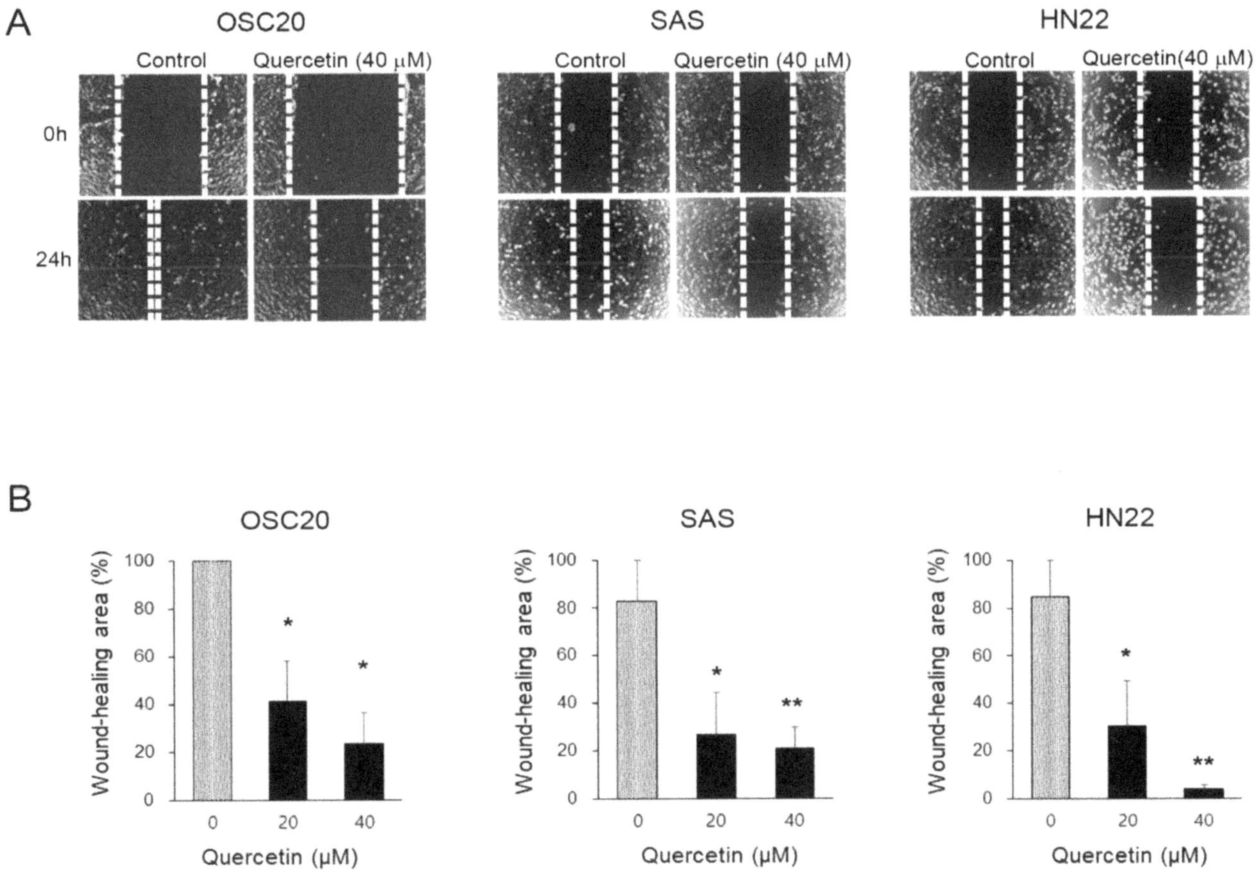

Figure 2. Cell migration ability assessed by a wound-healing assay. (**A**) Changes in the wound area were observed after 24 h. In the quercetin-treated cells, the wound area was less closed. This indicates a decrease in migration capacity. (**B**) The wound area was calculated and presented as a graph. Data are the means ± SEM. * $p < 0.05$ and ** $p < 0.01$ vs. the corresponding control (quercetin 0 μM).

2.3. Quercetin Regulated EMT and MMPs in OSCC Cells

The effects of quercetin treatment on EMT and the activity of ECM-degrading enzymes in OSCC cell lines were analyzed by Western blot or gelatin zymography. OSC20, SAS, and HN22 cells were treated with different concentrations of quercetin (0, 10, 20, and 40 μM) for 24 h. As shown in Figure 3A, quercetin, in a dose-dependent manner, increased the expression of epithelial markers, such as E-cadherin and claudin-1, while decreasing the expression of mesenchymal markers, such as fibronectin, vimentin, and alpha-smooth muscle actin (α-SMA). We observed that 40 μM of quercetin specifically downregulated the expression of the mesenchymal markers in OSCC cells. The activation of MMP-2 and MMP-9 was significantly decreased by quercetin treatment (Figure 3B). These results demonstrate that quercetin suppressed the expression levels of EMT inducers and MMPs in OSCC cells.

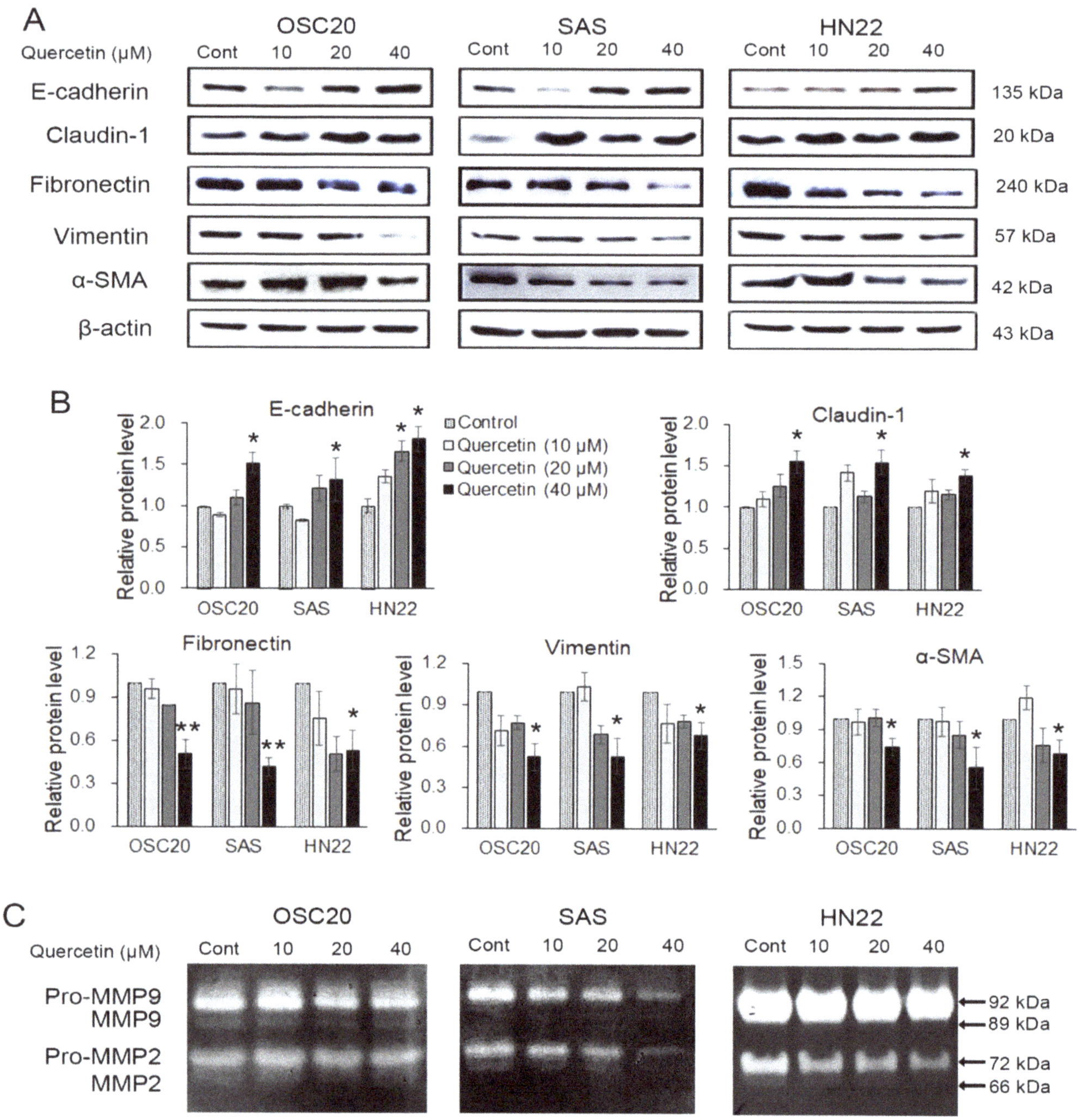

Figure 3. Quercetin is shown to induce regulation of epithelial-mesenchymal transition (EMT) and matrix metalloproteinase (MMP). (**A**) Western blotting was conducted to examine the changes in the EMT inducers. The results showed that the epithelial markers (E-cadherin and claudin-1) were upregulated, and the mesenchymal markers (fibronectin, vimentin, and alpha-smooth muscle actin (α-SMA)) were downregulated upon treatment with quercetin. (**B**) Quantitation of A. The band intensities of each target protein were measured using an image analyzer and presented as relative ratio. (**C**) Gelatin zymography shows the MMP-2 and MMP-9 activities in oral cancer cell lines (OSC20, SAS, and HN22 cells) upon quercetin treatment. Data are the means ± SEM. * $p < 0.05$, and ** $p < 0.01$ vs. the corresponding control (quercetin 0 μM).

2.4. Quercetin Regulated EMT-Activating Transcription Factors in OSCC Cells

EMT-activating transcription factors (EMT-TFs), such as Twist, Slug, and Snail 1, were observed by Western blot and immunofluorescence. Twist and Slug were significantly downregulated in quercetin-treated OSC20 and SAS cells compared to the untreated cells (Figure 4A,B). Slug was significantly downregulated in quercetin-treated HN22 cells compared to untreated cells, but Twist was unchanged (Figure 4A,B). Moreover, upon quercetin treatment, translocation of Twist and Slug expression was observed in the OSC20 and SAS cells by immunofluorescence (Figure 4C,D). The basal level of Twist was observed in the cytosol, and there was no translocation upon quercetin treatment in HN22 cells (Figure 4C). The basal levels of Slug were observed in the nucleus on untreated HN22 cells but were observed in the cytosol upon quercetin treatment (Figure 4D). These data strongly suggest that quercetin inhibits Slug activation by inducing its translocation into the cytoplasm.

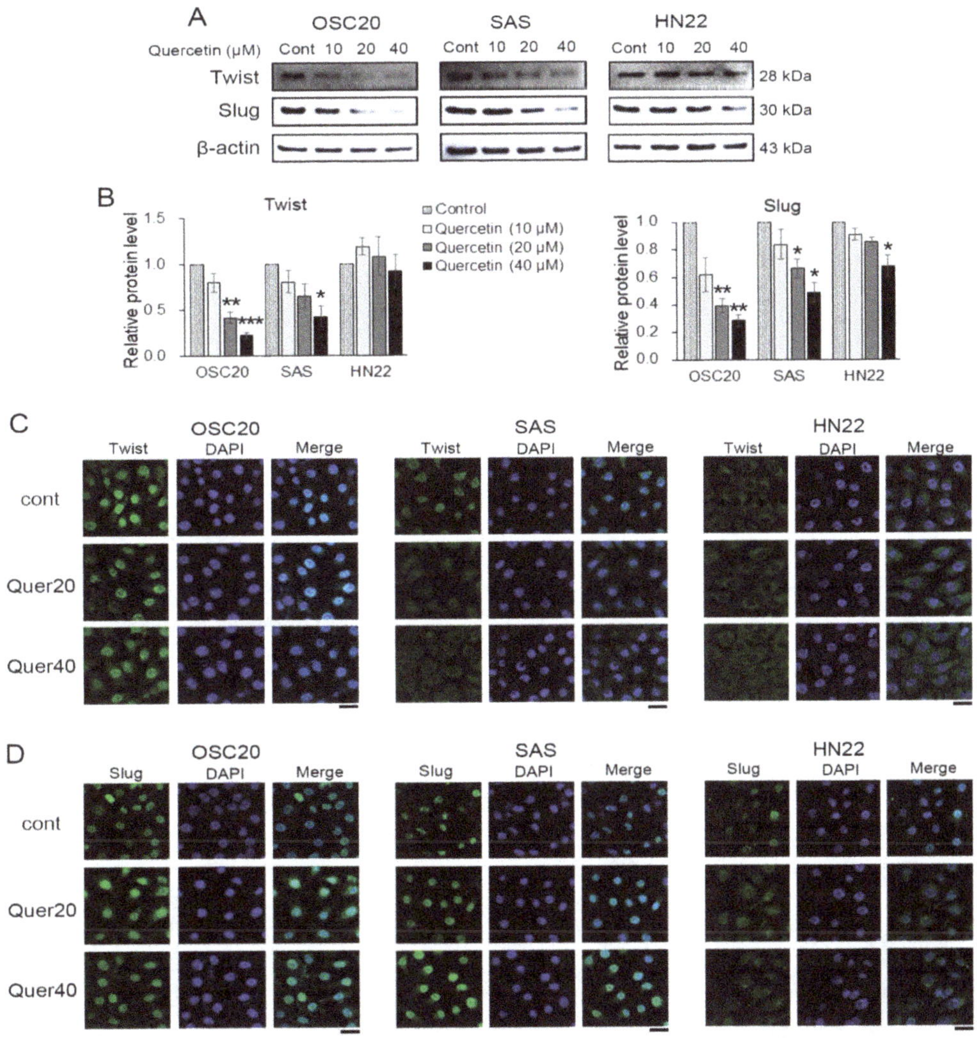

Figure 4. EMT-activating transcription factors were detected using Western blot and immunofluorescence. (**A**) The Western blot showed that quercetin downregulated EMT transcription factors at the protein level. (**B**) Quantitation of A. The band intensities of each target protein were measured using an image analyzer and presented as relative ratio. (**C**) Representative fluorescence microscopy images of Twist in OSCC cell lines. (**D**) Representative fluorescence microscopy images of Slug in OSCC cell lines. Scale bars: 20 μM. Data are the means ± SEM. * $p < 0.05$, ** $p < 0.01$, and *** $p < 0.001$ vs. the corresponding control (quercetin 0 μM).

2.5. Transforming Growth Factor β1 (TGF-β1) Induced EMT in Human Keratinocyte HaCaT Cells

Previous results indicated that quercetin exerts anticancer effects through the regulation of EMT in OSCC cells. To examine the viability effect of quercetin on human keratinocyte cells, HaCaT (immortal keratinocyte) and nHOK (primary normal human oral keratinocyte) cells were treated with various concentrations (0~160 μM) of quercetin for 24 h, and cell viability was determined by an MTT assay. Cell viability of HaCaT cells and nHOK cells was not changed by the low concentration (10–40 μM) of quercetin compared to the control group but was significantly reduced in 160 μM quercetin treatment ($p < 0.05$) (Figure 5A). The results show that quercetin had not much effect on cell viability of HaCaT and nHOK cells in the concentration range of 10–80 μM compared to the OSCC cell lines. To investigate whether quercetin also inhibits TGF-β1-induced EMT in human keratinocyte, HaCaT cells were treated with TGF-β1 (2 ng, 5 ng, and 10 ng) for 24 h. Changes in the expression of EMT inducers upon treatment with TGF-β1 were confirmed by Western blot (Figure 5B). The expression levels of the epithelial markers (E-cadherin and claudin-1) were decreased and those of the mesenchymal markers (fibronectin, vimentin, α-SMA, and Slug) were increased (Figure 5C–H). TGF-β1 (10 ng/mL) was determined to be the optimal concentration for the EMT induction in HaCaT cells. Thus, 10 ng/mL of TGF-β1 was used for the subsequent experiment.

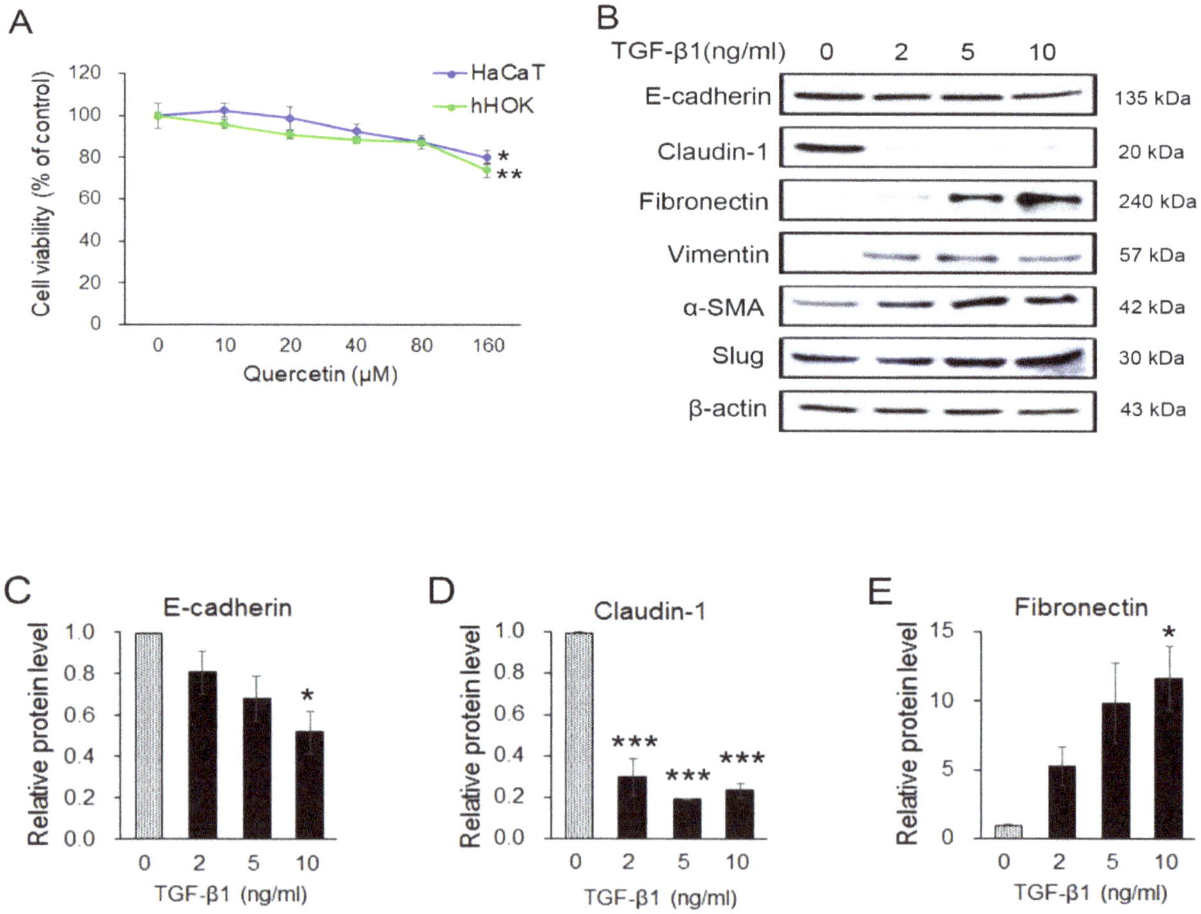

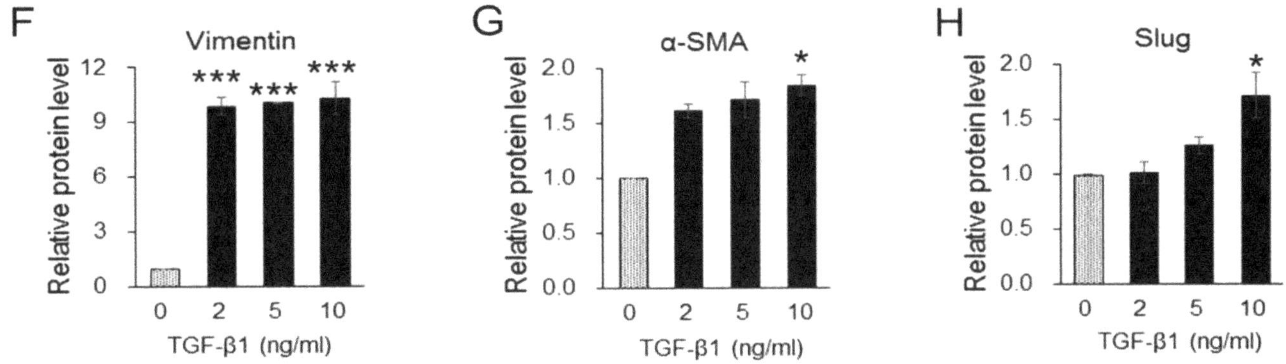

Figure 5. Quercetin was not toxic in normal keratocyte and transforming growth factor β1 (TGF-β1) stimulated EMT in HaCaT cells. (**A**) To examine the effect of quercetin on cell viability, an MTT assay was conducted on HaCaT and nHOK cells. Data are means ± SEM. # $p < 0.05$ vs. the corresponding control (quercetin 0 μM). (**B**) Expression of EMT-related markers such as in TGF-β1-treated HaCaT cells were analyzed by Western blotting. (**C–H**) Quantitation of B. The band intensities of each target protein were measured using an image analyzer and presented as relative ratio. Data are means ± SEM. * $p < 0.05$ and *** $p < 0.005$ vs. corresponding control (TGF-β1 0 ng/mL).

2.6. Quercetin Attenuated TGF-β1-induced EMT in HaCaT Cells

To investigate whether quercetin also inhibits TGF-β1-induced EMT in normal cells, HaCaT was treated with 10 ng of TGF-β1 for 24 h, followed by various concentrations of quercetin for 24 h without changing the media (Figure 6A). To observe the morphological changes of the treated HaCaT cells, phalloidin staining was conducted. Without treatment, the cells tended to grow together and exhibited a triangle–square shape. However, after treatment with 10 ng of TGF-β1, the HaCaT cells showed morphological changes to their spindle shapes and were spread out (Figure 6B). Additionally, when the cells were treated with TGF-β1 and quercetin together, as explained previously, the morphological changes recovered but the cells did not gather as before (Figure 6B). Western blot data show that quercetin regulated the TGF-β1-induced EMT markers. With regard to the epithelial markers (E-cadherin and claudin-1) of the induced EMT, there were no changes in recovery. In contrast, changes in the mesenchymal markers indicate that treatment with 40 μM quercetin leads to the greatest recovery. Thus, we determined the optimal concentration of quercetin as 40 μM for use in the subsequent experiment (Figure 6C–I). To evaluate the TGF-β1-induced EMT migration ability, a wound-healing assay was performed. The wound area was narrower in the TGF-β1-treated HaCaT cells than in the untreated HaCaT cells (Figure 6J,K). Further, quercetin seemed to inhibit the invasion of EMT-induced HaCaT cells (Figure 6L). The invasion assay also showed that the invasion ability improved upon TGF-β1 treatment. The number of cells that passed the Matrigel and membrane was less in the HaCaT cells treated with quercetin and TGF-β1 than in those treated with only TGF-β1 (Figure 6L). In conclusion, quercetin decreased the TGF-β1-induced EMT in HaCaT cells.

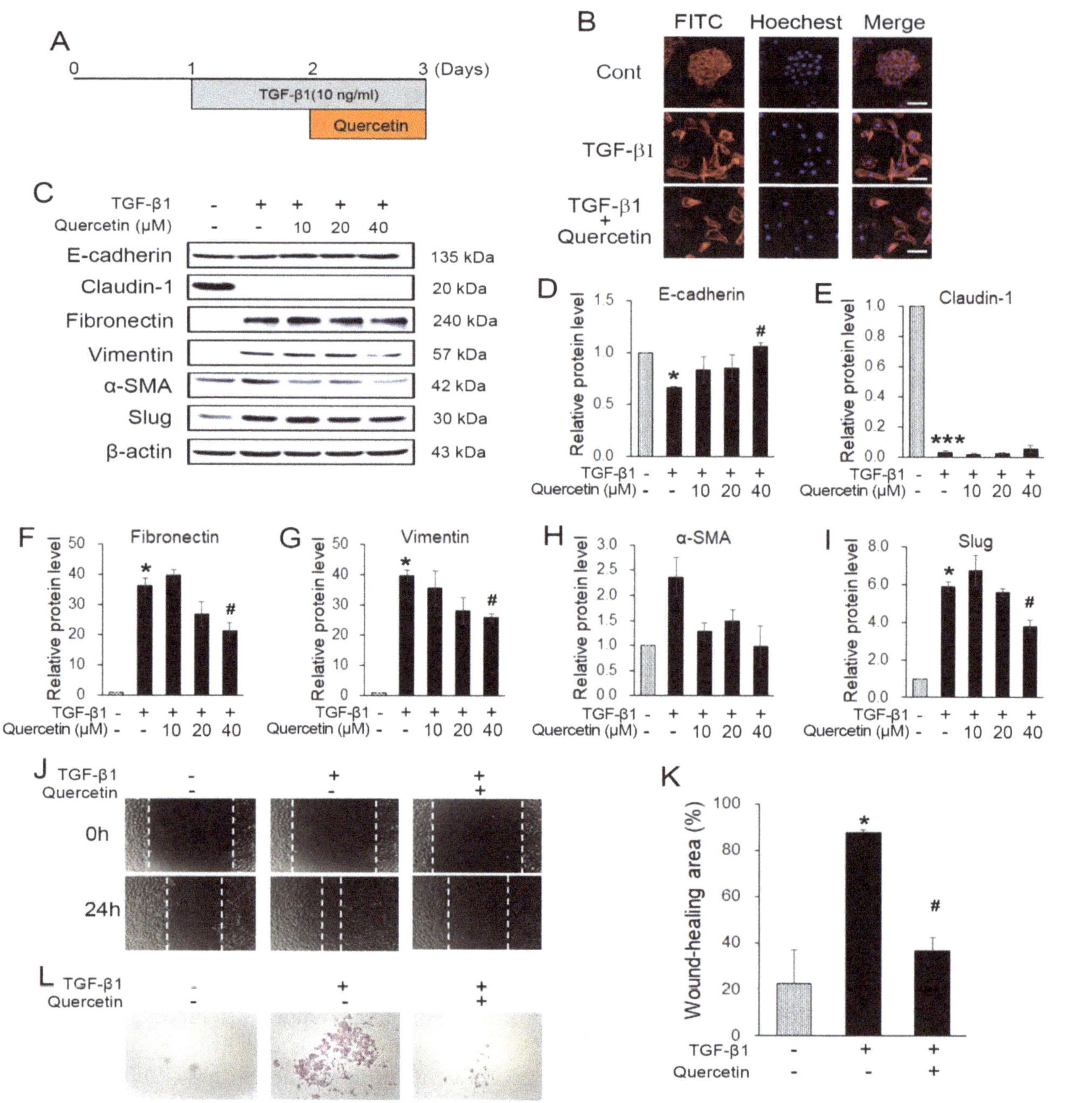

Figure 6. Quercetin inhibited TGF-β1-induced EMT. (**A**) Experimental setup. (**B**) Western blot results showed that quercetin also regulated TGF-β1-induced EMT markers. (**C**) Treatment of TGF-β1 also changed the morphology of HaCaT. Further, quercetin induced morphological recovery. Scale bars: 50 μM. (**D**–**I**) Quantification of hRPTECs viability by MTT assay. (**J**,**K**) A wound-healing assay was conducted to evaluate the TGF-β1-induced EMT migration ability; quercetin attenuated EMT-induced migration in HaCaT cells. (**L**) Quercetin inhibited the invasion capacity of EMT-induced HaCaT cells. Data are the means ± SEM. * $p < 0.05$, and *** $p < 0.001$ vs. the corresponding control (without TGF-β1 and quercetin); # $p < 0.05$ vs. the corresponding control (with TGF-β1 and without quercetin).

3. Discussion

Suppression of cancer metastasis is considered an effective strategy for preventing cancer progression. Many studies have reported that a variety of natural products and compounds exert antitumor effects by inducing apoptosis and cell cycle arrest in cancer cells and reducing their metastatic capacities [33,34]. Thus, the use of dietary biologically active compounds may be a safe and desirable approach for cancer treatment. Quercetin is a potent candidate for cancer treatment, because it is known to have a regulatory effect on apoptosis, migration, and invasion. However, quercetin has limited applications as a therapeutic agent due to problems such as low oral bioavailability (8~16%) and poor water solubility [35]. Numerous studies have used various cancer cell lines to study the anticancer effects of quercetin, and quercetin concentrations vary depending on the cell line and treatment time. Quercetin is used at 10–80 μM concentrations for 24 treatments in cancer cells because of its low bioactivity. Quercetin concentrations 10–80 μM are used under 24-h treatment conditions. Quercetin IC50 values of quercetin are 60–120 μM [36–38]. Especially, quercetin of 25–50 μM had anticancer effects in SAS cells, a typical oral cancer cell [39]. In this study, the anticancer effect of quercetin at 10, 20, 40, 80, and 160 μM was assessed in vitro by MTT assay in the OSCC cell line, such as OSC20, SAS, and HN22 cells. The optimal concentration of quercetin was determined to be 10–40 μM for assessing metastatic capacity in OSCC cells. The 10–40 μM quercetin concentration used in this study is commonly used for cancer cells under 24-h treatment conditions. Quercetin, a flavonoid found in many fruits, vegetables, and grains, has been shown to have an antitumor effect on OSCC cells via the induction of cell cycle arrest [29,40]. Quercetin treatment suppressed cell growth by inducing G2/M arrest and apoptosis in EGFR-overexpressing HSC-3 and TW206 oral cancer cells [30]. Our result show that quercetin inhibits the viability of OSCC cell lines, such as OSC20, SAS, and HN22 cells, in a dose-dependent manner by inducing cell cycle arrest at the G2/M phase (Figure 1A,B).

The EMT process contributes to greater interstitial cell adhesion profiles, as unregulated cellular or cell matrix adhesion and increased migration and invasion are required for the development of metastatic cancer [41]. The ability of cancer cells to migrate and invade is increased by the reduction of the expression of E-cadherin, a cell–cell adhesion molecule, whereas the expression of N-cadherin is decreased, which is inversely proportional to that of E-cadherin [42]. Quercetin regulates the expression of EMT markers, such as E-cadherin, vimentin, and β-catenin, in head and neck cancer-derived sphere cells and breast cancer cells [43,44]. In addition, quercetin prevented the EGF-induced expression of N-cadherin and vimentin and increased the expression of E-cadherin in prostate cells [45]. Based on these reports, it is assumed that quercetin treatment can modulate the expression of EMT-related markers. Additionally, quercetin suppressed cell viability, migration, and invasion by regulating miR-16/HOXA10, which inhibits the expression of MMP-2 and 9 in oral cancer cells [30]. Studies on the mechanism of action of quercetin in the metastasis of OSCCs are still insufficient. In this study, quercetin inhibited EMT by increasing the expression of E-cadherin and claudin-1 and decreasing the expression of fibronectin, vimentin, α-SMA, and Slug in OSCC cell lines (Figures 3 and 4). The activation of MMP-2 and MMP-9 was significantly decreased by quercetin treatment (Figure 3B). Thus, quercetin inhibits cell migration and invasion by regulating the expression of EMT-related genes in OSCC cell lines.

It has been found that transforming growth factor-beta 1 (TGF-β1) induces epithelial mesenchymal transition (EMT) in various cancer cells, promoting motility and invasiveness [46,47]. Additionally, TGF-β1 treatment reduces the enhanced expression of Snail1 and Twist1 and, subsequently, the expression of E-cadherin [47]. We observed whether quercetin reduced EMT-related factors increased by TGF- β1 treatment in human keratinocyte HaCaT cells. TGF-β1 can promote tumor formation by inducing mesenchymal metastasis (via EMT) in the epithelium in various cancer cells. The main TGF-β1-induced effectors in this process are EMT transcription inhibitors, such as Snail 1, Snail 2 (also known as Slug), ZEB1/2, and Twist. HaCaT cells showed morphological changes and induction of EMT-related markers upon TGF-β1 treatment (Figure 6B,C). Quercetin reduced TGF-β1-induced EMT expression in HaCaT cells.

Overall, our results strongly suggest that quercetin suppressed the viability of OSCC cells inducing cell cycle arrest in the G2/M phase (Figure 1). Significantly, our results demonstrate that quercetin suppresses the metastatic ability via EMT and MMP in OSCC cells and decreases the expression level of TGF-β1-induced EMT in human normal HaCaT cells. Thus, quercetin may provide a novel pharmacological approach for the treatment of OSCCs.

4. Materials and Methods

4.1. Reagents and Antibodies

Quercetin was purchased from Sigma-Aldrich (St. Louis, MO) and dissolved in DMSO (DUKSAN, Korea) to prepare stock solutions (100 mM). TGF-β1 was purchased from R&D Systems (Minneapolis, USA) and dissolved in 4 mM HCl containing 0.1% fatty acid-free bovine serum albumin to a concentration of 1.0 mg/mL to prepare stock solutions (20 μg/mL). 3-(4,5-dimethylthiazol-2-yl)-2,5-diphenyltetrazolium bromide (MTT) and thymidine were purchased from Sigma-Aldrich (St. Louis, MO). Antibodies against E-cadherin, vimentin, and Slug were purchased from Cell Signaling Technology (Danvers, MA, USA), whereas fibronectin was purchased from BD Bioscience (San Jose, CA, USA); α-smooth muscle actin was purchased from Abcam (Cambridge, MA, USA), and Twist and beta-actin were purchased from Santa Cruz Biotechnology (Santa Cruz, CA, USA).

4.2. Cell Culture and Treatment

Three OSCC cell lines (OSC20, SAS, and HN22 cells) and human keratinocyte cells such as HaCaT (immortal keratinocyte) and nHOK (primary normal human oral keratinocyte) were used in this study. OSC20 and SAS cells were grown in Dulbecco's modified Eagle's medium F-12, 1:1 mixture (Hyclone, UT, USA); HN22 and HaCaT cells were grown in Dulbecco's modified Eagle's medium with high glucose (DMEM; Hyclone); and nHOK (primary normal human oral keratinocyte) were cultured in KBM™ Gold Keratinocyte growth basal medium (Lonza, MD, USA, #CC-3103) containing KGM™-2 SingleQuots™ supplements (Lonza, MD, USA, #CC-4152) at 37 °C in 5% CO_2 and 95% O_2 in a humidified environment. Further, both media contained 10% fetal bovine serum (FBS; Hyclone) and 1% penicillin and streptomycin (Thermo Fisher, Waltham, MA, USA). In this study, the three OSCC cell lines were treated with various concentrations of quercetin for 24 h; the HaCaT cells were treated with 10 ng of TGF-β1 for 24 h and then treated with various concentrations of quercetin.

4.3. MTT Assay

An MTT (3-(4,5-dimethylthiazol-2-yl)-2,5-diphenyltetrazolium bromide) assay was conducted to evaluate the cytotoxicity of quercetin on cell viability. Each cell line was seeded at 1×10^4 cells per well in a 96-well plate and incubated with 10% FBS-containing media. However, the exception was that nHOK cells were seeded with 3×10^4 cells per well with serum-free media. After stabilization, the media was replaced with a media containing 10% FBS for 24 h. Then, the cells were treated with various concentrations of quercetin (10, 20, 40, 80, and 160 μM) with media containing 10% FBS. After 24 h, the media were replaced with MTT (500 μg/mL) in a fresh serum-free media, and the cells were incubated for 3 h at 37 °C. Then, the supernatant was removed, and 200 μL of dimethylsulfoxide (DMSO) was added to dissolve the MTT formazan. The absorbance of the plate was read at 570 nm using a Synergy HT micro plate reader (Bio-tek, Winooski, VT, USA).

4.4. Cell Cycle Analysis

A cell cycle analysis was conducted to observe the cell cycle's progression. Cells were seeded at a density of 5×10^5 cells in 60 mm dishes. After cell stabilization, the cells were treated with 40 μM of quercetin for 24 h. Then, the cells were detached using trypsin and washed with phosphate-buffered saline (PBS). The harvested cells were then fixed with 75% ethanol at 4 °C overnight; subsequently, they were centrifuged and incubated with 20 μL RNase A (10 mg/mL) in 1 mL PBS at 4 °C for 30 min. Lastly, cells were stained with 25 μg/mL PI at room temperature for 10 min in the dark. The DNA content was then analyzed using a BD FACSCanto II flow cytometer (BD Bioscience, San Joes, CA, USA).

4.5. Wound-Healing Assay

A wound-healing assay was conducted to evaluate cell migration ability. Cells were seeded in 6-well plates at 5×10^5 per well. At 80% confluence, the cells were treated with 1 mM thymidine for 2 h before reagent treatment. Then, a wound was made in the middle of the well using a sterile 200 µL pipette tip. Further, wells were washed three times with PBS. OSCC cell lines were incubated with media containing 1% FBS and 40 µM of quercetin for 24 h. HaCaT cells were incubated with media containing 1% FBS and 10 ng TGF-β1 for 24 h; then, 40 µM of quercetin was added continuously for 24 h without discarding the existing media. Images were captured using a microscope (Nikon Eclipse TS100, Japan; X100). The rate of reduction of the wound area was calculated as a percentage of the remaining wound area compared to the initial wound area.

4.6. Western Blot Analysis

After treatment, cells were washed three times with cold PBS and lysed with 1X RIPA buffer containing a protease inhibitor cocktail and phosphatase inhibitors. The lysed cells were centrifuged at 12,000 ×g for 24 h. Subsequently, the supernatant was collected. Using the method of Bradford, the protein concentration was quantified as 20 µg. Samples were separated on 10% SDS-polyacrylamide gels. Then, SDS-gels were transferred electrophoretically onto polyvinylidene fluoride membranes (Bio-Rad) using a wet transfer kit. The transferred membranes were blocked with 5% skim milk in Tris-buffered saline containing 0.1% Tween-20 for 1 h at room temperature. The membranes were incubated overnight at 4 °C with the primary antibodies against E-cadherin (cell signaling, #3195, 1:1000); claudin-1 (cell signaling, #4933, 1:1000); fibronectin (BD Bioscience, #610077, 1:1000); vimentin (cell signaling, #5741, 1:1000); α-SMA (Abcam, #ab5694, 1:000); slug (cell signaling, #9585, 1:1000); and Twist (Santa Cruz, #SC-81417, 1:500) and β-actin (Santa Cruz, #SC-47778, 1:4000). Continuously, the membranes were washed three times with 1X TNE buffer, and HRP-conjugated secondary antibodies (ENZO, #ADI-SAB-300-J, and #ADI-SAB-100-J, 1:8000) were applied for 3 h at room temperature. The antigen–antibody complexes were detected using a SuperSignal West–Femto reagent (Thermo Fisher, Waltham, MA, USA).

4.7. Gelatin Zymography

Gelatin zymography was conducted to detect matrix metalloproteinase (MMP) activity using the conditioned media. Each cell line was seeded at 5×10^5 cells per well in a 6-well plate with 10% FBS-containing media. After cell stabilization, the media were transformed into serum-free media and treated with different concentrations of quercetin for 24 h at 37 °C. Subsequently, the supernatant was collected and mixed with a sample buffer (50% 0.5 M Tris-HCl (pH 6.8), 40% glycerol, 8% SDS, and 0.01% bromophenol blue). Further, samples were loaded onto a 7.5% SDS-polyacrylamide gel containing 0.2% gelatin (Sigma). The gels were washed twice with PBS containing 2.5% Triton X-100 for 1 h and incubated with an incubation buffer at 37 °C for 48 h. Then, the gels were stained with Coomassie Blue R-250 (LPS solution, Dae Jeon, Korea) for 1 h. Progressively, the gels were destained with a destaining buffer (8% acetic acid and 4% methanol) until a clear zone was visible.

4.8. Immunofluorescence Staining

Cells were seeded at 2×10^5 cells onto a coverslip in a 6-well plate. In the case of OSCC, the cells were stained for transcription factor expression. The treated cells were fixed in 4% paraformaldehyde at room temperature for 15 min and washed three times with PBS for 10 min. Then, the cells were permeabilized by 0.02% Triton X-100 in PBS at room temperature for 20 min and washed with PBS. Diluted 1:100 primary antibodies (Slug and Twist) were applied to the cells overnight at 4 °C. On the following day, cells were washed three times with PBS, treated with fluorescein isothiocyanate (FITC)-conjugated secondary antibodies for 1 h at 37 °C, and washed three times. Then, 4 µg/mL Hoechst was used to stain the nuclei for 30 min at 37 °C. The treated HaCaT cells were stained to assess changes in their morphology. HaCaT cells were incubated with a phalloidin-conjugate working solution (1:100) and 4 μg/mL Hoechst instead of antibodies. Subsequently, the cells were washed and mounted on a slide glass. An image was then captured via confocal microscopy (LSM780, Carl Zeiss, Jena, Germany).

4.9. Invasion Assay

An 8 μM pore size Transwell (Corning Inc, Corning, NY, USA) was coated with 40 μL of Matrigel (BD Bioscience, San Joes, CA, USA), mixing the serum-free media at a ratio of 1:3 and air drying for 3 h at 37 °C. HaCaT cells were incubated for 24 h with or without 10 ng TGF-β1 and detached using trypsin. The cells were seeded in a Matrigel-coated Transwell culture chamber at 5×10^4 cells with serum-free media containing 10 ng TGF-β1, co-treated with TGF-β1 and quercetin (10 ng TGF-β1 and 40 μM) or without treatment. Then, 600 μL of culture medium containing 10% FBS was placed onto the lower chamber. The cells were next incubated at 37 °C in a 5% CO_2 atmosphere for 44 h. After incubation, the cells on the upper chamber were removed using a cotton swab. The cells passing through the Matrigel and membrane were fixed with cold methanol for 30 min and washed with PBS. The membrane was stained with Mayer's hematoxylin (Muto, Tokyo, Japan) and 1% Eosin Y solution (Muto). Photographs were captured under microscopy (Olympus BX51; 40X).

4.10. Statistical Analyses

Statistical analyses were performed by a one-way analysis of variance (ANOVA) followed by a Bonferroni post-test, whereby three or more experimental groups were compared. p-values of < 0.05 were considered statistically significant. All data are the means ± standard error of the mean (SEM).

Author Contributions: Conceptualization and methodology, H.J.K. and H.R.P.; Performing experiments and analyzing data, S.R.K., E.Y.L., and D.J.K.; Validation, H.J.K. and H.R.P.; Writing—Original draft preparation, H.J.K. and S.R.K.; and funding acquisition, H.R.P. All authors have read and agreed to the published version of manuscript.

References

1. Cooper, J.S.; Porter, K.; Mallin, K.; Hoffman, H.T.; Weber, R.S.; Ang, K.K. National Cancer Database report on cancer of the head and neck: 10-year update. *Head Neck.* **2009**, *31*, 748–758. [CrossRef] [PubMed]
2. Markopoulos, A.K. Current aspects on oral squamous cell carcinoma. *Open Dent. J.* **2012**, *6*, 126–130. [CrossRef] [PubMed]
3. Su, C.W.; Chang, Y.C.; Chien, M.H.; Hsieh, Y.H.; Chen, M.K.; Lin, C.W.; Yang, S.F. Loss of TIMP3 by promoter methylation of Sp1 binding site promotes oral cancer metastasis. *Cell Death Dis.* **2019**, *10*, 793. [CrossRef] [PubMed]
4. Tsantoulis, P.K.; Kastrinakis, N.G.; Tourvas, A.D.; Laskaris, G.; Gorgoulis, V.G. Advances in the biology of oral cancer. *Oral. Oncol.* **2007**, *43*, 523–534. [CrossRef]
5. Gasche, J.A.; Goel, A. Epigenetic mechanisms in oral carcinogenesis. *Future Oncol.* **2012**, *8*, 1407–1425. [CrossRef]
6. Galbiatti, A.L.; Padovani-Junior, J.A.; Maníglia, J.V.; Rodrigues, C.D.; Pavarino, É.C.; Goloni-Bertollo, E.M. Head and neck cancer: Causes, prevention and treatment. *Braz J. Otorhinolaryngol.* **2013**, *79*, 239–247. [CrossRef]
7. Sano, D.; Myers, J.N. Metastasis of squamous cell carcinoma of the oral tongue. *Cancer Metastasis Rev.* **2007**, *26*, 645–662. [CrossRef]
8. Pihlstrom, B.L.; Michalowicz, B.S.; Johnson, N.W. Periodontal diseases. *Lancet* **2005**, *366*, 1809–1820. [CrossRef]
9. Makita, H.; Tanaka, T.; Fujitsuka, H.; Tatematsu, N.; Satoh, K.; Hara, A.; Mori, H. Chemoprevention of 4-nitroquinoline 1-oxide-induced rat oral carcinogenesis by the dietary flavonoids chalcone, 2-hydroxychalcone, and quercetin. *Cancer Res.* **1996**, *56*, 4904–4909.
10. Mehrotra, R.; Yadav, S. Oral squamous cell carcinoma: Etiology, pathogenesis and prognostic value of genomic alterations. *Indian J. Cancer* **2006**, *43*, 60–66. [CrossRef]

11. Javed, F.; Warnakulasuriya, S. Is there a relationship between periodontal disease and oral cancer? A systematic review of currently available evidence. *Crit. Rev. Oncol Hematol.* **2016**, *97*, 197–205. [CrossRef] [PubMed]
12. American Cancer Society. Cancer Facts & Figures: 2018. Available online: https://www.cancer.org/content/dam/cancer-org/research/cancer-facts-and-statistics/annual-cancer-facts-and-figures/2018/cancer-facts-and-figures-2018.pdf (accessed on 26 February 2018).
13. Brabletz, T.; Kalluri, R.; Nieto, M.A.; Weinberg, R.A. EMT in cancer. *Nat. Rev. Cancer.* **2018**, *18*, 128–134. [CrossRef] [PubMed]
14. Bacac, M.; Stamenkovic, I. Metastatic cancer cell. *Annu. Rev. Pathol.* **2008**, *3*, 221–247. [CrossRef]
15. Valastyan, S.; Weinberg, R.A. Tumor metastasis: Molecular insights and evolving paradigms. *Cell* **2011**, *147*, 275–292. [CrossRef] [PubMed]
16. Yoon, S.O.; Park, S.J.; Yun, C.H.; Chung, A.S. Roles of matrix metalloproteinases in tumor metastasis and angiogenesis. *J. Biochem. Mol. Biol.* **2003**, *36*, 128–137. [CrossRef] [PubMed]
17. Kessenbrock, K.; Plaks, V.; Werb, Z. Matrix metalloproteinases: Regulators of the tumor microenvironment. *Cell* **2010**, *141*, 52–67. [CrossRef] [PubMed]
18. Gialeli, C.; Theocharis, A.D.; Karamanos, N.K. Roles of matrix metalloproteinases in cancer progression and their pharmacological targeting. *FEBS J.* **2011**, *278*, 16–27. [CrossRef] [PubMed]
19. Krisanaprakornkit, S.; Iamaroon, A. Epithelial-mesenchymal transition in oral squamous cell carcinoma. *ISRN Oncol.* **2012**, *681469*, 1–10. [CrossRef]
20. Khasigov, P.Z.; Podobed, O.V.; Gracheva, T.S.; Salbiev, K.D.; Grachev, S.V.; Berezov, T.T. Role of matrix metalloproteinases and their inhibitors in tumor invasion and metastasis. *Biochemistry* **2003**, *68*, 711–717.
21. Marunaka, Y.; Marunaka, R.; Sun, H.; Yamamoto, T.; Kanamura, N.; Inui, T.; Taruno, A. Actions of Quercetin, a Polyphenol, on Blood Pressure. *Molecules* **2017**, *22*, 209. [CrossRef]
22. Valentová, K.; Vrba, J.; Bancířová, M.; Ulrichová, J.; Křen, V. Isoquercitrin: Pharmacology, toxicology, and metabolism. *Food Chem Toxicol.* **2014**, *68*, 267–282.
23. Massi, A.; Bortolini, O.; Ragno, D.; Bernardi, T.; Sacchetti, G.; Tacchini, M.; De Risi, C. Research Progress in the Modification of Quercetin Leading to Anticancer Agents. *Molecules* **2017**, *22*, 1270. [CrossRef] [PubMed]
24. Kee, J.Y.; Han, Y.H.; Kim, D.S.; Mun, J.G.; Park, J.; Jeong, M.Y.; Um, J.Y.; Hong, S.H. Inhibitory effect of quercetin on colorectal lung metastasis through inducing apoptosis, and suppression of metastatic ability. *Phytomedicine* **2016**, *23*, 1680–1690. [CrossRef] [PubMed]
25. Rather, R.A.; Bhagat, M. Quercetin as an innovative therapeutic tool for cancer chemoprevention: Molecular mechanisms and implications in human health. *Cancer Med.* **2019**. [CrossRef] [PubMed]
26. Murakami, A.; Ashida, H.; Terao, J. Multitargeted cancer prevention by quercetin. *Cancer Lett.* **2008**, *269*, 315–325. [CrossRef]
27. Geoghegan, F.; Wong, R.W.; Rabie, A.B. Inhibitory effect of quercetin on periodontal pathogens in vitro. *Phytother Res.* **2010**, *24*, 817–820.
28. Palaska, I.; Papathanasiou, E.; Theoharides, T.C. Use of polyphenols in periodontal inflammation. *Eur J. Pharmacol.* **2013**, *720*, 77–83. [CrossRef]
29. Ma, Y.S.; Yao, C.N.; Liu, H.C.; Yu, F.S.; Lin, J.J.; Lu, K.W.; Liao, C.L.; Chueh, F.S.; Chung, J.G. Quercetin induced apoptosis of human oral cancer SAS cells through mitochondria and endoplasmic reticulum mediated signaling pathways. *Oncol. Lett.* **2018**, *15*, 9663–9672. [CrossRef]
30. Zhao, J.; Fang, Z.; Zha, Z.; Sun, Q.; Wang, H.; Sun, M.; Qiao, B. Quercetin inhibits cell viability, migration and invasion by regulating miR-16/HOXA10 axis in oral cancer. *Eur J. Pharmacol.* **2019**, *847*, 11–18. [CrossRef]
31. Li, X.; Guo, S.; Xiong, X.K.; Peng, B.Y.; Huang, J.M.; Chen, M.F.; Wang, F.Y.; Wang, J.N. Combination of quercetin and cisplatin enhances apoptosis in OSCC cells by downregulating xIAP through the NF-κB pathway. *J. Cancer.* **2019**, *10*, 4509–4521. [CrossRef]
32. Huang, C.Y.; Chan, C.Y.; Chou, I.T.; Lien, C.H.; Hung, H.C.; Lee, M.F. Quercetin induces growth arrest through activation of FOXO1 transcription factor in EGFR-overexpressing oral cancer cells. *J. Nutr. Biochem.* **2013**, *24*, 1596–1603. [CrossRef] [PubMed]
33. Surh, Y.J. Cancer chemoprevention with dietary phytochemicals. *Nat. Rev. Cancer.* **2003**, *3*, 768–780. [CrossRef] [PubMed]

34. Kim, H.J.; Kim, S.K.; Kim, B.S.; Lee, S.H.; Park, Y.S.; Park, B.K.; Kim, S.J.; Kim, J.; Choi, C.; Kim, J.S.; et al. Apoptotic effect of quercetin on HT-29 colon cancer cells via the AMPK signaling pathway. *J. Agric Food Chem.* **2010**, *58*, 8643–8650. [CrossRef] [PubMed]
35. Nam, J.S.; Sharma, A.R.; Nguyen, L.T.; Chakraborty, C.; Sharma, G.; Lee, S.S. Application of Bioactive Quercetin in Oncotherapy: From Nutrition to Nanomedicine. *Molecules* **2016**, *21*, 108. [CrossRef]
36. Hashemzaei, M.; Delarami, A.; Yari, A.; Heravi, R.E.; Tabrizian, K.; Taghdisi, S.M.; Sadegh, S.E.; Tsarouhas, K.; Kouretas, D.; Tzanakakis, G.; et al. Anticancer and apoptosis-inducing effects of quercetin in vitro and in vivo. *Oncol. Rep.* **2017**, *38*, 819–828. [CrossRef]
37. Yu, D.; Ye, T.; Xiang, Y.; Shi, Z.; Zhang, J.; Lou, B.; Zhang, F.; Chen, B.; Zhou, M. Quercetin inhibits epithelial-mesenchymal transition, decreases invasiveness and metastasis, and reverses IL-6 induced epithelial-mesenchymal transition, expression of MMP by inhibiting STAT3 signaling in pancreatic cancer cells. *Onco Targets Ther.* **2017**, *10*, 4719–4729. [CrossRef]
38. Cai, W.; Yu, D.; Fan, J.; Liang, X.; Jin, H.; Liu, C.; Zhu, M.; Shen, T.; Zhang, R.; Hu, W.; et al. Quercetin inhibits transforming growth factor β1-induced epithelial-mesenchymal transition in human retinal pigment epithelial cells via the Smad pathway. *Drug Des. Dev. Ther.* **2018**, *12*, 4149–4161. [CrossRef]
39. Lai, W.W.; Hsu, S.C.; Chueh, F.S.; Chen, Y.Y.; Yang, J.S.; Lin, J.P.; Lien, J.C.; Tsai, C.H.; Chung, J.G. Quercetin inhibits migration and invasion of SAS human oral cancer cells through inhibition of NF-κB and matrix metalloproteinase-2/-9 signaling pathways. *Anticancer Res.* **2013**, *33*, 1941–1950.
40. ElAttar, T.M.; Virji, A.S. Modulating effect of resveratrol and quercetin on oral cancer cell growth and proliferation. *Anticancer Drugs* **1999**, *10*, 187–193. [CrossRef]
41. Gupta, G.P.; Massagué, J. Cancer metastasis: Building a framework. *Cell* **2006**, *127*, 679–695. [CrossRef]
42. Thiery, J.P.; Sleeman, J.P. Complex networks orchestrate epithelial-mesenchymal transitions. *Nat. Rev. Mol. Cell. Biol.* **2006**, *7*, 131–142. [CrossRef] [PubMed]
43. Chang, W.W.; Hu, F.W.; Yu, C.C.; Wang, H.H.; Feng, H.P.; Lan, C.; Tsai, L.L.; Chang, Y.C. Quercetin in elimination of tumor initiating stem-like and mesenchymal transformation property in head and neck cancer. *Head Neck.* **2013**, *35*, 413–419. [CrossRef]
44. Srinivasan, A.; Thangavel, C.; Liu, Y.; Shoyele, S.; Den, R.B.; Selvakumar, P.; Lakshmikuttyamma, A. Quercetin regulates β-catenin signaling and reduces the migration of triple negative breast cancer. *Mol. Carcinog.* **2016**, *55*, 743–756. [CrossRef] [PubMed]
45. Bhat, F.A.; Sharmila, G.; Balakrishnan, S.; Arunkumar, R.; Elumalai, P.; Suganya, S.; Raja Singh, P.; Srinivasan, N.; Arunakaran, J. Quercetin reverses EGF-induced epithelial to mesenchymal transition and invasiveness in prostate cancer (PC-3) cell line via EGFR/PI3K/Akt pathway. *J. Nutr. Biochem.* **2014**, *25*, 1132–1139. [CrossRef]
46. Feng, J.; Song, D.; Jiang, S.; Yang, X.; Ding, T.; Zhang, H.; Luo, J.; Liao, J.; Yin, Q. Quercetin restrains TGF-β1-induced epithelial-mesenchymal transition by inhibiting Twist1 and regulating E-cadherin expression. *Biochem. Biophys. Res. Commun.* **2018**, *498*, 132–138. [CrossRef]
47. Zavadil, J.; Bottinger, E.P. TGF-beta and epithelial-to-mesenchymal transitions. *Oncogene* **2005**, *24*, 5764–5774. [CrossRef] [PubMed]

11

Reverse Transcriptase Inhibitors Nanosystems Designed for Drug Stability and Controlled Delivery

Fedora Grande *, Giuseppina Ioele *, Maria Antonietta Occhiuzzi, Michele De Luca, Elisabetta Mazzotta, Gaetano Ragno, Antonio Garofalo and Rita Muzzalupo

Department of Pharmacy, Health and Nutritional Sciences, University of Calabria, Via P. Bucci, 87036 Rende (CS), Italy; mariaantonietta.occhiuzzi@unical.it (M.A.O.); michele.deluca@unical.it (M.D.L.); mazzotta-elisabetta@libero.it (E.M.); gaetano.ragno@unical.it (G.R.); antonio.garofalo@unical.it (A.G.); rita.muzzalupo@unical.it (R.M.)

* Correspondence: fedora.grande@unical.it (F.G.); giuseppina.ioele@unical.it (G.I.)

Abstract: An in-depth analysis of nanotechnology applications for the improvement of solubility, distribution, bioavailability and stability of reverse transcriptase inhibitors is reported. Current clinically used nucleoside and non-nucleoside agents, included in combination therapies, were examined in the present survey, as drugs belonging to these classes are the major component of highly active antiretroviral treatments. The inclusion of such agents into supramolecular vesicular systems, such as liposomes, niosomes and lipid solid NPs, overcomes several drawbacks related to the action of these drugs, including drug instability and unfavorable pharmacokinetics. Overall results reported in the literature show that the performances of these drugs could be significantly improved by inclusion into nanosystems.

Keywords: HIV; antiretrovirals; nanoformulations; drug degradation; drug protection

1. Introduction

The human immunodeficiency virus (HIV), belonging to the lentivirus genus of the large family of retroviridae, is the etiological agent of AIDS. The infection causes severe consequences to the immune system including a loss of CD4+T lymphocytes that leads to an increased susceptibility to even fatal opportunistic infections. The identification of various antiretroviral drugs allowed defining efficacious therapeutic regimens for the prevention and treatment of the disease by the combined administration of two, three or more different drugs acting on crucial steps of viral replication. In particular, the targets of conventional drugs are proteins involved in the viral entry or specific enzymes necessary for the virus replication such as protease (PR), reverse transcriptase (RT) and integrase (IN). This approach known as HAART (highly active antiretroviral therapy) nowadays represents the most useful therapeutic treatment, even though it is affected by many drawbacks such as lifetime administration with a consequent reduced patients' compliance, severe side effects, and quick viral outbreak after drug resistance emergence. HAART was demonstrated to be particularly effective in cutting down the overall number of viral particles, but is unable to completely eradicate infection in sanctuary sites, such as the brain, liver and lymphatic system [1–5]. Moreover, HAART always includes one or more nucleoside and non-nucleoside reverse transcriptase inhibitors (NRTI and NNRTI, respectively), which, despite a high antiviral efficacy, unavoidably show important clinical drawbacks. Relevant information on common RTI is summarized in Table 1 [6,7].

Table 1. Relevant information of currently used RTI. *Year of FDA approval; LS = Lipid Solubility; OB = Oral Bioavailability; t/2 = Plasma Half-life.

Drug Class	Name (Acronym)	Year*	LS	OB (%)	t/2 (hours)	Side Effects
NRTIs	Stavudine (STV)	1996	low	86	1.3–1.4	Peripheral neuropathy, pancreatitis, asymptomatic acidosis, lipoatrophy, hepatic steatosis
	Zidovudine (AZT)	1986	low	60	0.5–3	Neutropenia, anemia, nausea, vomiting, asthenia, headache, insomnia, skin hyperpigmentation, acidosis, hepatic steatosis
	Lamivudine (3TC)	1995	low	86	5–7	Cough, diarrhea, fatigue, headache, malaise, nasal symptoms, lactic acidosis, hepatic steatosis
	Abacavir (ABV)	1998	low	83	0.8–1.5	Systemic respiratory hypersensitivity, gastrointestinal symptoms, fever, tiredness, sore throat
	Emtricitabine (FTC)	2006	low	93	8–10	Headache, nausea, upset stomach, diarrhea, trouble sleeping, dizziness, skin rash, strange dreams, cough, runny nose
	Zalcitabine (ZCT)	1992	low	85		Peripheral neuropathy, stomatitis, esophageal ulcerations, acidosis, hepatic steatosis
	Didanosine (DDN)	1991	low	30	2	Gastrointestinal intolerance, peripheral neuropathy, pancreatitis, asymptomatic acidosis, lipoatrophy, hepatic steatosis
	Tenofovir (TDF)	2001	low	25-39	12–15	Nausea, depression, confusion, headache, hitching, weakness, kidneys problems
NNRTIs	Nevirapine (NVR)	1996	moderate	92	25–30	Rash, Stevens-Johnson syndrome, elevated transaminases blood level, hepatitis, severe hypersensitivity reaction
	Efavirenz (EFV)	1998	high	50	40–55	Rash, Stevens-Johnson syndrome, sleep disturbances, dizziness, vertigo, depression, euphoria, difficulty concentrating, hallucination.
	Etravirine (ETV)	2008	high	–	30–40	Rash, Stevens-Johnson syndrome, toxic epidermal necrosis and multiform erythema, hypersensitivity reactions, hepatic failure
	Rilpivirine (RPV)	2011	high	50	19	Rash, depression, liver problems, mood changes

The above therapeutic strategy is not even capable of stimulating a lasting immune response of memory cells necessary to antagonize the infective agent [8]. Even after taking into account all these considerations, innovative therapeutic approaches based on both the identification of alternative drugs and innovative pharmaceutic formulations still have demanding requirements [9–11]. Nanotechnologies could help to reach this latter crucial point in order to increase cellular uptake, enhance drug distribution, prolong half-life and reduce side effects depending on the lower drug dosage in the nanosystem. In particular, application of nanoformulations consisting of a given drug and a supramolecular matrix such as niosomes, liposomes and solid lipid nanoparticles (SLN), already led to some improvements of pharmacokinetic and pharmacodynamic parameters. Very interesting results have been recorded in the anti-cancer research field where an altered microenvironment of cancer cells facilitates a selective drug delivery [12]. A similar approach could be adopted in the case of cells infected by HIV [13].

In the light of these findings, the incorporation of new or customary anti-HIV drugs into supramolecular carriers could be particularly effective in suppressing viral replication. This strategy is corroborated by the possibility of encapsulating drugs or genes to not only be delivered next to the infected cells but also to target reservoir tissues to eradicate latent HIV [14]. This innovative strategy is suitable for improving the distribution of both hydrophilic and hydrophobic small molecules, as well as macromolecular drugs, which can be driven toward specific tissues thanks to the reduced size of the nanoscale delivery systems. Antiretroviral drugs can be carried as nanoparticles for their potential to better reach macrophages, CD4+T cells and latent reservoirs organs, such as brain and lymph nodes, that are particularly responsible of viral survival. [15–19]. Drug delivery systems (DDS) for RTI, developed in the last few years, are described in this survey and depicted in Figure 1, while their main properties are summarized in Table 2.

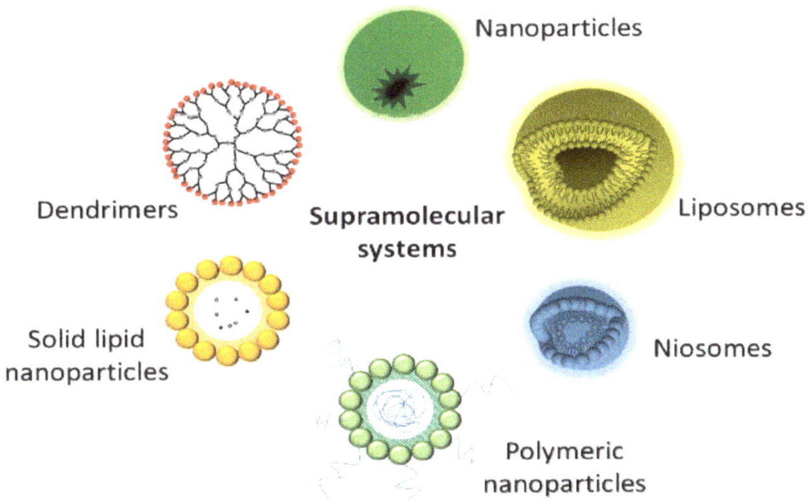

Figure 1. Drug delivery systems for RTI nanoformulations.

Table 2. Targets of DDS designed for anti-HIV therapy.

DDS		TARGET
Matrix	**Surface**	
Liposome NPs	Mannose	Liver, spleen, lung, brain, macrophages
Liposomes	Galactose	Liver
Chitosan NPs	Glycyrrhizin	Liver
NPs	Transferrin	Brain, endothelial cells
NPs	Serum albumin	Brain, liver, spleen
SLN	Phenylalanine	Blood brain barrier
Polymeric micelles	Anti-GP2 antibody	M-cell of gut-associated lymphoid tissue
Dendrimers	Tuftsin	Macrophages, monocytes, polymorph nuclear leukocytes

Once the supramolecular system reaches the site of action, a controlled drug release provides high local concentration and longer residence time, resulting in an improved antiviral effect (Figure 2). Furthermore, some nanomaterials possess themselves favorable biological effects. The nanotechnology approach has been advanced for many aspects dealing with HIV infection, namely theranostic, vaccine prophylaxis and gene therapy. This survey however focuses on studies describing NRTI and NNRTI based nanoformulations for prevention or treatment of HIV infection. Although these systems allow a remarkable improvement of the pharmacokinetics and pharmacodynamics of RTI, several drawbacks still need to be overcame. The major advantages and limitations of known nanosystems are listed in Table 3.

Table 3. Advantages and limitations of anti-HIV DDS.

DDS	Advantages	Limitations
Liposomes	Co-delivery of hydrophilic and lipophilic drug Selective uptake by mononuclear phagocytes Surface modification with target moiety of virus reservoir	Low drug loading capacity Physical and chemical instability Drug leakage Difficulty in sterilization Short half-life Poor scale up
Niosomes	Chemical stability Protection of drug from degradation Large uptake by mononuclear phagocytes and localization in virus reservoir organs Less expensive respect liposomes Functionalization with target ligand	Physical instability during the storage Difficulty in sterilization Difficulty in large-scale production
Polymeric NPs	High drug loading capacity Co-delivery of different drug for anti-HIV combination therapy Selective uptake by lymphoid organ Prolonged circulation time Surface functionalization with target moiety	Fast burst release Limited safe correlated to polymer toxicity High cost production
SLN	Higher stability and biological compatibility than liposomes and polymeric NPs Increase the bioavailability of poorly water soluble drug Avoidance of organic solvent Slow uptake by the RES Feasible-large scale production and sterilization Less expensive than polymeric and surfactant carriers	Low drug solubility in lipid matrix and loading capacity Drug leakage Particle growth Unpredictable gelation tendency
Dendrimers	Uniform particle size Large surface functional groups for the conjugation with target moieties	Toxicity problems

Several of these clinically used drugs show an undesirable stability profile when exposed to stressing conditions either in solution or in solid form [20,21]. Similarly, stress tests have been performed on supramolecular systems in order to confirm any improved stability, under different conditions [22]. In particular, studies published in the last few years on the RT inhibitors included in combined therapy have been taken into consideration [15,16,23].

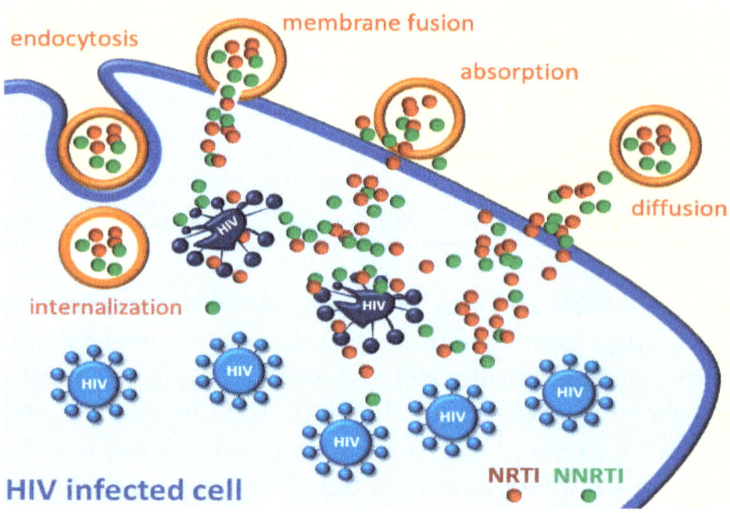

Figure 2. Representative delivery modalities for NRTI/NNRTI nanosystems to HIV reservoirs.

2. Drug Protection Nanosystems

Most of the protocols adopted for studying the drug stability are suggested by the ICH (International Conference on Harmonization) guidelines [24]. According to such rules, clearly defined drug storage conditions are required to prevent the degradation effects related to pH, temperature, light, air and humidity for either solution/suspension or commercial formulations/packaging [25]. The protection of sensitive drugs could often be assured by shielding with an adequate packaging [26]. When this simple precaution showed not to be sufficient, the stability of the drug, exposed to different environmental conditions, could be improved by suitable delivery devices, such as vesicular matrices (i.e., liposomes and niosomes), nanoparticles (NPs), and solid lipid nanoparticles (SLN).

Niosomal and liposomal vesicles consist of amphiphilic molecules and an aqueous compartment and differ for their structural chemical units. Both systems are very versatile. The hydrophilic drugs can be entrapped in their aqueous core while the lipophilic drugs can be partitioned into the bilayer domains. Liposomes are made of natural phospholipids, resulting in a greater stability, a low production cost and reduced toxicity [27–32], while niosomes are prepared by means of synthetic, non-ionic surfactants, as alkyl ethers, alkyl esters and pluronics copolymers, or fatty acid and amino acid compounds [31–33]. The preparation of these vesicles requires a simple procedure based on a gentle agitation or sonication of an aqueous solution of phospholipid/surfactant and drug mixtures taken from an ultracentrifugation or low-pressure gel filtration chromatography to purify the formed systems [34].

More recent SLN have been proposed as alternative formulations for both hydrophilic and hydrophobic drugs. These systems are colloidal carriers based on a solid phase lipid and a surfactant and are characterized by a spherical shape in which the lipid portion is always solid and the surfactant acts as a stabilizing factor [22,35–40]. Fatty acids, monoglycerides, diglycerides, triglycerides, waxes and steroids can be applied in the preparation of SLN in the absence of organic solvent [35]. Low cost, good physical stability, large scale production, no toxicity and high biodegradability represent the greatest advantages in the use of these formulations with respect to the liposomes matrices [41].

Nanoparticles systems are known promising carriers for the improvement of solubility and pharmacokinetics of drugs as well as vaccines, nucleic acids and therapeutic proteins. These delivery devices can influence therapeutic efficiency of a drug, enhance its protection from degradation and reduce dose-limiting side effects. A variety of hydrophobic or hydrophilic active molecules can be dissolved, encapsulated, absorbed or conjugated to polymeric nanoparticles following different techniques [42]. Several natural and biodegradable materials like chitosan have been proposed for the realization of anti-HIV drug nanosystems. An alternative approach, based on the formation of crystalline complex with a fixed range size, was attempted by inclusion of the pure drug into a hydrophobic synthetic polymer [43]. Polymeric nanoparticles based on poly(lactic acid) (PLA) or poly(lactide-*co*-glycolide) (PLGA) are reported as ideal delivery systems, showing an improved therapeutic efficacy with lower incidence of side effects [42,44–49].

A higher local concentration of active molecules is often reached by integration of classic antiretroviral drugs in different NPs of metals [50]. According to a relative inertness and low toxicity, silver or gold NPs have been explored in biomedicine as multifunctional scaffolds. In particular, the application of gold NPs has been employed to conjugate biomolecules on the outer surface. Alternative inorganic multifunctional materials, such as silver NPs coated with poly(vinyl)pyrrolidone, have also been exploited as drug carriers. [51].

Synthetic well-defined nanopolymers with a three-dimensional architecture, known as dendrimers, have been proposed for the vehiculation of several drugs. Generally, a dendrimer is a symmetric and hyper-branched macromolecule characterized by the presence of reactive groups in the central core, repeated branching units in the interior layers of the core and functional groups spanning from the outer surface. The drug molecule can be either entrapped inside the structure or linked to the external functional groups. This approach was proposed for the carrying of several anti HIV agents [52–55].

Some of these matrices are also able to improve the stability of drugs. Several studies described the use of niosomes, metal based and polymeric NPs to prevent the degradation effects caused by stressing conditions [33,50,56].

3. Nucleoside Reverse Transcriptase Inhibitors Nanosystems

The therapy based on the administration of nucleoside antiviral derivatives such as stavudine, zidovudine, lamivudine and emtricitabine represented a first and effective approach adopted for the management of HIV infection (Figure 3).

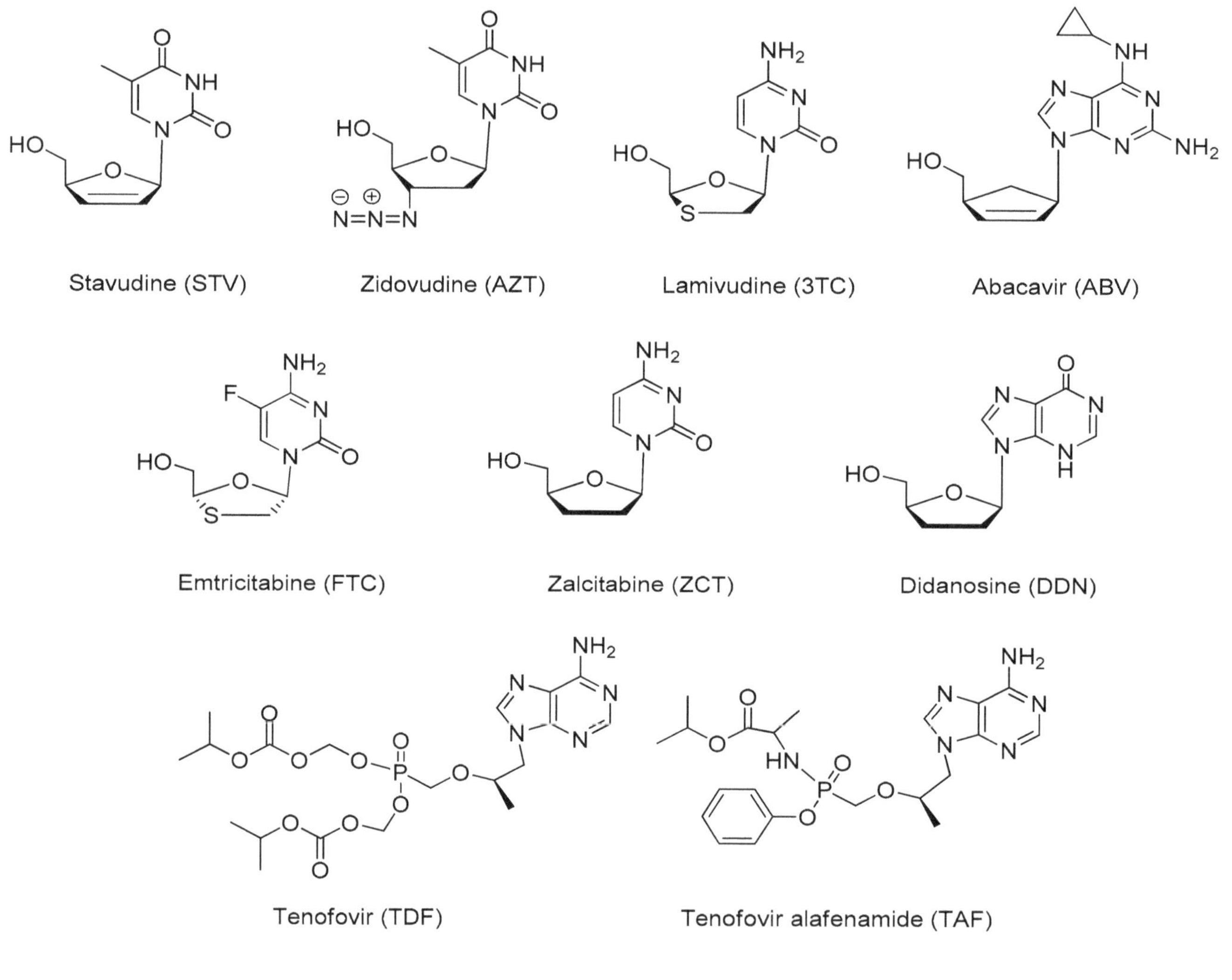

Figure 3. Chemical structures of NRTIs.

Due to the structural similarity to purine or pyrimidine nucleosides, the mode of action of these drugs consists of the competition for the incorporation into viral DNA, catalyzed by RT, so causing chain termination (Figure 4, panel b). Nowadays the most common nucleoside derivatives used in therapy are lamivudine, abacavir, emtricitabine, tenofovir and tenofovir alafenamide [57]. Stavudine and zidovudine, not yet recommended in first-line therapy, were early examples of NRTIs included in nanoformulations designed for limiting their severe side effects and improving pharmacokinetics.

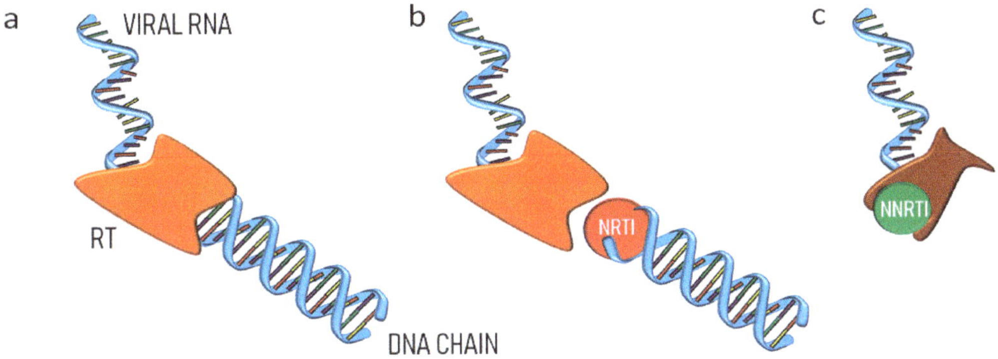

Figure 4. (**a**) RT catalyzes the conversion of viral RNA into pro-viral DNA before its incorporation into the target cell genome; (**b**) NRTIs are incorporated into the DNA causing chain termination; (**c**) NNRTIs bind the enzyme inhibiting its function.

3.1. *Stavudine*

Stavudine (1-((2R,5S)-5-(hydroxymethyl)-2,5-dihydrofuran-2-yl)-5-methylpyrimidine-2,4(1H, 3H)-dione, STV) is one of the most commonly used forms of NRT approved by FDA in 1996 and its use was recommended in association with other antiretroviral agents. The drug showed major side effects, such as high blood lactate, pancreatitis and hepatomegaly. STV was characterized by a serum half-life of 1h only, while that of its phosphorylated active metabolite was calculated as being 3.5 h [27]. Thus, STV loaded formulations able to concomitantly increase cellular uptake and sustain release should reduce unwanted effects. Accordingly, galactosyl or mannosyl coated liposomes loaded with STV were described. These formulations reached the desired results showing an increased *in vitro* anti-HIV activity together with a remarkable decrease of side effects. The efficacy was tested in a mononuclear phagocyte system, a major reservoir of HIV, proving advantages in terms of bio-stability, site-specific and ligand-mediated delivery, compared to free drug and uncoated liposomes [27,28]. More recently, STV-containing nanoformulations were proposed for the dual utilization to control the residual viremia as well as to target the reservoir sites. To achieve this aim, gelatin nanoformulations containing very low dosage of the drug were prepared through a simple desolvation process and loaded into soya lecithin based liposomes [29]. A study on STV degradation under different stress conditions (hydrolysis, oxidation, photolysis and thermal stress) was initially reported. A stability-indicating reversed-phase HPLC assay method showed the hydrolysis of the drug to thymine in acidic, neutral, alkaline and under oxidative stress conditions [20]. In order to improve the stability of this drug, STV-loaded SLN for intravenous injection were produced by high-pressure homogenization of drug lipid melt dispersed in hot surfactant solution [22]. This SLN formulation was also studied for its active delivery to lymphatic tissues by ex vivo cellular uptake evaluation in macrophages. Reported experiments confirmed an improved cellular uptake together with a prolonged activity next to the delivery site of the formulation compared to the simple drug solution. This could account for an efficient and safe therapeutic profile of the drug-carrier system [58].

3.2. *Zidovudine*

Zidovudine, also known as azidothymidine (1-((2R,4S,5S)-4-azido-5-(hydroxymethyl)tetra hydrofuran-2-yl)-5-methylpyrimidine-2,4(1H,3H)-dione, AZT), the first antiretroviral medication proposed to prevent and treat HIV/AIDS, has been approved in 1986. An extensive first pass metabolism often requires an in vein administration. This feature and a long list of severe side effects limit the use of this drug, which is however still present in many therapeutic anti-HIV regimens. Its incorporation into supramolecular matrices was extensively exploited in order to increase bioavailability and to reduce dose-dependent unwanted effects.

Positively and negatively charged liposomes based on stearylamine and diacetyl phosphate were used as AZT carriers. In order to enhance localization to lymph nodes and spleen, these systems were even coated with a site-specific mannose-terminated stearylamine ligand. Fluorescent microscopy images showed an enhanced uptake and localization of these liposomes in the target tissues [59]. In an early paper, a dispersed system comprising polyoxypropylene, polyoxyethylene, oleic acid, water and cetyl alcohol as surfactant, was described as a potential DDS. The release profile experimental analysis showed that the delivery of AZT could be controlled this way, in accordance with a mathematical theoretical approach [60]. This system has been proposed as a carrier, which potentially could overcome the main drawbacks of conventional pharmaceutical formulations [61].

AZT loaded in polymeric NPs based on PLA and poly(L-lactide)poly(ethyleneglycol) (PLA/PEG) were prepared by double emulsion solvent evaporation and thoroughly investigated *in vitro* for uptake into polymorphonuclear leucocytes of rat peritoneal exudate. The cells activation by NPs was assessed by a chemiluminescence assay suggesting a more favorable behavior of PLA vs. PLA/PEG complexes [62]. On the other hand, the drug release increased proportionally to the PEG amount in the blend [63]. AZT was encapsulated in alginate-glutamic acid amide based NPs obtained by an emulsion solvent evaporation method. The polymeric NPs were coated with pluronic F-68 to favor cellular internalization through the endocytosis mechanism. As a result, the antiviral drug loaded in these nanosystems was released in a prolonged manner. Intracellular uptake and cell viability assays also confirmed an efficient uptake of AZT in glioma cell lines [64]. Solid lipid NPs based on modified stearic acid and *Aloe vera* extract were described as an alternative drug delivery carrier for controlled release and targeting of AZT. The plant extract was used because of its high content of polysaccharides that showed synergistic antiretroviral activity with AZT. The described nanocarriers did not interact with plasma proteins and showed high drug loading and entrapment efficiency. Moreover, fluorescent microscopy images suggested that the natural gel facilitated the cellular uptake of AZT in brain cells [36]. The drug proved to decompose when exposed to light or under hydrolytic conditions, while it was more stable toward oxidation agents and thermal stress [65]. In particular, the acid degradation induced the formation of a pyrimidine derivative endowed with higher toxicity when compared to AZT, as demonstrated by a mutagenicity and an aerobic biodegradability assay [21]. Recently, three novel prodrugs of AZT, obtained by functionalization with dicarboxylic acids, were designed in order to enhance pharmacokinetics, chemical stability and affinity for human serum albumin [66].

3.3. *Lamivudine*

The oral agent lamivudine, (4-amino-1-((2S,5R)-2-(hydroxymethyl)-1,3-oxathiolan-5-yl)pyrimidin-2(1H)-one, 3TC), an analog of nucleoside cytidine, was approved by FDA for the combined therapy with AZT in 1995 and for monotherapy in 2002. However, the emergence of drug resistance, associated to the gene mutation of RT, limited its clinical application [67,68].

Several nanocarriers were prepared by mixing biodegradable networks (i.e. PEG, pluronic-polyethyleneimmine (PEI), glycyrrhizin conjugated chitosan, mannosylated-PLGA) or dendritic networks (i.e. starPEG-PEI, poly(amidoamine)dendrimer-PEI-PEG) or nanogels with AZT or didanosine triphosphates under a freeze-drying method, to specifically deliver the antiviral agent next to macrophages in the CNS.

All nano-NRTIs demonstrated high efficacy in inhibiting HIV at low μM drug concentration. The major cause of NRTI neurotoxicity, consisting in the mitochondrial DNA depletion, was also reduced 3-fold compared to uncoated NRTIs [69]. Acid or alkaline conditions as well as an oxidative environment caused the degradation of the drug into five different products. On the other hand, light exposure or thermal stress did not affect drug stability [70,71].

More recently, a mass spectrometry study evidenced the formation of an additional degradation product when the solid drug was exposed to oxidative conditions [72]. 3TC was incorporated into polymethacrylic acid NPs in different drug/polymer ratio by nanoprecipitation method in order to overcome some drug limitations, such as accumulation during multi dose therapy and poor patient compliance. These polymers offer several advantages, including high stability and simple preparation route compared to remaining colloidal carriers. Moreover, these nanocarriers were shown to increase drug bioavailability and optimize the release time to the target site without significant chemical interactions between the drug and matrix [73]. An alternative encapsulation for 3TC was exploited by using PLGA NPs coated with bovine serum albumin through a double emulsion procedure. It was then demonstrated that PLGA NPs were rapidly internalized into the human liver cells after oral administration, at different drug concentrations, confirming their high potential as ideal 3TC delivery systems [74]. The PLGA/3TC system was also investigated for the formulation of a thermosensitive vaginal gel. The system was obtained in the form of NPs by the formation of an amide bond between the biodegradable polymer and the free amine group of the drug. An analogue formulation was prepared using emtricitabine as an alternative NRTI. The NPs were finally incorporated into a thermosensitive gel for vaginal administration. The nanoformulations showed to be non-toxic in HeLa cells assay up to a 100 μg/mL concentration. Similar preparations containing fluorescent NPs were found to be active for up to 5 days, suggesting a potential long-lasting application in therapy [75]. A similar approach was adopted for the achievement of transdermal formulation of PLGA/3TC complex. NPs obtained resulted in an ideal spherical shape and an external smooth shell. The high drug entrapment rate resulted in an improved physical stability of the drug together with an efficient delivery after skin permeation. This last property was enhanced after microneedles skin pre-treatment [76]. Mannosylated-PLGA NPs were prepared to ensure an efficient delivery of 3TC into brain macrophages. The experimental data confirmed the increased drug release from nanocarriers and this effect may be due to the presence of sugar receptors on the luminal surface of blood-brain barrier (BBB) [77]. 3TC was also entrapped into PLA/chitosan (CS) NPs by an emulsion technique. The drug was efficaciously entrapped and protected at low values of pH, while it was rapidly released at higher pH values, thus allowing the drug to be selectively absorbed in the intestinal tract. These NPs were also proven to be non-toxic in a mouse fibroblasts model. Efficient biomedical applications could be accordingly envisaged for such an inclusion system [78].

Similar results were obtained for 3TC-CS NPs prepared by ionic gelation of CS with tripolyphosphate anions. These formulations offer several advantages with respect to conventional dosage forms of the drug, particularly in terms of bioavailability [79]. The CS functionalization with glycyrrhizin was realized for a liver targeting and a 3TC controlled release. In fact, the results of this research confirmed a lower drug release and an augmented level of 3TC in hepatocyte tissues, if compared with CS NPs or the free-drug solution [80]. Successively, 3TC was loaded into poly(ε-caprolactone) through a double emulsion spray-drying method giving rise to NPs with spherical morphology. This system also proved to be effective in improving drug bioavailability and reducing side effects [81]. Multiple drugs combined in a single nanosystem showed significant advantages over therapy based on a single drug. Accordingly, an example of polymeric NPs based on methyl methacrylate or ε-caprolactone was designed for the release of four different anti HIV drugs, AZT, 3TC, nevirapine and the IN inhibitor raltegravir [82]. In a recent paper, the incorporation of 3TC into CS with sodium alginate/calcium chloride by the above gelation method, in different experimental conditions, was described and showed an impressive drug release rate lasting up to 24 h. The method proved to furnish highly homogenous particles capable of improve bioavailability together with a constant drug release, following a first order mechanism, with diffusion of the drug after swelling of the polymer [83].

Protein-based NPs were prepared using lactoferrin for the controlled release of 3TC combined with AZT and EFV, after its application for a single DDS. The lactoferrin possesses itself antiviral activity and therefore acts synergistically with the entrapped drugs. The assessment of pharmacokinetic profile for each entrapped drug and *in vitro* data suggested that these NPs are able to release drugs intracellularly in a controlled and sustained manner [84,85].

Alternative nanotechnologies used for anti-HIV drugs release included the use of inorganic components such as iron or silica. Preliminary results suggested a potential application for these new formulations. In particular, chemical-physical characterization of SiO2 NPs coated with magnetic

Fe_2O_3 loaded with 3TC were investigated for their pharmacokinetic and cytotoxic profiles showing more favorable features compared to the free drug [86].

A similar preparation was attempted for 3TC and zalcitabine both in form of triphosphosphates. Preliminary results showed that these nanosystems of dideoxynucleoside triphosphates/SiO2 NPs were useful transport systems for delivering these drugs to target cells with increased antiviral efficiency [87].

Moreover, the co-encapsulation of 3TC and AZT, both in form of triphosphates, into iron carboxylate mesoporous NPs gave biocompatible systems endowed with peculiar delivery properties. In particular, the drugs were released with different kinetics: 3TC showed accelerated release, while AZT was released more slowly. This vector protected drug from degradation, conferring at the same time improved *in vitro* anti-HIV activity. In fact, these formulations contribute to stabilizing the drugs since no alterations were detected after two-month storage and freeze-drying reconstitution [50]. High drug bioavailability and patient compliance were recorded after the administration of the of 3TC encapsulated into a new gum odina based biopolymer obtained by a multiple water-in-oil-in-water emulsion approach. The long-term stability study showed the improvement of the stability of the emulsions after a 90-day storage compared to a similar emulsion comprising Tween 80 as a stabilizer [88]. 3TC was also loaded in nanovesicles based on phospholipids or non-ionic surfactants (niosomes and liposomes). The best components and reparation methods able to produce formulations with suitable size, improved drug encapsulation efficiency and release profile were formulated for these systems [89,90].

3.4. *Abacavir*

Abacavir ((1S,4R)-4-(2-amino-6-(cyclopropylamino)-9H-purin-9-yl)cyclopent-2-en-1-yl)methanol, ABV) introduced in 1998, represented an alternative nucleoside derivative administered orally in solid or solution form for the prevention and treatment of HIV infection. Similarly to other nucleoside analogs, its use is recommended in combination therapy because of its severe side effects like hypersensitivity, liver damage and lactic acidosis, which all preclude monotherapy. ABV and its congener 3TC, after transformation into the corresponding thiol ending ester derivatives, were conjugated to glucose-coated gold NPs, which were investigated for their pH dependent drug release performances. This drug-delivery system was in turn studied for new multifunctional devices since such gold NPs, themselves endowed with microbicide properties, proved useful for the loading of more than one active agent differently targeting the viral replication cycle, and therefore representing a multivalent therapeutic approach [51]. Albumin NPs loaded with ABV sulfate were prepared by solvation method and studied for their mechanism of drug release. Results obtained revealed a remarkable drug loading capacity together with a sustained and controlled release within 24 h in HIV reservoir organs [91]. A myristoylated ABV prodrug entrapped into poloxamers was evaluated for the pharmacokinetic properties after injection in mice. Comparison of such nanoformulation with the free drug was performed on human monocyte-derived macrophages by proton nuclear magnetic resonance studies in terms of anti-HIV activity.

As a result, an efficacy comparable to that of the native drug was detected for the encased polymer, which showed a two-week lasting release [92]. A detailed study described the formation of innovative nanocarriers named ProTide (PROdrug and nucleoTIDE) obtained by the loading of L-alanine and L-phenylalanine ester phosphoramidates of ABV into PLGA and poloxamer NPs. Such formulations showed sustained retention and antiretroviral activities for up to one month [93].

3.5. *Emtricitabine*

Emtricitabine (4-amino-5-fluoro-1-((2S,5R)-2-(hydroxymethyl)-1,3-oxathiolan-5-yl)pyrimidin-2(1H)-one, FTC), is a deoxycytidine nucleoside analog approved in 2006 for anti-HIV therapy. Even if it showed reduced side effects when compared to other NRTIs, FTC is largely used in triple or quadruple drug combinations.

A customary PLGA nanoformulation of this water soluble drug was achieved through the water-in-oil-in-water emulsion method and showed a sustained release profile in rats, with adequate drug concentration up to two weeks [94,95]. The large volume distribution, beside a short plasma half-life, suggests the use of FTC in alternative formulations, such as PLGA NPs. This particular administration form proved to be able in enhancing drug stability and intracellular retention time, as demonstrated by an ex vivo endosomal assay. A once-biweekly dosing for HIV infection prevention or treatment was accordingly hypothesized [96]. In addition, eight degradation products were separated and characterized by LC–MS/MS from ABV sulfate when subjected to forced degradation under hydrolysis, oxidation, photolysis and thermal stressing conditions [97]. More recently, a solution state study showed the formation of eleven degradation products [98].

The thermal decomposition of FTC was well investigated by applying different methods. FTC largely decomposed to small molecules and insoluble substances. A small amount decomposed to 5-fluorocytosine due to an oxidation reaction [99]. When the drug was exposed to the action of acids or bases as well as oxidative stress conditions, an additional degradation product was detected [100].

3.6. *Tenofovir*

Tenofovir disoproxil fumarate ((R)-(((((1-(6-amino-9H-purin-9-yl)propan-2-yl)oxy)methyl) phosphoryl)bis(oxy))bis(methylene) diisopropyl dicarbonate, TDF) is a more recently approved NRTI (2001) used in the treatment of chronic hepatitis B and in the prevention and treatment of HIV infection. Successively its prodrug tenofovir alafenamide fumarate ((isopropyl 2-((((((R)-1-(6-amino-9H-purin-9-yl)propan-2-yl)oxy)methyl)(phenoxy)phosphoryl)amino)propanoate, TAF) was laun-ched in the market due to its more favorable properties after oral administration. TAF has greater antiviral activity and better distribution into lymphoid tissues than TDF. Both drugs are recommended in combination therapy along with other antiretroviral agents.

3.6.1. Tenofovir SLN

Lipid NPs loaded with NRTI and NNRTI agents including TDF or TAF were extensively studied for the improvement of bioavailability and long lasting drug release. Several lipid matrices were designed and showed a very promising behavior under different experimental conditions [37,101,102]. Toxic effects of TDF loaded in nanoemulsions on liver and kidney were assessed using an animal model. Although any behavioral toxicity and mortality were not detected, moderate alterations were however observed on both organs [103]. Extensive chemical-physical studies were performed on hybrid inclusion complexes obtained by encasement of TDF into lipid and polymer matrices by engineered melt emulsification-probe sonication technique. The carrier obtained by combining TDF, lauric acid and pemulen polymer was shown to promote a noteworthy increase of TDF trans-nasal flux, so potentially useful for nasal administration [104]. Nanocarriers based on a hydrogel-core and a lipid-shell were designed for the controlled loading and topical vaginal release of TDF and maraviroc, a virus entry inhibitor. These nanolipogels proved to be efficient systems and robust carriers for the encapsulation and the prolonged *in vivo* release of antiretroviral drugs, showing solubility concerns that are useful during the prevention and treatment of HIV infection [105].

3.6.2. Tenofovir/Dendrimers Complexes

A drug combination including TDF into dendrimers was designed for the evaluation in an *in vitro* model of semen-enhanced viral infection. The results obtained suggested that this therapeutic strategy could bypass the detrimental effects of amyloid fibrils, present in semen, which seem responsible of the failure of topical vaginal gels action [54]. An approach to the treatment of neuro-AIDS was based on the use of co-encapsulated drugs into ultra-small iron oxide NPs with the addition of dextran sulfate. The inclusion complex of TDF and vorinostat, a latency-breaking agent, was assembled by magnetically guided layer-by-layer method and a noteworthy blood–brain barrier transmigration of drugs was then observed. This strategy, aimed to the activation of latent virus and its simultaneous killing, would result in a high efficacy to eradicate completely the infection from the CNS [106]. Nanosystems such as carbosilane dendrimers seem themselves able to inhibit HIV replication with a potential as local antiviral agents. Nevertheless, the concomitant administration of specific antiretroviral agents led to a potent synergistic activity. TDF, along with AZT and EFV or with maraviroc was encapsulated into anionic carbosilane dendrimers, bringing sulfated and naphthyl sulfonated groups to generate potential microbicides to prevent the sexual transmission of HIV [55,107–110]. An innovative therapeutic strategy could be based on the TDF prolonged release from NPs obtained by hyaluronic acid (HA) cross-linked with adipic acid dihydrazide. This nanosystem did not show detectable toxicity under the control of hyaluronidase enzyme. Comparative experiments with a simple TDF/HA gel suggested an essential role of the enzyme during the HA degradation and TDF release. The potential of these formulations for topical delivery of antiviral agents for the prevention of sexually transmitted diseases was accordingly hypothesized [111].

3.6.3. Chitosan based TDF Nanoparticles

TDF was also used as a model drug in a CS based nanopreparation coated with sodium acetate, an aggregation-preventing agent, realized by the freeze-drying method. The NPs cytotoxic profile on macrophages was assessed by neutral red, resazurin, nitrite oxide and cytokines assays. Satisfactory encapsulation rate together with a good stability of the colloidal dispersions was observed for the formulation. Moreover, a sustained drug release beside a lack of cytotoxicity and a pro-inflammatory effect was recorded [112]. Further improvements in terms of mucoadhesive performance were obtained by a formulation based on TDF-loaded CS NPs dispersed in vaginal thermogels [113]. CS based oral NPs loaded with TDF were prepared by the ionic gelation technique and studied for their potential in preventing esterase metabolism and facilitate active transport uptake. Both processes were affected as confirmed by *in vitro* experiments. Moreover, data obtained suggested that a clathrin-mediated mechanism is involved in the enhancement of drug oral absorption [114]. A triple combination of TDF, FTC and bictegravir, an integrase inhibitor, was loaded into trimethyl CS to generate a nanoconjugate with improved cellular uptake. The efficiency of the nanocarrier was determined by spectrophotometry while XTT and ELISA tests were used to determine cytotoxicity and anti-retroviral efficiency, respectively. As a result, this formulation proved to inhibit viral replication at lower concentrations than the free drugs combination, without a significant cytotoxicity, therefore resulting in a lower drug resistance [115]. Colloids based on polyelectrolyte complexes of CS and chondroitin sulfate were loaded with TDF and examined for the stability at physiological conditions. This property was assured by the use of Zn(II) throughout the formulation procedure. *In vitro* studies did not reveal toxicity of such NPs on human peripheral blood mononuclear cells, while a remarkable dose-dependent antiretroviral activity was detected [116]. TDF was loaded into thiolated CS core/shell nanofibers in order to investigate the rate of drug loading, mucoadhesion properties and *in vivo* safety. The formulation was fabricated by assembling poly(ethylene oxide) with the CS component and PLA by a coaxial electrospinning technique. An enhanced drug loading together with a prolonged drug release and an increased mucoadhesion were assessed by in vitro studies, whereas a significant toxicity was not detected in neither *in vitro* nor *in vivo* experimental models. These new formulations could be therefore considered promising tools for the local delivery of microbicide agents [117].

3.6.4. Alternative Polymeric TDF NPs

An original formulation to be used for vaginal administration was fabricated by oil-in-water emulsification of the inclusion product of TFV into PLGA and sodium deoxycholate as an ion-pairing agent and a thermosensitive gel. Sustained release properties in humanized BLT mice were shown for these nanoformulations when instilled locally [118]. Similar results were obtained by loading TFV into PLGA/stearylamine and incorporating such NPs into a hydroxypropyl methylcellulose/PVA-based film [119,120]. TAF and FTC entrapped NPs were prepared for subcutaneous administration during pre-exposure prophylaxis. Drugs were included into the PLGA/PVA system and investigated for their long-acting potency detectable even after 14 days by a humanized mice model [121,122]. A similar approach was exploited for the incorporation of TAF and elvitegravir, an integrase inhibitor, during the fabrication of devices to be used during vaginal prevention [123,124]. The drug absorption following oral administration were also positively affected by the use of TAF/PGLA loaded NPs, as highlighted by a statistical model study [125]. Formulations containing mono- or by-layered films of PVA and pectin were coupled with Eudragit NPs loaded with TDF/FTC, by nano spray-drying technique. These systems were designed for vaginal use with a better patient compliance. The time of disintegration and drug release was evaluated in a simulated vaginal fluid, showing favorable results. The by-layered films equipped with NPs loaded with drugs showed the best performances in terms of drug release delay. Moreover, this topic formulation was shown particularly safe by MTT and lactate dehydrogenase assays using different cervical cell lines [126]. Multifunctional magneto-plasmonic liposomes charged with TDF were obtained with the aim to study guided systems for enhancing efficiency of antiviral treatment. The distribution of such a hybrid system can be monitored by image technique and activated magnetically into the brain. The gold shell of such nanocomplexes can be followed by computed tomography. This way, these particular systems proved to be efficient against HIV in infected microglia cells after adequately crossing the BBB [127]. A nanosuspension of drug combination particles consisting of TDF, ritonavir and lopinavir, two protease inhibitors, and lipids were prepared for the development of innovative topical formulations. This system was highly efficient in targeting lymphocytes during anti-HIV therapy with a long-lasting action after a single subcutaneous administration [128]. Similar results were described after the addition of 3TC to the previously combination to give a four-drug components nanosuspension [129]. Similar results were obtained for alternative combinations of TDF and other RTI. In all cases, a persistent drug concentration was detected after single subcutaneous injection in different HIV reservoir cells [130,131]. A stability study was performed on TAF and compared with the stress degradation behavior of TDF. Gastrointestinal stability studies were conducted on both drugs, showing the formation of six degradation products. These studies revealed a higher stability of TAF, except for with the acid condition, where the drug was extensively degraded [132].

4. Non-Nucleoside Reverse Transcriptase Inhibitors Nanosystems

An alternative approach to anti-HIV treatment with RTIs is represented by the combined therapy using both NRTIs and NNRTIs, exploiting the synergism of the two distinct classes of drugs. Accordingly, the multi-therapy is nowadays the most widely adopted strategy for the treatment of HIV infection in the clinic. NNRTI act directly by binding the enzyme, so preventing its DNA polymerase function. In fact, their heterogeneous structures do not resemble those of nucleobases, the natural substrate of RT (Figure 4, panel c).

After a first generation NNRTI drugs introduced in the 90s (i.e. nevirapine, delavirdine, efavirenz) approved for anti-HIV therapy, recently some new and effective compounds entered the market (i.e. etravirine, rilpivirine). Some more interesting compounds are currently under clinical investigation. The structures of representative NNTRI are reported in Figure 5.

4.1. Nevirapine

Nevirapine (11-cyclopropyl-4-methyl-5H-dipyrido[3,2-b:2′,3′-e][1,4]diazepin-6(11H)-one, NVR) was the first NNRTI approved by FDA in 1996 for the treatment of HIV infection. In order to improve the pharmacokinetics of this hydrophobic drug, NVR was loaded into liposomes prepared by thin film hydration and extrusion method to give uniform spherical vesicles. The matrix, obtained from egg phospholipid and cholesterol, proved to release the drug during 22 h at physiological pH values. The presence of proteins into the medium or the exposition of the system to ultrasounds greatly impair the delivery mode of the drug. However, this encapsulation method could optimize the efficacy of NVR in terms of drug stability and controlled release to the target tissues [30]. Transferrin grafted PLGA NPs have been designed in order to facilitate NVR in crossing vascular endothelial cells of the human brain. This particular nanosystem allowed a favorable drug loading with a desired controlled release, so proving to act as an efficient carrier to promote vascular diffusion of the compound [133]. Nanoparticles of PLA/PEG, the surface of which was modified with serum albumin, were prepared to improve release of the drug to the target tissues. This favorable feature was measured after i.v. injection in rats, showing an improved bioavailability, cellular uptake and drug accumulation in the brain, liver and spleen, compared to pure drug solution or uncoated nanoformulations. Moreover, no additional cytotoxicity was recorded. The capability to cross the BBB makes these formulations potentially useful for the treatment of AIDS related dementia [134,135]. The stability of NVP was well investigated by a stability-indicating ultra-high performance liquid chromatography (UHPLC) method. Drug product efficacy, safety and quality were verified in different degradation conditions by using acids, bases, water, metal ions, heat, light and oxidation agents. The tests were applied on the pure compound and on its tablet formulation leading to the formation of five degradation products [136]. A physically stable formulation of NVP was prepared by forming a crystalline inclusion complex with biodegradable and hydrophobic poly(ε-caprolactone). Compared to pure NVP crystals, the formulation assured a sustained drug release at physiological conditions in PBS solution up to 6 weeks, due to the reduction of drug solubility [43].

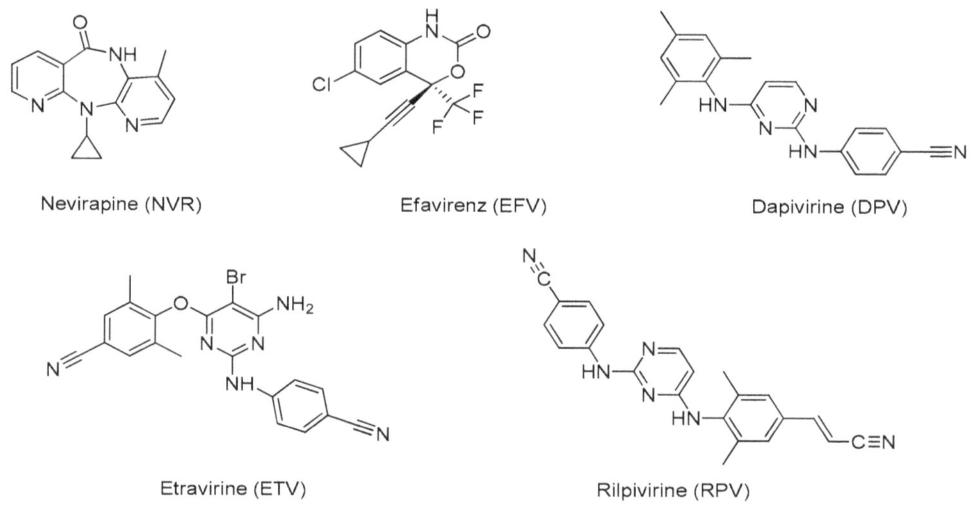

Figure 5. Chemical structures of NNRTI.

4.2. *Efavirenz*

Efavirenz, ((S)-6-chloro-4-(cyclopropylethynyl)-4-(trifluoromethyl)-1H-benzo[d][1,3]oxazin-2(4H)-one, EFV) was approved in 1998 and is largely utilized with other drugs for anti-HIV association therapies. However, its potential was limited by a low bioavailability due to its high lipophilicity and other drawbacks related to irritant effects on mucosae [137,138]. A strategy devoted to the improvement of EFV pharmacokinetics resides in its incorporation into SLN, which should drive the delivery of the drug next to the lymphoid system and brain [38]. Phenylalanine anchored SLN (PA-SLN) were used to encapsulate EFV and the resulting nanocomplex was tested for its potential to cross BBB. Phenylalanine was chosen in order to exploit the aromatic amino acid transporter active within the barrier. The nanocomplex showed good entrapment efficiency and a favorable drug release, with a remarkable accumulation in brain assuring a long-lasting therapeutic effect [139].

4.2.1. Efavirenz SLN

SLN of selected lipids as matrix medium and EFV were prepared with the addition of a surfactant by high-pressure homogenization technique and evaluated *in vivo* for their enhanced bioavailability and brain targeting. In particular, such properties were assessed after an intranasal administration route, which could be useful for therapy devoted to the complete eradication of HIV [39]. As an example, EFV was loaded into SLN assembled with the use of mono- and tri-glycerides with the aid of a surfactant. This particular formulation allowed the drug to partly by-pass liver metabolism after oral administration and in doing so increasing bioavailability and accumulation into spleen [140]. A prolonged drug release together with a lower incidence of side effects, consequent to a reduced drug dosage, was achieved after EFV incorporation into SLN.

4.2.2. Polymeric EFV NPs

Efavirenz was loaded into NPs based on methacrylate polymers, which conferred an increased drug uptake in monocytes and macrophages [141,142]. Emulsion or nanoprecipitation methods allowed loading EFV into biodegradable PLGA NPs. The effects of the resulting formulations administered in combination with other free or encapsulated anti-HIV drugs were investigated. As a result, the new formulations proved more efficient compared to the free drugs and also a noteworthy synergistic effect was recorded for encapsulated EFV combined with TDF, a second NRTI [143]. EFV was dispersed with α-tocopherol polyethylene glycol succinate and PVA by an emulsion-templated freeze-drying technique to realize solid inclusion NPs. Dry monoliths charged with these NPs proved to be stable for several months. Their reconstitution in water furnished nanodispersions, which showed reduced cytotoxicity together with an improved bioavailability and pharmacokinetics [49]. A nanoformulation was obtained by combining EFV with cellulose acetate phthalate, acting as an HIV entry inhibitor, by the nanoprecipitation method. The resulting NPs were formulated into a thermosensitive gel, which resulted in an efficient nanomicrobicide for long-term HIV prophylaxis [144]. Polymeric micelles based on pluronic F127 loaded with EFV and bio-conjugated with anti-M-cell-specific antibodies were prepared in order to evaluate their preferential target delivery to gut micro fold cells of lymphoid tissue, one of the major HIV reservoirs in the body. The efficiency of such nanosystem was showed to be higher than the free drug and a possible oral application by enteric-coated capsule was accordingly hypothesized [145]. EFV was loaded into eudragit, pluronic and alginate sodium polymeric based NPs by solvent evaporation method. Cytotoxicity and antiviral characterization was investigated by syncytium inhibition assay. The polymeric nanocarrier was proven to be more effective than the pure free drug by an enhanced drug dissolution and bio-distribution, especially after BBB crossing. A reduced toxicity was also detected [146,147]. NPs to be used during intranasal administration were prepared by the encasement of EFV into CS grafted hydroxypropyl beta cyclodextrin matrices. The results obtained confirmed a better CNS access due to an improved cellular permeation consequent to both a higher drug solubility and a concomitant beneficial action of CS on cell membrane [148]. Rectal polymeric formulations were prepared by incorporation of EFV into PLGA NPs coated with PEG. This particular form assured a prolonged drug residence in the lower colon with a long lasting prophylactic action against HIV transmission [149]. A better BBB crossing together with a reduction of side effects incidence was attempted by the preparation of transferrin functionalized PLGA NPs loaded with EFV. Although a higher deposition rate of the drug to the targeted site was recorded, the formulation did not improve drug membrane permeation [150]. Lactoferrin NPs were fabricated for oral or vaginal administration giving raise to significant results in terms of drug release and bioavailability. A combination of EFV and curcumin was also attempted in order to reach synergism for the two-microbicide agents. The results obtained confirmed an improved pharmacokinetic profile for the drug combination nanoformulation with respect to free drugs [151,152].

4.2.3. Efavirenz/Dendrimer Complexes

EFV was incorporated into t-Boc–glycine and mannose conjugated dendrimer-based poly(propyleneimine) (PPI). These branched three-dimensional polymers were shown to be less toxic than free PPI and could allow the drug to reach monocytes and macrophages, both reservoirs of HIV in the body. In fact, it is known that inhibitors targeting only lymphocytes are ineffective in completely eradicating the infection. These formulations demonstrated to be particularly effective since they are able to promote a significant increase of EFV cellular uptake [153]. The same authors loaded EFV into dendrimer-based PPI complexed with tuftsin (Tu). This latter is a tetrapeptide coming from the cleavage of immunoglobulin G and showed to be capable of selectively target and activate macrophages, monocytes and polymorph nuclear leukocytes. This strategy would help EFV in avoiding unwanted effects acting in a synergistic fashion with the peptide. Such an option was suggested by the fact that the TuPPI complex showed no toxicity and prolonged EFV cellular uptake in HIV infected macrophages with respect to uninfected cells [154].

4.2.4. Alternative Supramolecular EFV NPs

Vesicular systems consisting of gold NPs entrapped inside the aqueous core were loaded with EFV in the bilayer membrane. The niosomes so formed were dispersed in carrageenan/hyaluronic acid/poloxamer based thermogel after coating with an opportunely functionalized mannose, in order to combine the action of the protein and the sugar for an effective prophylactic vaginal application. A remarkable inhibition of viral transmission as well as a drastic reduction of side effects was recorded [31]. A soya lecithin/cholesterol and PEG liposomal DDS was designed in order to overcome the limited solubility, dissolution rate and bioavailability of EFV [32]. Similar results were achieved by the entrapment of EFV into boron nitride and carbon nanotubes as delivery vehicles. Both the systems showed a favorable behavior. Between the two distinct formulations, carbon nanotubes assured a higher drug adsorption [155]. Enhanced solubility and dissolution of the drug were also obtained by inclusion complex with hydroxypropyl-β-cyclodextrin. The solubility of the complex was further increased by the addition of l-Arginine [156]. Degradation behavior of the drug in water solution was assessed by HPLC analyses, detecting a total twelve degradation products under acidic conditions. Alkaline stress resulted in the formation of only two degradation products, whereas oxidative and photolytic conditions did not promote any degradation of the drug. All the degradation derivatives showed remarkable toxicity, including carcinogenicity, mutagenicity and skin irritation, as confirmed by *in silico* experiments [72]. The thermal behavior of glass EFV was evaluated in different experimental conditions, showing a good stability only at room temperature [157].

4.3. Dapivirine

Dapivirine (4-((4-(mesitylamino)pyrimidin-2-yl)amino)benzonitrile, DPV) is a new, sparingly soluble NNRTI, under investigation for vaginal application during the prevention of HIV sexual transmission. This compound was shown to be a noncompetitive inhibitor of RT that is particularly useful for topic treatments. In order to improve efficacy, a microbicide film for vaginal delivery was formulated by loading DPV into PLGA NPs and the nanosystems were in turn coupled to a PVA in a cellulose based platform film using solvent casting technique. TDF was also added to the formulation to achieve a synergist antiviral effect. A rapid release of active principles was accordingly recorded suggesting an ideal behavior of such a formulation as prophylactic microbicide [158,159]. Some advantages were also obtained by alternative formulations of this drug. In particular, surface-engineered poly(ε-caprolactone) NPs were manufactured and evaluated in pig vaginal and rectal mucosa, resulting in favorable drug release properties [160]. Physical–chemical properties of these nanocarriers were evaluated upon one-year storage to a variable temperature range. Colloidal instability affected the *in vitro* drug release of the NPs, although no detectable degradation was observed for the entrapped drug [56].

4.4. Etravirine

Etravirine (4-((6-amino-5-bromo-2-((4-cyanophenyl)amino)pyrimidin-4-yl)oxy)-3,5-dimethyl-benzonitrile, ETV) is a NNRTI approved in 2008 for monotherapy against HIV, also clinically used in combination with other antiviral agents in antiretroviral treatment-experienced adult patients with onset of resistance. A combination of ETV, maraviroc and raltegravir was loaded into PLGA by emulsion-solvent evaporation technique. The antiviral potency of the resulting NPs was compared to the free triple drug combination in an *in vitro* cells assay and on a macaque cervicovaginal explant model *in vivo*. The nanoformulation provided a prolonged release by extension of the half-life of drugs, leading to an enhanced synergistic antiviral action [161]. An innovative approach for the design of NPs overcoming the drawback, consisting in low drug retention and massive leakage, was undertaken by the preparation of NP-releasing nanofiber vaginal devices. Mucoadhesive PVA fibers coupled to PEGylated NPs should ensure an adequate retention together with a rapid mucus diffusion. These composite nanoformulations proved to assure a sustained ETV release for up to seven days [162].

4.5. Rilpivirine

Rilpivirine ((E)-4-((4-((4-(2-cyanovinyl)-2,6-dimethylphenyl)amino)pyrimidin-2-yl)amino) benzonitrile, RPV) is a second-generation NNRTI, approved in 2011, possessing increased potency, longer half-life and lesser side-effects with respect to former non-nucleoside agents, today mainly used in combination with other anti-HIV drugs [163]. RPV met therapeutic success either in combination with other anti-HIV agents or in long-acting injectable nanoformulations during maintenance therapy. Its use could also be advantageous for the prophylactic treatment of high-risk uninfected individuals [164,165]. In two separate papers, the potential use of long acting RPV NPs associated with cabotegravir, an HIV integrase inhibitor, was described and an innovative monthly dosing therapeutic regimen was accordingly proposed. Recently, the result of a phase IIb study was reported on the effectiveness of this combination nanoformulation in maintaining adequate drug concentration in plasma or vaginal mucus for up to one month [166–168]. RPV-loaded PLGA NPs were fabricated by emulsion-solvent evaporation method. A sustained release in plasma as well as faster clearance were observed in animal models, suggesting a prophylactic use after the preparation of thermosensitive gels as well as long acting injectable nanosuspensions [169].

Biodistribution of tri-modal theranostic NPs was studied by single-photon emission computed tomography, magnetic resonance imaging and fluorescence techniques. These devices were prepared by the incorporation of Indium radiolabeled, europium doped cobalt-ferrite particles and RPV loaded into a poly(ε-caprolactone) matrix included into a lipid shell. A sustained drug release and antiretroviral activity were observed in HIV infected macrophages. These multi-functional NPs represent a platform for the monitoring and optimization of the antiretroviral drug pharmacokinetic profile [170].

5. Conclusions

There is a high level of interest in nanotechnologies for their relevant roles in the design and development of innovative anti-HIV formulations either for oral or topical administration. In the first case, a more specific targeted delivery together with a sustained release represents the major goal in the field. Mucoadhesive performance, prolonged retention time and improved patients' compliance were desired for vaginal or rectal application of microbicide nanoformulated antiretroviral agents. A large number of diversely assembled nanocarriers loaded with different classes of antiviral drugs were then developed and deeply investigated to improve both pharmacokinetic characteristics and stability behavior. Overall results demonstrated a potential success of such an approach for monotherapy, even though more profitable applications were recorded for the combination therapy, the most diffused method nowadays. In fact, anti-HIV therapeutic regimens today comprise multiple daily doses of more drugs acting at different stages of viral replication, which lead to poor patient compliance. Although the use of protease, integrase and viral entry inhibitors has become customary, NRTIs and NNRTIs remain pivotal tools during the infection management. In the light of these findings, this overview focuses mainly on the application of nanotechnology applied to RTI as vehicles for challenging virus eradication from depot organs and/or as a platform for the design of modern prophylactic devices for stable or stressing conditions.

Author Contributions: Conceptualization: F.G., G.I.; Supervision: R.M., A.G.; Writing-original draft preparation: M.A.O., E.M., M.D.L., F.G.; Writing-review and editing: A.G., G.R., F.G., G.I., R.M. All authors agree with the final version of the manuscript. The authors declare that the content of this paper has not been published or submitted for publication elsewhere.

References

1. Vandamme, A.M.; Van Vaerenbergh, K.; De Clercq, E. Anti-human immunodeficiency virus drug combination strategies. *Antivir. Chem. Chemoth.* **1998**, *9*, 187–203. [CrossRef] [PubMed]
2. Lisziewicz, J.; Toke, E.R. Nanomedicine applications towards the cure of HIV. *Nanomed-Nanotechnol.* **2013**, *9*, 28–38. [CrossRef] [PubMed]
3. Bangsberg, D.R.; Hecht, F.M.; Charlebois, E.D.; Zolopa, A.R.; Holodniy, M.; Sheiner, L.; Bamberger, J.D.; Chesney, M.A.; Moss, A. Adherence to protease inhibitors, HIV-1 viral load, and development of drug resistance in an indigent population. *Aids* **2000**, *14*, 357–366. [CrossRef] [PubMed]
4. Schrager, L.K.; D'Souza, M.P. Cellular and anatomical reservoirs of HIV-1 in patients receiving potent antiretroviral combination therapy. *JAMA* **1998**, *280*, 67–71. [CrossRef] [PubMed]
5. Richman, D.D. HIV chemotherapy. *Nature* **2001**, *410*, 995–1001. [CrossRef] [PubMed]
6. Yilmaz, A.; Price, R.W.; Gisslen, M. Antiretroviral drug treatment of CNS HIV-1 infection. *J. Antimicrob. Chemother.* **2012**, *67*, 299–311. [CrossRef]
7. Guidelines for the Use of Antiretroviral Agents in Adults and Adolescents with HIV. Available online: http://aidsinfo.nih.gov/guidelines/html/1/adult-and-adolescent-treatment-guidelines/0 (accessed on 10 April 2019).
8. Rohit, S.; Ramesh, J.; Karan, G.; Raman, K.; Anil, K.S. Nanotechnological interventions in HIV drug delivery and therapeutics. *Biointerface Res. Appl. Chem.* **2014**, *4*, 820–831.
9. Harrigan, P.R.; Hogg, R.S.; Dong, W.W.; Yip, B.; Wynhoven, B.; Woodward, J.; Brumme, C.J.; Brumme, Z.L.; Mo, T.; et al. Predictors of HIV drug-resistance mutations in a large antiretroviral-naive cohort initiating triple antiretroviral therapy. *J. Infect. Dis.* **2005**, *191*, 339–347. [CrossRef] [PubMed]
10. Chun, T.W.; Davey, R.T., Jr.; Engel, D.; Lane, H.C.; Fauci, A.S. Re-emergence of HIV after stopping therapy. *Nature* **1999**, *401*, 874–875. [CrossRef] [PubMed]
11. Marsden, M.D.; Zack, J.A. Eradication of HIV: current challenges and new directions. *J. Antimicrob. Chemother.* **2009**, *63*, 7–10. [CrossRef] [PubMed]
12. Nie, S.; Xing, Y.; Kim, G.J.; Simons, J.W. Nanotechnology applications in cancer. *Annu. Rev. Biomed. Eng.* **2007**, *9*, 257–288. [CrossRef] [PubMed]
13. Mazzuca, P.; Caruso, A.; Caccuri, F. HIV-1 infection, microenvironment and endothelial cell dysfunction. *New. Microbiol.* **2016**, *39*, 163–173. [PubMed]
14. Mahajan, S.D.; Aalinkeel, R.; Law, W.C.; Reynolds, J.L.; Nair, B.B.; Sykes, D.E.; Yong, K.T.; Roy, I.; Prasad, P.N.; Schwartz, S.A. Anti-HIV-1 nanotherapeutics: promises and challenges for the future. *Int. J. Nanomed.* **2012**, *7*, 5301–5314. [CrossRef] [PubMed]
15. Vyas, T.K.; Shah, L.; Amiji, M.M. Nanoparticulate drug carriers for delivery of HIV/AIDS therapy to viral reservoir sites. *Expert Opin. Drug Deliv.* **2006**, *3*, 613–628. [CrossRef]
16. Amiji, M.M.; Vyas, T.K.; Shah, L.K. Role of nanotechnology in HIV/AIDS treatment: potential to overcome the viral reservoir challenge. *Discov. Med.* **2006**, *6*, 157–162.
17. Ferrari, M. Cancer nanotechnology: opportunities and challenges. *Nat. Rev. Cancer* **2005**, *5*, 161–171. [CrossRef] [PubMed]
18. Farokhzad, O.C. Nanotechnology for drug delivery: the perfect partnership. *Expert Opin. Drug Deliv.* **2008**, *5*, 927–929. [CrossRef] [PubMed]
19. Farokhzad, O.C.; Langer, R. Impact of nanotechnology on drug delivery. *ACS Nano* **2009**, *3*, 16–20. [CrossRef] [PubMed]
20. Dunge, A.; Sharda, N.; Singh, B.; Singh, S. Establishment of inherent stability of stavudine and development of a validated stability-indicating HPLC assay method. *J. Pharm. Biomed. Anal.* **2005**, *37*, 1115–1119. [CrossRef] [PubMed]
21. Devrukhakar, P.S.; Shiva Shankar, M.; Shankar, G.; Srinivas, R. A stability-indicating LC-MS/MS method for zidovudine: Identification, characterization and toxicity prediction of two major acid degradation products. *J. Pharm. Biomed. Anal.* **2017**, *7*, 231–236. [CrossRef]
22. Shegokar, R.; Singh, K.K.; Muller, R.H. Production & stability of stavudine solid lipid nanoparticles–from lab to industrial scale. *Int. J. Pharm.* **2011**, *416*, 461–470. [PubMed]
23. Nowacek, A.; Gendelman, H.E. NanoART, neuroAIDS and CNS drug delivery. *Nanomedicine (Lond)* **2009**, *4*, 557–574. [CrossRef] [PubMed]

24. *ICH Q1A(R2)- Stability Testing of New Drug Substances and Products*; International Council for Harmonisation of Technical Requirements for Pharmaceuticals for Human Use (ICH): Geneve, Switzerland, 2003.
25. Tonnesen, H.H. *Photostability of Drugs and Drug Formulations*; CRC Press: New York, NY, USA, 2004.
26. De Luca, M.; Ioele, G.; Spatari, C.; Ragno, G. Photostabilization studies of antihypertensive 1,4-dihydropyridines using polymeric containers. *Int. J. Pharm.* **2016**, *505*, 376–382. [CrossRef] [PubMed]
27. Garg, M.; Asthana, A.; Agashe, H.B.; Agrawal, G.P.; Jain, N.K. Stavudine-loaded mannosylated liposomes: *in-vitro* anti-HIV-I activity, tissue distribution and pharmacokinetics. *J. Pharm. Pharmacol.* **2006**, *58*, 605–616. [CrossRef] [PubMed]
28. Garg, M.; Dutta, T.; Jain, N.K. Reduced hepatic toxicity, enhanced cellular uptake and altered pharmacokinetics of stavudine loaded galactosylated liposomes. *Eur. J. Pharm. Biopharm.* **2007**, *67*, 76–85. [CrossRef]
29. Nayak, D.; Boxi, A.; Ashe, S.; Thathapudi, N.C.; Nayak, B. Stavudine loaded gelatin liposomes for HIV therapy: Preparation, characterization and *in vitro* cytotoxic evaluation. *Mater. Sci. Eng. C Mater. Biol. Appl.* **2017**, *73*, 406–416. [CrossRef] [PubMed]
30. Ramana, L.N.; Sethuraman, S.; Ranga, U.; Krishnan, U.M. Development of a liposomal nanodelivery system for nevirapine. *Int. J. Biomed. Sci.* **2010**, *17*, 57. [CrossRef] [PubMed]
31. Malik, T.; Chauhan, G.; Rath, G.; Kesarkar, R.N.; Chowdhary, A.S.; Goyal, A.K. Efaverinz and nano-gold-loaded mannosylated niosomes: a host cell-targeted topical HIV-1 prophylaxis via thermogel system. *Artif. Cells Nanomed. Biotechnol.* **2018**, *46*, 79–90. [CrossRef] [PubMed]
32. Rao, M.R.P.; Babrekar, L.S. Liposomal Drug Delivery for Solubility and Bioavailability Enhancement of Efavirenz. *Indian J. Pharm. Sci.* **2018**, *80*, 1115–1124.
33. Abdelkader, H.; Alani, A.W.; Alany, R.G. Recent advances in non-ionic surfactant vesicles (niosomes): self-assembly, fabrication, characterization, drug delivery applications and limitations. *Drug Deliv.* **2014**, *21*, 87–100. [CrossRef] [PubMed]
34. Khan, R.; Irchhaiya, R. Niosomes: a potential tool for novel drug delivery. *J. Pharm. Investig.* **2016**, *46*, 195–204. [CrossRef]
35. Naseri, N.; Valizadeh, H.; Zakeri-Milani, P. Solid Lipid Nanoparticles and Nanostructured Lipid Carriers: Structure, Preparation and Application. *Adv. Pharm. Bull.* **2015**, *5*, 305–313. [CrossRef]
36. Joshy, K.S.; Chandra, P.S.; Nandakumar, K.; Sandeep, K.; Sabu, T.; Laly, A.P. Evaluation of *in-vitro* cytotoxicity and cellular uptake efficiency of zidovudine-loaded solid lipid nanoparticles modified with Aloe Vera in glioma cells. *Mater. Sci. Eng. C Mater. Biol. Appl.* **2016**, *66*, 40–50.
37. Freeling, J.P.; Koehn, J.; Shu, C.; Sun, J.; Ho, R.J. Anti-HIV drug-combination nanoparticles enhance plasma drug exposure duration as well as triple-drug combination levels in cells within lymph nodes and blood in primates. *AIDS Res. Hum. Retroviruses* **2015**, *31*, 107–114. [CrossRef] [PubMed]
38. Mishra, N.; Mishra, M.; Padh, H. Formulation Development and Optimization of Efavirenz Loaded SLNs and NLCs using Plackett- Burman Design and its Statistical Elucidation. *Int. J. Pharm. Res. Health Sci.* **2018**, *6*, 2379–2388.
39. Gupta, S.; Kesarla, R.; Chotai, N.; Misra, A.; Omri, A. Systematic Approach for the Formulation and Optimization of Solid Lipid Nanoparticles of Efavirenz by High Pressure Homogenization Using Design of Experiments for Brain Targeting and Enhanced Bioavailability. *Biomed. Res. Int.* **2017**, *2017*, 5984014. [CrossRef] [PubMed]
40. Madhusudhan, A.; Bhagavanth, R.G.; Venkatesham, M.; Veerabhadram, G. Design and Evaluation of Efavirenz loaded Solid Lipid Nanoparticles to Improve the Oral Bioavailability. *Int. J. Pharm. Pharm. Sci.* **2012**, *2*, 84–89.
41. Pardeshi, C.; Rajput, P.; Belgamwar, V.; Tekade, A.; Patil, G.; Chaudhary, K.; Sonje, A. Solid lipid based nanocarriers: an overview. *Acta Pharm.* **2012**, *62*, 433–472. [CrossRef]
42. Date, A.A.; Destache, C.J. A review of nanotechnological approaches for the prophylaxis of HIV/AIDS. *Biomaterials* **2013**, *34*, 6202–6228. [CrossRef]
43. Yang, X.; Yu, B.; Zhong, Z.; Guo, B.H.; Huang, Y. Nevirapine-polycaprolactone crystalline inclusion complex as a potential long-acting injectable solid form. *Int. J. Pharm.* **2018**, *543*, 121–129. [CrossRef] [PubMed]
44. Cao, S.; Woodrow, K.A. Nanotechnology approaches to eradicating HIV reservoirs. *Eur. J. Pharm. Biopharm.* **2018**, *138*, 48–63. [CrossRef] [PubMed]

45. Singh, L.; Kruger, H.G.; Maguire, G.E.M.; Govender, T.; Parboosing, R. The role of nanotechnology in the treatment of viral infections. *Therap. Adv. Infect. Dis.* **2017**, *4*, 105–131. [CrossRef] [PubMed]
46. Parboosing, R.; Maguire, G.E.; Govender, P.; Kruger, H.G. Nanotechnology and the treatment of HIV infection. *Viruses* **2012**, *4*, 488–520. [CrossRef] [PubMed]
47. das Neves, J.; Amiji, M.M.; Bahia, M.F.; Sarmento, B. Nanotechnology-based systems for the treatment and prevention of HIV/AIDS. *Adv. Drug Deliv. Rev.* **2010**, *62*, 458–477. [CrossRef] [PubMed]
48. Patel, B.K.; Parikh, R.H.; Patel, N. Targeted delivery of mannosylated-PLGA nanoparticles of antiretroviral drug to brain. *Int. J. Nanomed.* **2018**, *13*, 97–100. [CrossRef] [PubMed]
49. McDonald, T.O.; Giardiello, M.; Martin, P.; Siccardi, M.; Liptrott, N.J.; Smith, D.; Roberts, P.; Curley, P.; Schipani, A.; Khoo, S.H.; et al. Antiretroviral solid drug nanoparticles with enhanced oral bioavailability: production, characterization, and *in vitro-in vivo* correlation. *Adv. Healthc. Mater.* **2014**, *3*, 400–411. [CrossRef] [PubMed]
50. Marcos-Almaraz, M.T.; Gref, R.; Agostoni, V.; Kreuz, C.; Clayette, P.; Serre, C.; Couvreurb, P.; Horcajada, P. Towards improved HIV-microbicide activity through the co-encapsulation of NRTI drugs in biocompatible metal organic framework nanocarriers. *J. Mater. Chem. B* **2017**, *5*, 8563–8569. [CrossRef]
51. Chiodo, F.; Marradi, M.; Calvo, J.; Yuste, E.; Penades, S. Glycosystems in nanotechnology: Gold glyconanoparticles as carrier for anti-HIV prodrugs. *Beilstein J. Org. Chem.* **2014**, *10*, 1339–1346. [CrossRef]
52. Peng, J.; Wu, Z.; Qi, X.; Chen, Y.; Li, X. Dendrimers as potential therapeutic tools in HIV inhibition. *Molecules* **2013**, *18*, 7912–7929. [CrossRef]
53. Ionov, M.; Ciepluch, K.; Klajnert, B.; Glinska, S.; Gomez-Ramirez, R.; de la Mata, F.J.; Munoz-Fernandez, M.A.; Bryszewska, M. Complexation of HIV derived peptides with carbosilane dendrimers. *Colloids Surf. B Biointerfaces* **2013**, *101*, 236–242. [CrossRef]
54. Garcia-Broncano, P.; Cena-Diez, R.; de la Mata, F.J.; Gomez, R.; Resino, S.; Munoz-Fernandez, M.A. Efficacy of carbosilane dendrimers with an antiretroviral combination against HIV-1 in the presence of semen-derived enhancer of viral infection. *Eur. J. Pharmacol.* **2017**, *811*, 155–163. [CrossRef] [PubMed]
55. Cena-Diez, R.; Vacas-Cordoba, E.; Garcia-Broncano, P.; de la Mata, F.J.; Gomez, R.; Maly, M.; Munoz-Fernandez, M.A. Prevention of vaginal and rectal herpes simplex virus type 2 transmission in mice: mechanism of antiviral action. *Int. J. Nanomed.* **2016**, *11*, 2147–2162. [PubMed]
56. das Neves, J.; Amiji, M.; Bahia, M.F.; Sarmento, B. Assessing the physical-chemical properties and stability of dapivirine-loaded polymeric nanoparticles. *Int. J. Pharm.* **2013**, *456*, 307–314. [CrossRef] [PubMed]
57. Nucleoside Reverse Transcriptase Inhibitors (NRTIs or nukes). Available online: https://www.hiv.va.gov/patient/treat/nrtis.asp (accessed on 10 April 2019).
58. Shegokar, R.; Singh, K.K. Stavudine entrapped lipid nanoparticles for targeting lymphatic HIV reservoirs. *Pharmazie* **2011**, *66*, 264–271. [PubMed]
59. Kaur, C.D.; Nahar, M.; Jain, N.K. Lymphatic targeting of zidovudine using surface-engineered liposomes. *J. Drug Target* **2008**, *16*, 798–805. [CrossRef] [PubMed]
60. Weibull, W. A statistical distribution function of wide applicability. *J. Appl. Mech.* **1951**, *18*, 293–297.
61. Carvalho, F.C.; Sarmento, V.H.; Chiavacci, L.A.; Barbi, M.S.; Gremiao, M.P. Development and *in vitro* evaluation of surfactant systems for controlled release of zidovudine. *J. Appl. Mech.* **2010**, *99*, 2367–2374. [CrossRef]
62. Mainardes, R.M.; Gremiao, M.P.; Brunetti, I.L.; da Fonseca, L.M.; Khalil, N.M. Zidovudine-loaded PLA and PLA-PEG blend nanoparticles: influence of polymer type on phagocytic uptake by polymorphonuclear cells. *J. Pharm. Sci.* **2009**, *98*, 257–267. [CrossRef] [PubMed]
63. Mainardes, R.M.; Gremiao, M.P. Nanoencapsulation and characterization of zidovudine on poly(L-lactide) and poly(L -lactide)-poly(ethylene glycol)-blend nanoparticles. *J. Nanosci. Nanotechnol.* **2012**, *12*, 8513–8521. [CrossRef] [PubMed]
64. Joshy, K.S.; Susan, M.A.; Snigdha, S.; Nandakumar, K.; Laly, A.P.; Sabu, T. Encapsulation of zidovudine in PF-68 coated alginate conjugate nanoparticles for anti-HIV drug delivery. *Int. J. Biol. Macromol.* **2018**, *107*, 929–937. [CrossRef] [PubMed]
65. Dunge, A.; Sharda, N.; Singh, B.; Singh, S. Validated specific HPLC method for determination of zidovudine during stability studies. *J. Pharm. Biomed. Anal.* **2005**, *37*, 1109–1114. [CrossRef]

66. Schenfeld, E.M.; Ribone, S.R.; Quevedo, M.A. Stability and plasmatic protein binding of novel zidovudine prodrugs: Targeting site ii of human serum albumin. *Eur. J. Pharm. Sci.* **2018**, *115*, 109–118. [CrossRef] [PubMed]
67. Perry, C.M.; Faulds, D. Lamivudine. A review of its antiviral activity, pharmacokinetic properties and therapeutic efficacy in the management of HIV infection. *Drugs* **1997**, *53*, 657–680. [CrossRef]
68. Vogenthaler, N.S. Lamivudine and second-line antiretroviral regimens. *Clin. Infect. Dis.* **2007**, *44*, 1387. [CrossRef] [PubMed]
69. Vinogradov, S.V.; Poluektova, L.Y.; Makarov, E.; Gerson, T.; Senanayake, M.T. Nano-NRTIs: efficient inhibitors of HIV type-1 in macrophages with a reduced mitochondrial toxicity. *Antivir. Chem. Chemother.* **2010**, *21*, 1–14. [CrossRef] [PubMed]
70. Bedse, G.; Kumar, V.; Singh, S. Study of forced decomposition behavior of lamivudine using LC, LC-MS/TOF and MS(n). *J. Pharm. Biomed. Anal.* **2009**, *49*, 55–63. [CrossRef]
71. Konari, N.S.; Jacob, J.T. Stability indicating validated UPLC technique for the simultaneous analysis of raltegravir and lamivudine in pharmaceutical dosage forms. *HIV AIDS Rev.* **2016**, *15*, 161–169. [CrossRef]
72. Kurmi, M.; Sahu, A.; Singh, D.K.; Singh, I.P.; Singh, S. Stability behaviour of antiretroviral drugs and their combinations. 8: Characterization and in-silico toxicity prediction of degradation products of efavirenz. *J. Pharm. Biomed. Anal.* **2018**, *148*, 170–181. [CrossRef] [PubMed]
73. Tamizhrasi, S.; Shukla, A.; Shivkumar, T.; Rathi, V.; Rathi, J.C. Formulation and evaluation of lamivudine loaded polymethacrylic acid nanoparticles. *Int. J. Pharmtech Res.* **2009**, *1*, 411–415.
74. Bing, W.; Guan Qun, C.; Zheng Wei, M.; Yu Ying, Z.; Da Hai, Y.; Chang You, G. Preparation and cellular uptake of PLGA particles loaded with lamivudine. *Chin. Sci. Bull.* **2012**, *57*, 3985–3993.
75. Rajca, A.; Li, Q.; Date, A.; Belshan, M.; Destache, C. Thermosensitive Vaginal Gel Containing PLGA-NRTI conjugated nanoparticles for HIV prophylaxis. *NSTI-Nanotech* **2013**, *3*, 293–296.
76. Ramadan, E. Transdermal microneedle–mediated delivery of polymeric lamivudine loaded nanoparticles. *J. Pharm. Technol. Drug Res.* **2016**, 5. [CrossRef]
77. Hatami, E.; Mu, Y.; Shields, D.N.; Chauhan, S.C.; Kumar, S.; Cory, T.J.; Yallapu, M.M. Mannose-decorated hybrid nanoparticles for enhanced macrophage targeting. *Biochem. Biophys. Rep.* **2019**, *17*, 197–207. [CrossRef]
78. Dev, A.; Binulal, N.S.; Anitha, A.; Nair, S.V.; Furuike, T.; Tamura, H.; Jayakumar, R. Preparation of poly(lactic acid)/chitosan nanoparticles for anti-HIV drug delivery applications. *Carbohydr. Polym.* **2010**, *80*, 833–838. [CrossRef]
79. Nesalin, J.A.J.; Smith, A.A. Stability study of chitosan nanoparticles containing some antiretroviral drugs. *Res. J. Pharm. Biol. Chem. Sci.* **2014**, *5*, 193–203.
80. Deepak, M.; Nivrati, J.; Vaibhav, R.; Ashish, K.J. Glycyrrhizin conjugated chitosan nanoparticles for hepatocyte-targeted delivery of lamivudine. *J. Pharm. Pharmacol.* **2014**, *66*, 1082–1093.
81. Tshweu, L.; Katata, L.; Kalombo, L.; Swai, H. Nanoencapsulation of water-soluble drug, lamivudine, using a double emulsion spray-drying technique for improving HIV treatment. *J. Nanopart. Res.* **2013**, *15*. [CrossRef]
82. Oluwaseun, O.; Namita, K.; Kahli, A.S.; Oleg, B.; Simeon, A.; Ayele, G.; Winston, A.A.; Sergei, N.; Emmanuel, O.A. Antiretroviral Drugs-Loaded Nanoparticles Fabricated by Dispersion Polymerization with Potential for HIV/AIDS Treatment. *Inf. Dis. Res. Treat.* **2016**, *9*, 21–32.
83. Pravalika, R.P.; Madhava, R.B.; Prakash, D.J.; Latha, K.; Prashanthi, D. Formulation and characterisation of chitosan based lamivudine nanoparticles. *Eur. J. Pharm. Med. Res.* **2017**, *4*, 377–383.
84. Kumar, P.; Lakshmi, Y.S.; C, B.; Golla, K.; Kondapi, A.K. Improved Safety, Bioavailability and Pharmacokinetics of Zidovudine through Lactoferrin Nanoparticles during Oral Administration in Rats. *PLoS ONE* **2015**, *10*, e0140399. [CrossRef]
85. Kumar, P.; Lakshmi, Y.S.; Kondapi, A.K. Triple Drug Combination of Zidovudine, Efavirenz and Lamivudine Loaded Lactoferrin Nanoparticles: an Effective Nano First-Line Regimen for HIV Therapy. *Pharm. Res.* **2017**, *34*, 257–268. [CrossRef] [PubMed]
86. Shahabadia, N.; Khorshidia, A.; Zhalehc, H.; Kashaniand, S. Synthesis, characterization, cytotoxicity and DNA binding studies of Fe3O4@ SiO2 nanoparticles coated by an antiviral drug lamivudine. *J. Drug Deliv. Sci. Technol.* **2018**, *46*, 55–65. [CrossRef]

87. Vasilyeva, S.V.; Shtil, A.A.; Petrova, A.S.; Balakhnin, S.M.; Achigecheva, P.Y.; Stetsenko, D.A.; Silnikov, V.N. Conjugates of phosphorylated zalcitabine and lamivudine with SiO2 nanoparticles: Synthesis by CuAAC click chemistry and preliminary assessment of anti-HIV and antiproliferative activity. *Bioorg. Med. Chem.* **2017**, *25*, 1696–1702. [CrossRef] [PubMed]
88. Kumar, J.A.; Kumar, A.N.; Arnab, D.; Debmalya, M.; Amalesh, S. Development of lamivudine containing multiple emulsions stabilizedby gum odina. *Future J. Pharm. Sci.* **2018**, *4*, 71–79.
89. Suma, U.S.; Parthiban, S.; Senthil, K.G.P.; Tamiz, M.T. Effect of span-80 in the formulation lamivudine niosomal gel. *Asian J. Res. Biol. Pharm. Sci.* **2015**, *4*, 35–45.
90. Godbole, M.D.; Mathur, V. Selection of phospholipid and method of formulation for optimum entrapment and release of lamivudine from liposome. *J. Drug Deliv. Ther.* **2018**, *8*, 175–183. [CrossRef]
91. Wilson, B.; Paladugu, L.; Priyadarshini, S.R.; Jenita, J.J. Development of albumin-based nanoparticles for the delivery of abacavir. *Int. J. Biol. Macromol.* **2015**, *81*, 763–767. [CrossRef] [PubMed]
92. Corbo, C.; Molinaro, R.; Parodi, A.; Toledano Furman, N.E.; Salvatore, F.; Tasciotti, E. The impact of nanoparticle protein corona on cytotoxicity, immunotoxicity and target drug delivery. *Nanomedicine (Lond.)* **2016**, *11*, 81–100. [CrossRef]
93. Lin, Z.; Gautam, N.; Alnouti, Y.; McMillan, J.; Bade, A.N.; Gendelman, H.E.; Edagwa, B. ProTide generated long-acting abacavir nanoformulations. *Chem. Commun.* **2018**, *54*, 8371–8374. [CrossRef]
94. Singh, G.; Pai, R.S. Pharmacokinetics and *in vivo* biodistribution of optimized PLGA nanoparticulate drug delivery system for controlled release of emtricitabine. *Drug Deliv.* **2014**, *21*, 627–635. [CrossRef] [PubMed]
95. Singh, G.; Pai, R.S. Optimization (central composite design) and validation of HPLC method for investigation of emtricitabine loaded poly(lactic-*co*-glycolic acid) nanoparticles: *in vitro* drug release and *in vivo* pharmacokinetic studies. *Sci. World J.* **2014**, *2014*, 583090. [CrossRef] [PubMed]
96. Mandal, S.; Belshan, M.; Holec, A.; Zhou, Y.; Destache, C.J. An Enhanced Emtricitabine-Loaded Long-Acting Nanoformulation for Prevention or Treatment of HIV Infection. *Antimicrob. Agents Chemother.* **2017**, 61. [CrossRef]
97. Rao, R.N.; Vali, R.M.; Ramachandra, B.; Raju, S.S. Separation and characterization of forced degradation products of abacavir sulphate by LC-MS/MS. *J. Pharm. Biomed. Anal.* **2011**, *54*, 279–285. [CrossRef] [PubMed]
98. Kurmi, M.; Sahu, A.; Singh, S. Stability behaviour of antiretroviral drugs and their combinations. 5: Characterization of novel degradation products of abacavir sulfate by mass and nuclear magnetic resonance spectrometry. *J. Pharm. Biomed. Anal.* **2017**, *134*, 372–384. [CrossRef] [PubMed]
99. Wang, X.J.; Youa, J.; Yub, F. Study on the thermal decomposition of emtricitabine. *J. Anal. Appl. Pyrolysis* **2015**, *115*, 344–352. [CrossRef]
100. Kurmi, M.; Singh, S. Stability behavior of antiretroviral drugs and their combinations. 7: Comparative degradation pathways of lamivudine and emtricitabine and explanation to their differential degradation behavior by density functional theory. *J.Pharm. Biomed. Anal.* **2017**, *142*, 155–161. [CrossRef]
101. Duan, J.; Freeling, J.P.; Koehn, J.; Shu, C.; Ho, R.J. Evaluation of atazanavir and darunavir interactions with lipids for developing pH-responsive anti-HIV drug combination nanoparticles. *J. Pharm. Sci.* **2014**, *103*, 2520–2529. [CrossRef] [PubMed]
102. Freeling, J.P.; Koehn, J.; Shu, C.; Sun, J.; Ho, R.J. Long-acting three-drug combination anti-HIV nanoparticles enhance drug exposure in primate plasma and cells within lymph nodes and blood. *Aids* **2014**, *28*, 2625–2627. [CrossRef] [PubMed]
103. Peter, A.I.; Naidu, E.C.; Akang, E.; Ogedengbe, O.O.; Offor, U.; Rambharose, S.; Kalhapure, R.; Chuturgoon, A.; Govender, T.; Azu, O.O. Investigating Organ Toxicity Profile of Tenofovir and Tenofovir Nanoparticle on the Liver and Kidney: Experimental Animal Study. *Toxicol. Res.* **2018**, *34*, 221–229. [CrossRef] [PubMed]
104. Pokharkar, V.B.; Jolly, M.R.; Kumbhar, D.D. Engineering of a hybrid polymer-lipid nanocarrier for the nasal delivery of tenofovir disoproxil fumarate: physicochemical, molecular, microstructural, and stability evaluation. *Eur. J. Pharm. Sci.* **2015**, *71*, 99–111. [CrossRef]
105. Ramanathan, R.; Jiang, Y.; Read, B.; Golan-Paz, S.; Woodrow, K.A. Biophysical characterization of small molecule antiviral-loaded nanolipogels for HIV-1 chemoprophylaxis and topical mucosal application. *Acta Biomater.* **2016**, *36*, 122–131. [CrossRef] [PubMed]
106. Jayant, R.D.; Atluri, V.S.; Agudelo, M.; Sagar, V.; Kaushik, A.; Nair, M. Sustained-release nanoART formulation for the treatment of neuroAIDS. *Int. J. Nanomed.* **2015**, *10*, 1077–1093. [CrossRef]

107. Vacas-Cordoba, E.; Galan, M.; de la Mata, F.J.; Gomez, R.; Pion, M.; Munoz-Fernandez, M.A. Enhanced activity of carbosilane dendrimers against HIV when combined with reverse transcriptase inhibitor drugs: searching for more potent microbicides. *Int. J. Nanomed.* **2014**, *9*, 3591–3600.
108. Briz, V.; Sepulveda-Crespo, D.; Diniz, A.R.; Borrego, P.; Rodes, B.; de la Mata, F.J.; Gomez, R.; Taveira, N.; Munoz-Fernandez, M.A. Development of water-soluble polyanionic carbosilane dendrimers as novel and highly potent topical anti-HIV-2 microbicides. *Nanoscale* **2015**, *7*, 14669–14683. [CrossRef]
109. Sepulveda-Crespo, D.; Sanchez-Rodriguez, J.; Serramia, M.J.; Gomez, R.; De La Mata, F.J.; Jimenez, J.L.; Munoz-Fernandez, M.A. Triple combination of carbosilane dendrimers, tenofovir and maraviroc as potential microbicide to prevent HIV-1 sexual transmission. *Nanomedicine (Lond)* **2015**, *10*, 899–914. [CrossRef]
110. Sepulveda-Crespo, D.; Gomez, R.; De La Mata, F.J.; Jimenez, J.L.; Munoz-Fernandez, M.A. Polyanionic carbosilane dendrimer-conjugated antiviral drugs as efficient microbicides: Recent trends and developments in HIV treatment/therapy. *Nanomed.- Nanotechnol. Biol. Med.* **2015**, *11*, 1481–1498. [CrossRef] [PubMed]
111. Agrahari, V.; Zhang, C.; Zhang, T.; Li, W.; Gounev, T.K.; Oyler, N.A.; Youan, B.B. Hyaluronidase-sensitive nanoparticle templates for triggered release of HIV/AIDS microbicide *in vitro*. *AAPS J.* **2014**, *16*, 181–193. [CrossRef]
112. Ngo, A.N.; Ezoulin, M.J.; Murowchick, J.B.; Gounev, A.D.; Youan, B.B. Sodium Acetate Coated Tenofovir-Loaded Chitosan Nanoparticles for Improved Physico-Chemical Properties. *Pharm. Res.* **2016**, *33*, 367–383. [CrossRef]
113. Timur, S.S.; Sahin, A.; Aytekin, E.; Ozturk, N.; Polat, K.H.; Tezel, N.; Gursoy, R.N.; Calis, S. Design and *in vitro* evaluation of tenofovir-loaded vaginal gels for the prevention of HIV infections. *Pharm. Dev. Technol.* **2018**, *23*, 301–310. [CrossRef] [PubMed]
114. Shailender, J.; Ravi, P.R.; Reddy Sirukuri, M.; Dalvi, A.; Keerthi Priya, O. Chitosan nanoparticles for the oral delivery of tenofovir disoproxil fumarate: formulation optimization, characterization and ex vivo and *in vivo* evaluation for uptake mechanism in rats. *Drug Dev. Ind. Pharm.* **2018**, *44*, 1109–1119. [CrossRef]
115. Shohani, S.; Mondanizadeh, M.; Abdoli, A.; Khansarinejad, B.; Salimi-Asl, M.; Ardestani, M.S.; Ghanbari, M.; Haj, M.S.; Zabihollahi, R. Trimethyl Chitosan Improves Anti-HIV Effects of Atripla as a New Nanoformulated Drug. *Curr. HIV Res.* **2017**, *15*, 56–65. [CrossRef] [PubMed]
116. Wu, D.; Ensinas, A.; Verrier, B.; Primard, C.; Cuvillier, A.; Champier, G.; Paul, S.; Delair, T. Zinc-Stabilized Chitosan-Chondroitin Sulfate Nanocomplexes for HIV-1 Infection Inhibition Application. *Mol. Pharm.* **2016**, *13*, 3279–3291. [CrossRef] [PubMed]
117. Meng, J.; Agrahari, V.; Ezoulin, M.J.; Zhang, C.; Purohit, S.S.; Molteni, A.; Dim, D.; Oyler, N.A.; Youan, B.C. Tenofovir Containing Thiolated Chitosan Core/Shell Nanofibers: *In Vitro* and *in Vivo* Evaluations. *Mol. Pharm.* **2016**, *13*, 4129–4140. [CrossRef] [PubMed]
118. Destache, C.J.; Mandal, S.; Yuan, Z.; Kang, G.; Date, A.A.; Lu, W.; Shibata, A.; Pham, R.; Bruck, P.; Rezich, M.; et al. Topical Tenofovir Disoproxil Fumarate Nanoparticles Prevent HIV-1 Vaginal Transmission in a Humanized Mouse Model. *Antimicrob. Agents Chemother.* **2016**, *60*, 3633–3639. [CrossRef] [PubMed]
119. Machado, A.; Cunha-Reis, C.; Araujo, F.; Nunes, R.; Seabra, V.; Ferreira, D.; das Neves, J.; Sarmento, B. Development and *in vivo* safety assessment of tenofovir-loaded nanoparticles-in-film as a novel vaginal microbicide delivery system. *Acta Biomater.* **2016**, *44*, 332–340. [CrossRef]
120. Cunha-Reis, C.; Machado, A.; Barreiros, L.; Araujo, F.; Nunes, R.; Seabra, V.; Ferreira, D.; Segundo, M.A.; Sarmento, B.; das Neves, J. Nanoparticles-in-film for the combined vaginal delivery of anti-HIV microbicide drugs. *J. Control. Release* **2016**, *243*, 43–53. [CrossRef] [PubMed]
121. Mandal, S.; Kang, G.; Prathipati, P.K.; Fan, W.; Li, Q.; Destache, C.J. Long-acting parenteral combination antiretroviral loaded nano-drug delivery system to treat chronic HIV-1 infection: A humanized mouse model study. *Antiviral Res.* **2018**, *156*, 85–91. [CrossRef] [PubMed]
122. Mandal, S.; Kang, G.; Prathipati, P.K.; Zhou, Y.; Fan, W.; Li, Q.; Destache, C.J. Nanoencapsulation introduces long-acting phenomenon to tenofovir alafenamide and emtricitabine drug combination: A comparative pre-exposure prophylaxis efficacy study against HIV-1 vaginal transmission. *J. Control. Release* **2019**, *294*, 216–225. [CrossRef] [PubMed]
123. Mandal, S.; Prathipati, P.K.; Kang, G.; Zhou, Y.; Yuan, Z.; Fan, W.; Li, Q.; Destache, C.J. Tenofovir alafenamide and elvitegravir loaded nanoparticles for long-acting prevention of HIV-1 vaginal transmission. *Aids* **2017**, *31*, 469–476. [CrossRef]

124. Prathipati, P.K.; Mandal, S.; Pon, G.; Vivekanandan, R.; Destache, C.J. Pharmacokinetic and Tissue Distribution Profile of Long Acting Tenofovir Alafenamide and Elvitegravir Loaded Nanoparticles in Humanized Mice Model. *Pharm. Res.* **2017**, *34*, 2749–2755. [CrossRef] [PubMed]
125. Shailender, J.; Ravi, P.R.; Saha, P.; Dalvi, A.; Myneni, S. Tenofovir disoproxil fumarate loaded PLGA nanoparticles for enhanced oral absorption: Effect of experimental variables and *in vitro*, *ex vivo* and *in vivo* evaluation. *Colloids Surf. B Biointerfaces* **2017**, *158*, 610–619. [CrossRef] [PubMed]
126. Cautela, M.P.; Moshe, H.; Sosnik, A.; Sarmento, B.; das Neves, J. Composite films for vaginal delivery of tenofovir disoproxil fumarate and emtricitabine. *Eur. J. Pharm. Biopharm.* **2018**, *138*, 3–10. [CrossRef] [PubMed]
127. Tomitaka, A.; Arami, H.; Huang, Z.; Raymond, A.; Rodriguez, E.; Cai, Y.; Febo, M.; Takemura, Y.; Nair, M. Hybrid magneto-plasmonic liposomes for multimodal image-guided and brain-targeted HIV treatment. *Nanoscale* **2017**, *10*, 184–194. [CrossRef]
128. Kraft, J.C.; McConnachie, L.A.; Koehn, J.; Kinman, L.; Sun, J.; Collier, A.C.; Collins, C.; Shen, D.D.; Ho, R.J.Y. Mechanism-based pharmacokinetic (MBPK) models describe the complex plasma kinetics of three antiretrovirals delivered by a long-acting anti-HIV drug combination nanoparticle formulation. *J. Control. Release* **2018**, *275*, 229–241. [CrossRef]
129. McConnachie, L.A.; Kinman, L.M.; Koehn, J.; Kraft, J.C.; Lane, S.; Lee, W.; Collier, A.C.; Ho, R.J.Y. Long-Acting Profile of 4 Drugs in 1 Anti-HIV Nanosuspension in Nonhuman Primates for 5 Weeks After a Single Subcutaneous Injection. *J. Pharm. Sci.* **2018**, *107*, 1787–1790. [CrossRef]
130. Koehn, J.; Iwamoto, J.F.; Kraft, J.C.; McConnachie, L.A.; Collier, A.C.; Ho, R.J.Y. Extended cell and plasma drug levels after one dose of a three-in-one nanosuspension containing lopinavir, efavirenz, and tenofovir in nonhuman primates. *Aids* **2018**, *32*, 2463–2467. [PubMed]
131. Perazzolo, S.; Shireman, L.M.; Koehn, J.; McConnachie, L.A.; Kraft, J.C.; Shen, D.D.; Ho, R.J.Y. Three HIV Drugs, Atazanavir, Ritonavir, and Tenofovir, Coformulated in Drug-Combination Nanoparticles Exhibit Long-Acting and Lymphocyte-Targeting Properties in Nonhuman Primates. *J. Pharm. Sci.* **2018**, *107*, 3153–3162. [CrossRef] [PubMed]
132. Golla, V.M.; Kurmi, M.; Shaik, K.; Singh, S. Stability behaviour of antiretroviral drugs and their combinations. 4: Characterization of degradation products of tenofovir alafenamide fumarate and comparison of its degradation and stability behaviour with tenofovir disoproxil fumarate. *J. Pharm. Biomed. Anal.* **2016**, *131*, 146–155. [CrossRef] [PubMed]
133. Kuo, Y.C.; Lin, P.I.; Wang, C.C. Targeting nevirapine delivery across human brain microvascular endothelial cells using transferrin-grafted poly(lactide-co-glycolide) nanoparticles. *Nanomedicine (Lond)* **2011**, *6*, 1011–1026. [CrossRef] [PubMed]
134. Shegokar, R.; Singh, K.K. Nevirapine nanosuspensions for HIV reservoir targeting. *Die Pharmazie* **2011**, *66*, 408–415.
135. Shegokar, R.; Singh, K.K. Surface modified nevirapine nanosuspensions for viral reservoir targeting: *In vitro* and *in vivo* evaluation. *Int. J. Pharm.* **2011**, *421*, 341–352. [CrossRef] [PubMed]
136. Reis, N.F.; de Assis, J.C.; Fialho, S.L.; Pianetti, G.A.; Fernandes, C. Stability-indicating UHPLC method for determination of nevirapine in its bulk form and tablets: identification of impurities and degradation kinetic study. *J. Pharm. Biomed. Anal.* **2016**, *126*, 103–108. [CrossRef]
137. Aungst, B.J.; Nguyen, N.H.; Taylor, N.J.; Bindra, D.S. Formulation and food effects on the oral absorption of a poorly water soluble, highly permeable antiretroviral agent. *J. Pharm. Sci.* **2002**, *91*, 1390–1395. [CrossRef] [PubMed]
138. Csajka, C.; Marzolini, C.; Fattinger, K.; Decosterd, L.A.; Fellay, J.; Telenti, A.; Biollaz, J.; Buclin, T. Population pharmacokinetics and effects of efavirenz in patients with human immunodeficiency virus infection. *Clin. Pharmacol. Ther.* **2003**, *73*, 20–30. [CrossRef]
139. Vyas, A.; Jain, A.; Hurkat, P.; Jain, A.; Jain, S.K. Targeting of AIDS related encephalopathy using phenylalanine anchored lipidic nanocarrier. *Colloids Surf. B Biointerfaces* **2015**, *131*, 155–161. [CrossRef]
140. Makwana, V.; Jain, R.; Patel, K.; Nivsarkar, M.; Joshi, A. Solid lipid nanoparticles (SLN) of Efavirenz as lymph targeting drug delivery system: Elucidation of mechanism of uptake using chylomicron flow blocking approach. *Int. J. Pharm.* **2015**, *495*, 439–446. [CrossRef] [PubMed]

141. Gaur, P.K.; Mishra, S.; Bajpai, M.; Mishra, A. Enhanced Oral Bioavailability of Efavirenz by Solid Lipid Nanoparticles: In Vitro Drug Release and Pharmacokinetics Studies. *BioMed Res. Int.* **2014**, *2014*, 363404. [CrossRef]
142. Vedha Hari, B.N.; Dhevendaran, K.; Narayanan, N. Development of Efavirenz nanoparticle for enhanced efficiency of anti-retroviral therapy against HIV and AIDS. In Proceedings of the First International Science Symposium on HIV and Infectious Diseases (HIV SCIENCE 2012), Chennai, India, 20–22 January 2012; Springer-Verlag GmbH: Heidelberg, Germany, 2012.
143. Chaowanachan, T.; Krogstad, E.; Ball, C.; Woodrow, K.A. Drug synergy of tenofovir and nanoparticle-based antiretrovirals for HIV prophylaxis. *PLoS ONE* **2013**, *8*, e61416. [CrossRef]
144. Date, A.A.; Shibata, A.; McMullen, E.; La Bruzzo, K.; Bruck, P.; Belshan, M.; Zhou, Y.; Destache, C.J. Thermosensitive Gel Containing Cellulose Acetate Phthalate-Efavirenz Combination Nanoparticles for Prevention of HIV-1 Infection. *J. Biomed. Nanotechnol.* **2015**, *11*, 416–427. [CrossRef]
145. Roy, U.; Ding, H.; Pilakka-Kanthikeel, S.; Raymond, A.D.; Atluri, V.; Yndart, A.; Kaftanovskaya, E.M.; Batrakova, E.; Agudelo, M.; Nair, M. Preparation and characterization of anti-HIV nanodrug targeted to microfold cell of gut-associated lymphoid tissue. *Int. J. Nanomed.* **2015**, *10*, 5819–5835. [CrossRef] [PubMed]
146. Haria, V.B.N.; Lu, C.L.; Narayananc, N.; Wang, R.R.; Zheng, Y.T. Engineered polymeric nanoparticles of Efavirenz: Dissolution enhancement through particle size reduction. *Chem. Eng. Sci.* **2016**, *155*, 366–375. [CrossRef]
147. Hari, B.N.V.; Narayanan, N.; Dhevendaran, K.; Ramyadevi, D. Engineered nanoparticles of Efavirenz using methacrylate co-polymer (Eudragit-E100) and its biological effects in-vivo. *Mater. Sci. Eng. C. Mater. Biol. Appl.* **2016**, *67*, 522–532. [CrossRef] [PubMed]
148. Belgamwar, A.; Khan, S.; Yeole, P. Intranasal chitosan-g-HPbetaCD nanoparticles of efavirenz for the CNS targeting. *Artif. Cells Nanomed. Biotechnol.* **2018**, *46*, 374–386. [CrossRef] [PubMed]
149. Nunes, R.; Araujo, F.; Barreiros, L.; Bartolo, I.; Segundo, M.A.; Taveira, N.; Sarmento, B.; das Neves, J. Noncovalent PEG Coating of Nanoparticle Drug Carriers Improves the Local Pharmacokinetics of Rectal Anti-HIV Microbicides. *ACS Appl. Mater. Interfaces* **2018**, *10*, 34942–34953. [CrossRef] [PubMed]
150. Martins, C.; Araújo, F.; Gomes, M.J.; Fernandes, C.; Nunes, R.; Li, W.; Santos, H.A.; Borges, F.; Sarmento, B. Using microfluidic platforms to develop CNS-targeted polymeric nanoparticles for HIV therapy. *Eur. J. Pharm. Biopharm.* **2018**, *138*, 111–124. [CrossRef] [PubMed]
151. Kumar, P.; Lakshmi, Y.S.; Kondapi, A.K. An oral formulation of efavirenz-loaded lactoferrin nanoparticles with improved biodistribution and pharmacokinetic profile. *HIV Med.* **2017**, *18*, 452–462. [CrossRef] [PubMed]
152. Lakshmi, Y.S.; Kumar, P.; Kishore, G.; Bhaskar, C.; Kondapi, A.K. Triple combination MPT vaginal microbicide using curcumin and efavirenz loaded lactoferrin nanoparticles. *Sci. Rep.* **2016**, *6*, 25479. [CrossRef]
153. Dutta, T.; Agashe, H.B.; Garg, M.; Balakrishnan, P.; Kabra, M.; Jain, N.K. Poly (propyleneimine) dendrimer based nanocontainers for targeting of efavirenz to human monocytes/macrophages *in vitro*. *J. Drug Target.* **2007**, *15*, 89–98. [CrossRef] [PubMed]
154. Dutta, T.; Garg, M.; Jain, N.K. Targeting of efavirenz loaded tuftsin conjugated poly(propyleneimine) dendrimers to HIV infected macrophages *in vitro*. *Eur. J. Pharm. Sci.* **2008**, *34*, 181–189. [CrossRef]
155. Hong, X.; Long, L.; Guohong, F.; Xiangfeng, C. DFT study of nanotubes as the drug delivery vehicles of Efavirenz. *Comput. Theor. Chem.* **2018**, *1131*, 57–68.
156. Suvarna, V.; Thorat, S.; Nayak, U.; Sherje, A.; Murahari, M. Host-guest interaction study of Efavirenz with hydroxypropyl-β-cyclodextrin and L-arginine by computational simulation studies: Preparation and characterization of supramolecular complexes. *J. Mol. Liq.* **2018**, *259*, 55–64. [CrossRef]
157. Moura Ramos, J.J.; Piedade, M.F.M.; Diogo, H.P.; Viciosa, M.T. Thermal Behavior and Slow Relaxation Dynamics in Amorphous Efavirenz: A Study by DSC, XRPD, TSDC, and DRS. *J. Pharm. Sci.* **2019**, *108*, 1254–1263. [CrossRef] [PubMed]
158. das Neves, J.; Sarmento, B.; Amiji, M.M.; Bahia, M.F. Development and validation of a rapid reversed-phase HPLC method for the determination of the non-nucleoside reverse transcriptase inhibitor dapivirine from polymeric nanoparticles. *J. Pharm. Biomed. Anal.* **2010**, *52*, 167–172. [CrossRef] [PubMed]
159. Akil, A.; Devlin, B.; Cost, M.; Rohan, L.C. Increased Dapivirine tissue accumulation through vaginal film codelivery of dapivirine and Tenofovir. *Mol. Pharm.* **2014**, *11*, 1533–1541. [CrossRef] [PubMed]

160. das Neves, J.; Araújo, F.; Andrade, F.; Michiels, J.; Ariën, K.K.; Vanham, G.; Amiji, M.; Bahia, M.F.; Sarmento, B. *In Vitro* and *Ex Vivo* Evaluation of Polymeric Nanoparticles for Vaginal and Rectal Delivery of the Anti-HIV Drug Dapivirine. *Mol. Pharm.* **2013**, *10*, 2793–2807. [CrossRef] [PubMed]
161. Jiang, Y.; Cao, S.; Bright, D.K.; Bever, A.M.; Blakney, A.K.; Suydam, I.T.; Woodrow, K.A. Nanoparticle-Based ARV Drug Combinations for Synergistic Inhibition of Cell-Free and Cell-Cell HIV Transmission. *Mol. Pharm.* **2015**, *12*, 4363–4374. [CrossRef] [PubMed]
162. Krogstad, E.A.; Ramanathan, R.; Nhan, C.; Kraft, J.C.; Blakney, A.K.; Cao, S.; Ho, R.J.Y.; Woodrow, K.A. Nanoparticle-releasing nanofiber composites for enhanced *in vivo* vaginal retention. *Biomaterials* **2017**, *144*, 1–16. [CrossRef]
163. Goebel, F.; Yakovlev, A.; Pozniak, A.; Vinogradova, E.; Boogaerts, G.; Hoetelmans, R.; de Béthune, M.P.; Peeters, M.; Woodfall, B. Short-term antiviral activity of TMC278 – a novel NNRTI – in treatment-naive HIV-1-infected subjects. *Aids* **2006**, *20*, 1721–1726. [CrossRef] [PubMed]
164. Jackson, A.; McGowan, I. Long-acting rilpivirine for HIV prevention. *Curr. Opin. HIV AIDS* **2015**, *10*, 253–257. [CrossRef] [PubMed]
165. Viciana, P. Rilpivirine: The Key for Long-term Success. *AIDS Rev.* **2017**, *19*, 156–166. [CrossRef]
166. Spreen, W.R.; Margolis, D.A.; Pottage, J.C. Long-acting injectable antiretrovirals for HIV treatment and prevention. *Curr. Opin. HIV AIDS* **2013**, *8*, 565–571. [CrossRef] [PubMed]
167. Margolis, D.A.; Boffito, M. Long-acting antiviral agents for HIV treatment. *Curr. Opin. HIV AIDS* **2015**, *10*, 246–252. [CrossRef] [PubMed]
168. Ferretti, F.; Boffito, M. Rilpivirine long-acting for the prevention and treatment of HIV infection. *Curr. Opin. HIV AIDS* **2018**, *13*, 300–307. [CrossRef] [PubMed]
169. Kovarova, M.; Council, O.D.; Date, A.A.; Long, J.M.; Nochi, T.; Belshan, M.; Shibata, A.; Vincent, H.; Baker, C.E.; Thayer, W.O.; et al. Nanoformulations of Rilpivirine for Topical Pericoital and Systemic Coitus-Independent Administration Efficiently Prevent HIV Transmission. *PLoS Pathog.* **2015**, *11*, e1005075.
170. Ottemann, B.M.; Helmink, A.J.; Zhang, W.; Mukadam, I.; Woldstad, C.; Hilaire, J.R.; Liu, Y.; McMillan, J.M.; Edagwa, B.J.; Mosley, R.L.; et al. Bioimaging predictors of rilpivirine biodistribution and antiretroviral activities. *Biomaterials* **2018**, *185*, 174–193. [CrossRef] [PubMed]

12

The Antiproliferative Activity of Oxypeucedanin via Induction of G_2/M Phase Cell Cycle Arrest and p53-Dependent MDM2/p21 Expression in Human Hepatoma Cells

So Hyun Park, Ji-Young Hong, Hyen Joo Park and Sang Kook Lee *

College of Pharmacy, Natural Products Research Institute, Seoul National University, Seoul 08826, Korea; hanirela@snu.ac.kr (S.H.P.); jyhong7876@snu.ac.kr (J.-Y.H.); phj00@snu.ac.kr (H.J.P.)
* Correspondence: sklee61@snu.ac.kr

Abstract: Oxypeucedanin (OPD), a furocoumarin compound from *Angelica dahurica* (Umbelliferae), exhibits potential antiproliferative activities in human cancer cells. However, the underlying molecular mechanisms of OPD as an anticancer agent in human hepatocellular cancer cells have not been fully elucidated. Therefore, the present study investigated the antiproliferative effect of OPD in SK-Hep-1 human hepatoma cells. OPD effectively inhibited the growth of SK-Hep-1 cells. Flow cytometric analysis revealed that OPD was able to induce G_2/M phase cell cycle arrest in cells. The G_2/M phase cell cycle arrest by OPD was associated with the downregulation of the checkpoint proteins cyclin B1, cyclin E, cdc2, and cdc25c, and the up-regulation of p-chk1 (Ser345) expression. The growth-inhibitory activity of OPD against hepatoma cells was found to be p53-dependent. The p53-expressing cells (SK-Hep-1 and HepG2) were sensitive, but p53-null cells (Hep3B) were insensitive to the antiproliferative activity of OPD. OPD also activated the expression of p53, and thus leading to the induction of MDM2 and p21, which indicates that the antiproliferative activity of OPD is in part correlated with the modulation of p53 in cancer cells. In addition, the combination of OPD with gemcitabine showed synergistic growth-inhibitory activity in SK-Hep-1 cells. These findings suggest that the anti-proliferative activity of OPD may be highly associated with the induction of G_2/M phase cell cycle arrest and upregulation of the p53/MDM2/p21 axis in SK-HEP-1 hepatoma cells.

Keywords: oxypeucedanin; *Angelica dahurica*; antiproliferation; G_2/M phase cell cycle arrest; p53; SK-Hep-1; hepatoma cells

---

1. Introduction

Hepatocellular carcinoma (HCC) is the sixth most frequently diagnosed cancer and the second most common cause of death from cancer [1]. Approximately 30 to 40% of patients with HCC diagnosed at early stages are potentially effectively treated by surgical therapies such as hepatectomy or liver transplantation [2]. However, the disease diagnosed at an advanced stage or re-progression stage after treatment has poor prognosis due to the fundamental liver disease and lack of other treatment options [2–4]. In accordance, any systemic therapy has not effectively contributed to survival for patients with advanced HCC [5]. Therefore, it is necessary to procure potential chemotherapeutic agents for the treatment of advanced HCC cells.

Angelica dahurica (Umbelliferae) is an indigenous plant mainly distributed in Korea, China, and Russia. The root of *Angelica dahurica* has been used for the control of hysteria, bleeding, menstrual disorder, neuralgia and pain as a traditional medicine in Korea. Previous phytochemical studies revealed that the plant is a rich source of furanocoumarins, including oxypeucedanin [6]. Oxypeucedanin (OPD)

(Figure 1), a coumarin-type major constituent of the root of *Angelica dahurica*, has been reported to have several biological activities, including anti-mutagenic, uterus contraction, blood pressure increase, and cytotoxic and antiproliferative effects against cancer cells [7–9].

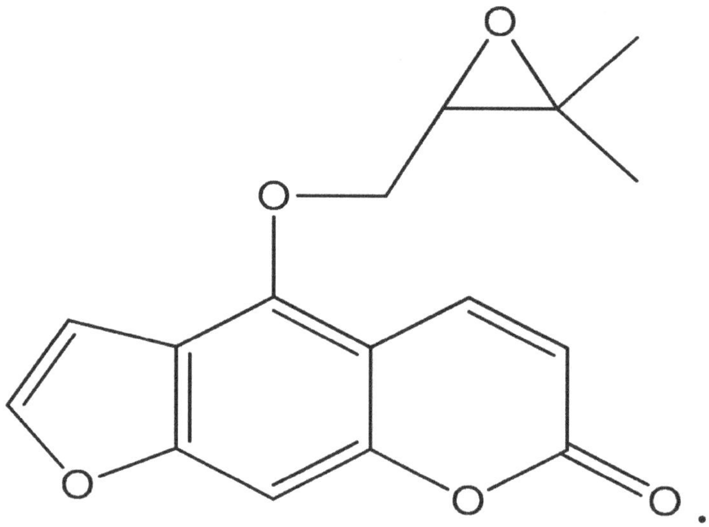

Figure 1. Chemical structure of oxypeucedanin (OPD).

When the DNA damage stimulus comes to the cells, the response of the cellular system is complex and finely controlled. The cellular response involves the functions of gene products that recognize DNA damage signals and activate processes such as the inhibition of proliferation, the stimulation of repair mechanisms, or the induction of apoptosis [10–12]. Generally, the cellular response to DNA damage and the disturbance to replication involve the activation of checkpoints, following signal transduction pathways for regulation of cell cycle progression and cell division [10,11]. Deficiency in these checkpoint responses can induce cell death, genomic instability, or predisposition to cancer [12–14]. In addition, cell cycle progression is finely regulated by cell cycle regulatory proteins and checkpoint proteins depending on the specific cell cycle phase. In particular, the G_2/M phase of the cell cycle is governed by the expression of key G_2/M transition regulatory proteins and the ATR/Chk1 signaling pathways. p53, a tumor suppressor, is also considered to be involved in the transcriptional regulation of a large number of growth-arrest and apoptosis-related genes [15].

Although several biological activities of OPD have been previously reported, the precise molecular mechanism of OPD related to its antiproliferative activity against human liver cancer cells has not been fully elucidated. In the present study, the growth-inhibitory activity and the underlying mechanisms of action of OPD were investigated in SK-Hep-1 human hepatoma cells.

2. Results

2.1. Antiproliferative Effects of Oxypeucedanin (OPD) in SK-Hep-1 Human Hepatoma Cells

To primarily evaluate whether OPD shows potential growth-inhibitory effects on human cancer cells, the anti-proliferative activity of OPD was determined in a panel of human cancer cell lines. As summarized in Table 1, OPD inhibited the growth of human cancer cells. Among the cell lines tested, SK-Hep-1 human hepatoma cells were the most sensitive to OPD. Therefore, further study on the mechanism of action of OPD in the regulation of cell proliferation was conducted in SK-Hep-1 cells. In addition, since OPD was shown to have the anti-proliferative activity against SK-Hep-1 cells, the isolated OPD analogs from the roots of *Angelica dahurica* were also evaluated for their antiproliferative activity in SK-Hep-1 cells. Among the test compounds, OPD was the most active growth inhibitor against SK-Hep-1 cells (Table 2).

Table 1. Anti-proliferative effects of furanocoumarins from *Angelica dahurica* on various human cancer cells.

Compounds	MDA-MB-231 [a]	T47D	SNU638	SK-Hep-1	A549
Isoimperatorin	>100	>100	90.2	>100	>100
Byakangelicol	74.7 [b]	46.0	50.0	72.1	41.1
Oxypeucedanin	50.8	95.5	50.4	32.4	46.3

[a] Cancer cell line: MDA-MB-231 (breast), T47D (breast), SK-Hep-1 (liver), A549 (lung), SNU638 (stomach), [b] IC_{50} value: μM.

Table 2. Anti-proliferative effects of oxypeucedanin analogs on SK-Hep-1 cells.

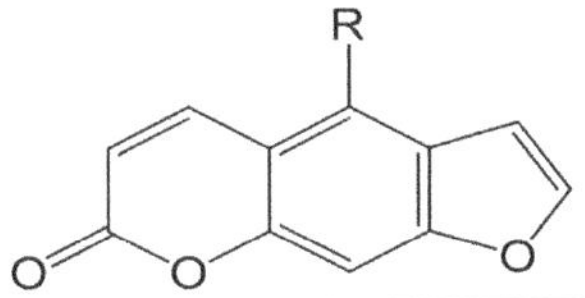

Compounds	R	IC_{50} (μM)
Oxypeucedanin	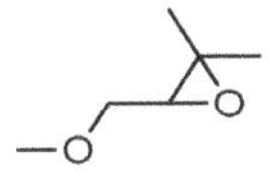	32.4
Isooxypeucedanin	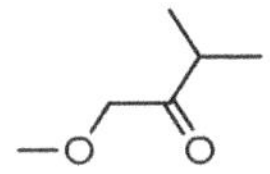	91.5
Oxypeucedanin hydrate	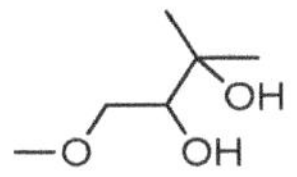	81.0
Oxypeucedanin methanolate	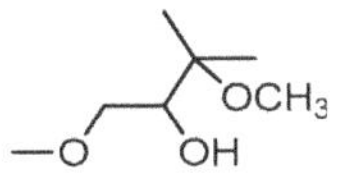	77.4

Since the anti-proliferative activity of OPD was found in SK-Hep-1 human hepatoma cells for 72 h, the growth-inhibitory activity of OPD was also investigated for 24 or 48 h in SK-Hep-1 cells. As shown in Figure 2, OPD exhibited growth-inhibitory activity against SK-Hep-1 human hepatoma cells in a concentration- and time-dependent manner.

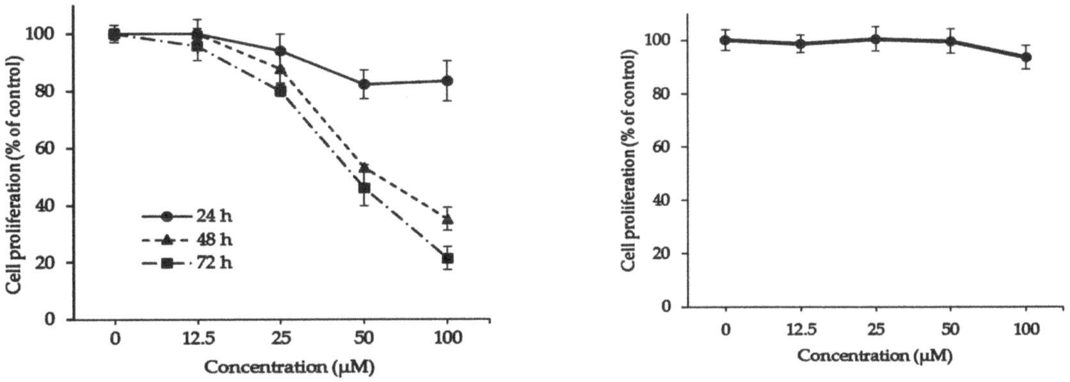

Figure 2. Anti-proliferative effects of OPD in SK-Hep-1 human hepatoma cells (left) and MRC5 human normal cell line (right). SK-Hep-1 cells were cultured in a 96-well plate and treated with the indicated concentrations of OPD for 24–72 h. MRC5 cells were cultured in a 96-well plate and treated with the indicated concentrations of OPD for 72 h. The cell proliferative activity was determined using the SRB assay. The % cell proliferation value was calculated by the mean absorbance of samples/absorbance of the vehicle-treated control as described in the Materials and Methods. Data are presented as the means ± S.E. (n = 3).

The IC_{50} value of OPD with a 72 h treatment was 32.4 μM. In addition, the growth-inhibitory activity of OPD was also determined in a normal cell line. OPD was unable to affect the growth rate of MRC5 normal human lung fibroblast cells (IC_{50} >100 μM). These data suggest that OPD may be able to selectively inhibit the proliferation of human hepatoma cancer cells compared to normal cells. Under the same experimental conditions, the IC_{50} value of etoposide, a positive control, was 0.3 μM.

2.2. *Effects of OPD on the Cell Cycle Distribution of SK-Hep-1 Cells*

To further elucidate the anti-proliferative mechanisms of OPD in SK-Hep-1 cells, the cells were treated with the indicated concentrations of OPD for 24 h, and flow cytometry analysis was performed with PI staining. As shown in Figure 3A, OPD enhanced the accumulation of the G_2/M phase peak from 22.66% (control) to 35.90% (75 μM). These data suggest that the antiproliferative activity of OPD in SK-Hep-1 cells is in part associated with the induction of G_2/M phase cell cycle arrest. To further investigate whether the G_2/M phase cell cycle arrest by OPD is correlated with the regulation of the checkpoint proteins, the expression of the G_2/M cell cycle regulatory proteins was determined by western blot analysis. Since OPD did not show significant cytotoxicity at the test concentration up to 100 μM for 24 h (Figure 2), the cells were treated with OPD (50, 75, or 100 μM) for 24 h, and then the checkpoint protein expression related to G_2/M phase cell cycle regulation was measured in SK-Hep-1 cells. As shown in Figure 3B, the expression levels of Chk1, p-cdc25c (Ser198), cdc25c, cyclin B1, cdc2, and p-cdc2 (Thr161) were downregulated, but the levels of p-Chk1 (Ser345) were upregulated by OPD treatment. Chk1 (checkpoint kinase 1) is a multifunctional protein kinase that coordinates the response to specific types of DNA damage [16]. Cdc25 is a protein phosphatase responsible for dephosphorylating and activating cdc2, a pivotal step in directing the cells toward mitosis [17]. When DNA damage ocurrs, the Chk1 phosphorylates cdc25c, which then leads to translocation of cdc25c from the cytoplasm to the nucleus, where cdc25c can interact with cdc2/cyclin B during mitosis [18,19]. Moreover, the activity of the cdc2-cyclin B1 complex is dependent on the phosphorylation/dephosphorylation status of cdc2 [11,13,20]. The entry of eukaryotic cells into mitosis is regulated by cdc2 activation, including the binding of cdc2 to cyclin B1 and its phosphorylation at the Thr161 residue. In this study, we found that cdc25c was inactivated by phosphor-Chk1 with OPD treatment, and the activation of the cdc2-cyclin B1 complex was also suppressed by OPD in a concentration-dependent manner, indicating the induction of G_2/M phase cell cycle arrest by OPD. These findings suggest that the activation of Chk1 and sequential regulation of signal transduction pathways by OPD may be due to the induction of G_2/M phase cell cycle arrest by OPD in SK-Hep-1 cells.

(A)

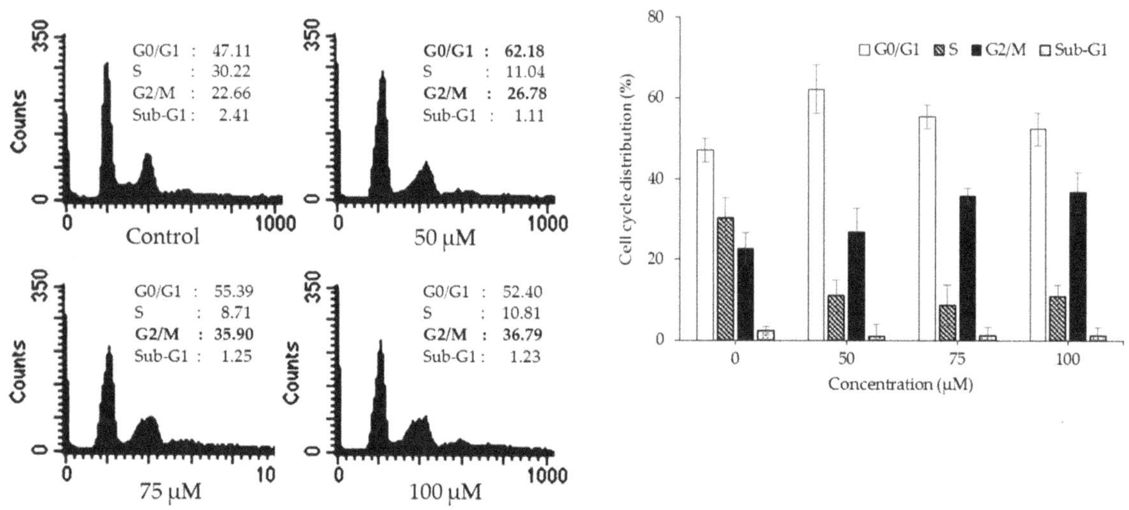

Figure 3. *Cont.*

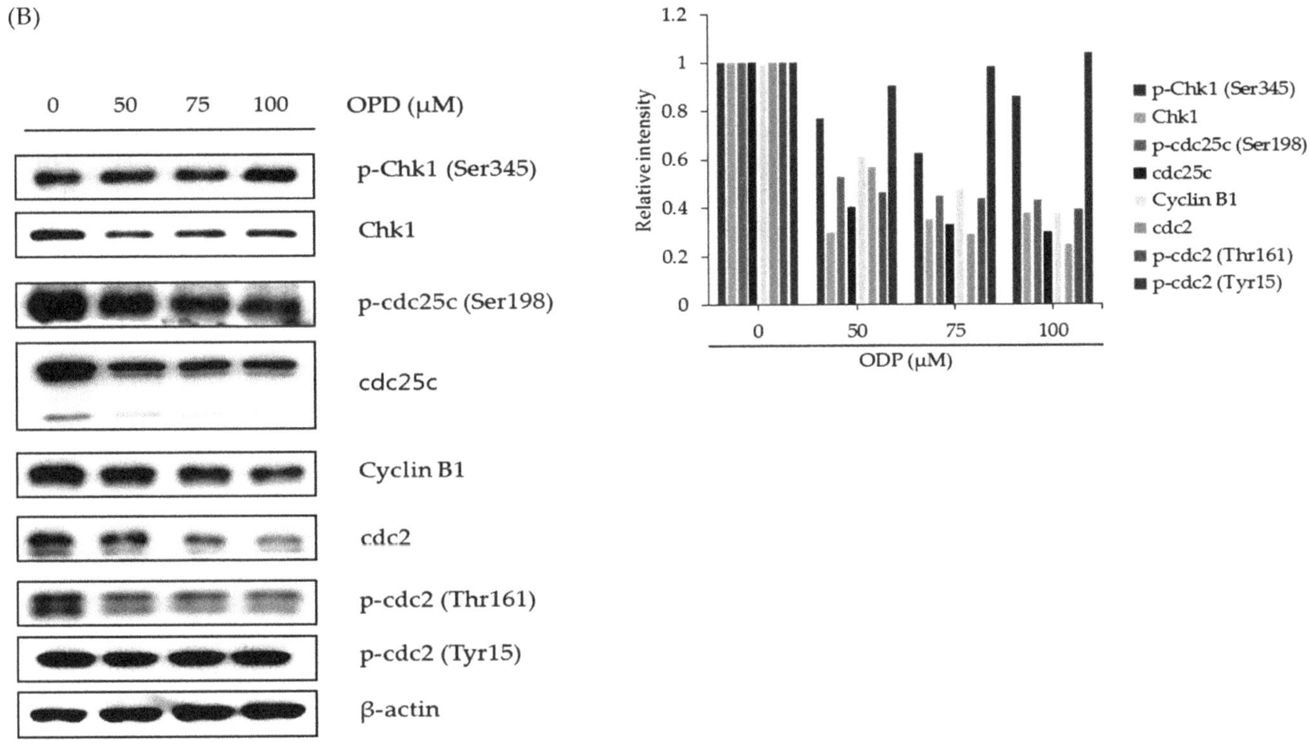

Figure 3. Effects of OPD on the regulation of cell cycle distribution in SK-Hep-1 cells. (**A**) SK-Hep-1 cells were treated with various concentrations of OPD for 24 h. Both adherent and floating cells were collected, fixed with 70% cold ethanol overnight, and then incubated with RNase A and PI for 30 min. The cell cycle distribution was analyzed by flow cytometry. (**B**) The cells were treated with the indicated concentrations of OPD for 24 h, and the expression of cell cycle regulatory proteins was determined by western blot analysis. β-Actin was used as an internal control.

2.3. Effects of OPD on the Regulation of p53-associated Signaling Pathways in SK-Hep-1 Cells

To further validate the association of p53-mediated signaling molecules in the anti-proliferative activity of OPD in SK-Hep-1 cells, the cells was treated with OPD for 24 h, and then the expression of p53-associated molecules were determined by western blot analysis. OPD significantly enhanced the protein expression of p53, p-p53(Ser15), MDM2, p21, and GADD45α in the cells (Figure 4A). Previous studies have reported that the phosphorylation of p53 at Ser15 or Ser20 upregulates p53 stability by disrupting the interaction between p53 and MDM2 [21,22]. Because OPD is able to induce the stability of p53, the accumulation of p53 by OPD may subsequently enhance its downstream target genes, including MDM2, p21, and GADD45α, in the cells. In addition, the expression of p53-associated proteins was also monitored for up to 48 h with treatment with 50 μM OPD and was found to be up-regulated after 4 h of treatment in SK-Hep-1 cells (Figure 4B). Further study was designed to confirm whether the cellular localization of p53 is affected by treatment of cells with OPD. Generally, in the nucleus, MDM2-mediated ubiquitination led to the transportation of p53 into the cytoplasm or its degradation by the 26S proteasome [21,22]. As an important transcriptional factor, the stability and nuclear localization of p53 are considered essential for its tumor suppressor activity [23]. Therefore, we determined the levels of p53 and MDM2 protein expression in both the cytosol and nucleus fraction following treatment with OPD in SK-Hep-1 cells. As shown in Figure 4C, the levels of p53 protein expression were upregulated and localized in the nucleus upon OPD treatment for 24 h in a concentration-dependent manner. The levels of MDM2 protein expression were also shown to be upregulated in the nucleus by OPD treatment in the cells. To further confirm the effects of OPD on the expression of p53-associated proteins, OPD treatment of cells was conducted in the absence or presence of caffeine. Because caffeine is known as an ATR/Chk1 kinase inhibitor [24,25], the effect of caffeine on the enhanced p53-associated protein expression by OPD was investigated in the cells.

As expected, treatment with OPD (50 μM) for 24 h led to a significant upregulation of p53, p21, and MDM2 expression in the absence of caffeine, but the pretreatment with caffeine for 2 h alleviated the enhancement of p53-associated protein expression by OPD in SK-Hep-1 cells (Figure 4D). Although the expression of p53-associated proteins was downregulated by the pretreatment with caffeine, OPD also exhibited a slight upregulation of p53 and p21 expression in the presence of caffeine (Figure 4D). These data suggest that the induction of G_2/M phase cell cycle arrest by OPD seems to be associated with not only the ATR/Chk1 signaling pathway but also the regulation of p53-mediated pathways. Further study examined the maintenance of p53 stability by OPD with the cotreatment of cycloheximide (CHX), a protein synthesis inhibitor [26], in SK-Hep-1 cells. As shown in Figure 4E, OPD significantly suppressed the degradation of p53 in the presence of cycloheximide, suggesting that the half-life of p53 degradation was sustained by OPD treatment compared to vehicle-treated control cells. However, the rate of MDM2 degradation was not greatly affected by the down-regulation of p53 turnover with OPD treatment of cells.

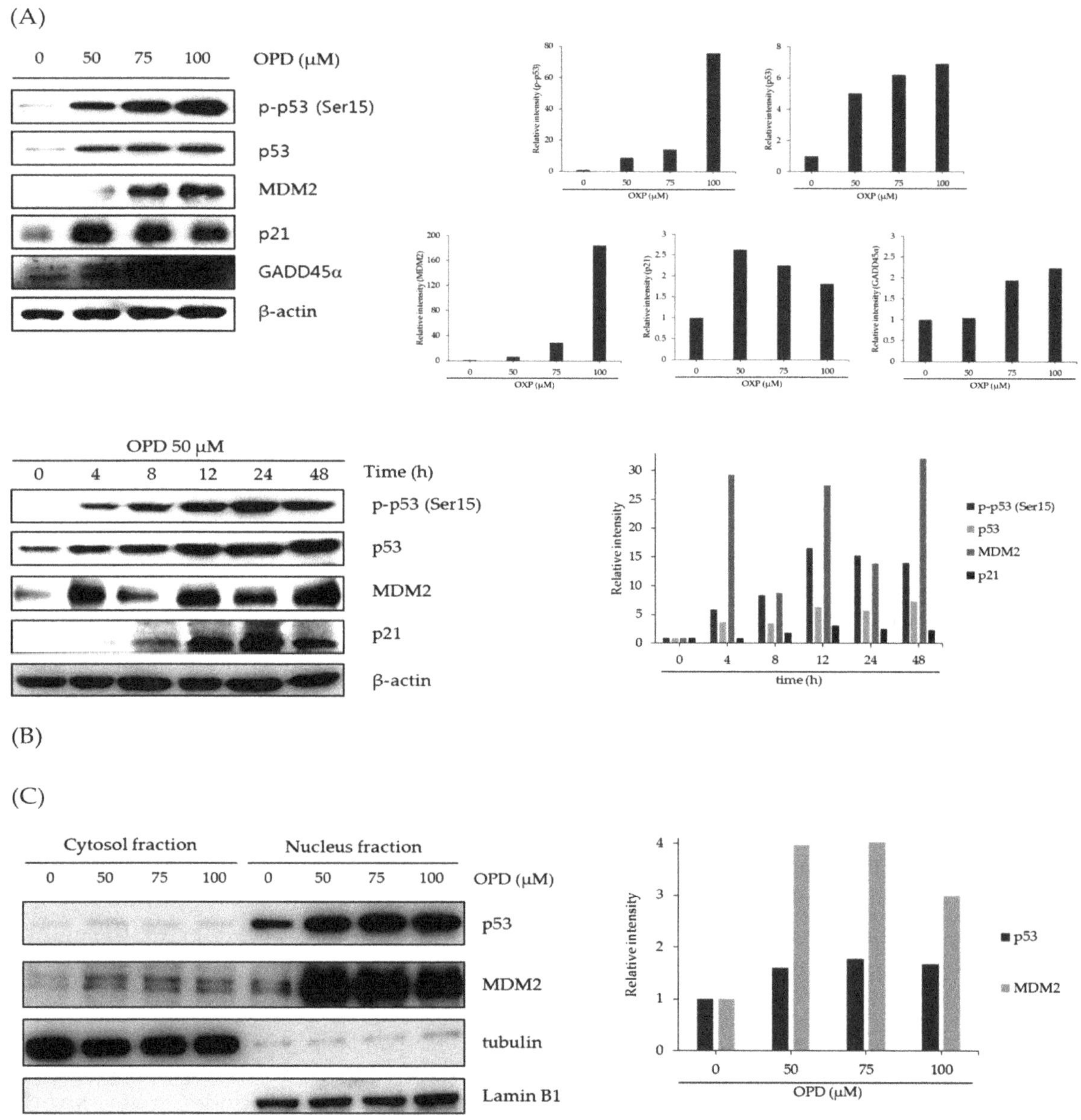

Figure 4. *Cont.*

(D)

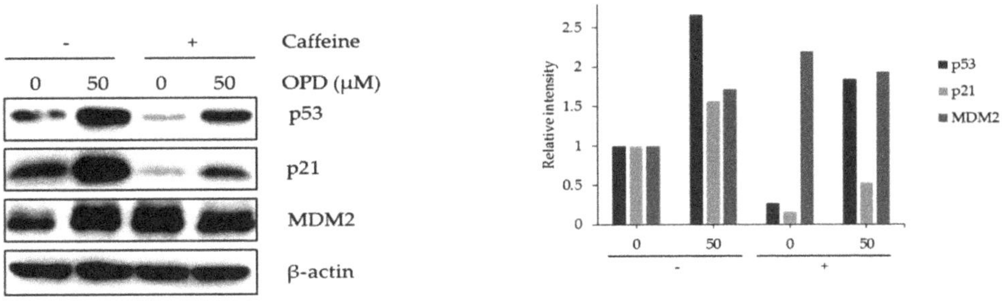

(E)

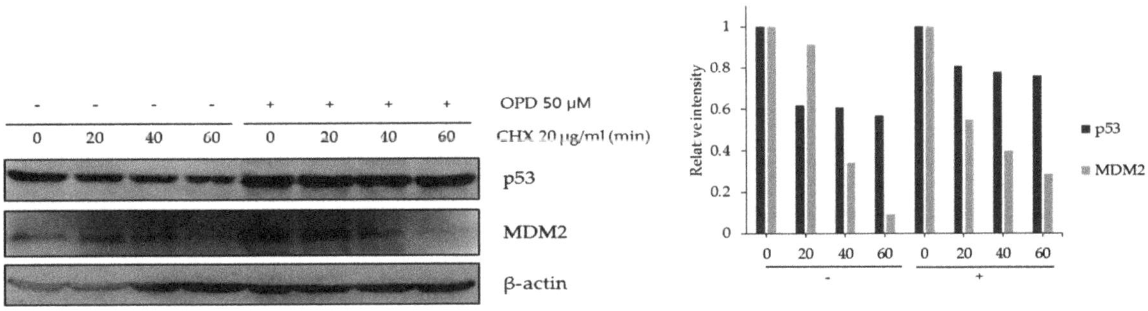

Figure 4. Effects of OPD on the regulation of p53-associated signaling pathways. (**A**) SK-Hep-1 cells were treated with the indicated concentrations of OPD for 24 h. The expression level of proteins was analyzed by western blot. β-Actin was used as an internal control. (**B**) SK-Hep-1 cells were treated with 50 μM OPD for various time points up to 48 h. The expression level of proteins was analyzed by western blot. β-Actin was used as an internal control. (**C**) SK-Hep-1 cells were treated with various concentrations of OPD for 24 h. After cells were harvested, the proteins were separated into cytosolic and nuclear fractions as described in the Materials and Methods. The protein expression levels were analyzed by western blot. β-Actin was used as an internal control. (**D**) SK-Hep-1 cells were pretreated for 2 h with 1 mM caffeine, and then cultured with 50 μM OPD for an additional 24 h. The expression level of proteins was analyzed by western blot. β-Actin was used as an internal control. (**E**) SK-Hep-1 cells were treated with 50 μM OPD for 24 h and then treated in the absence or presence of 20 μg/mL cycloheximide. The cells were harvested at 0, 20, 40, and 60 min. The expression level of proteins was analyzed by western blot, and the band density was quantified using the NIH ImageJ software (Bethesda, MD).

2.4. Effects of OPD on Cell Proliferation Depending on the p53 Status in Hepatoma Cells

Since p53 seems to be highly associated with the anti-proliferative activity of OPD in SK-Hep-1 cells, the effects of p53 status on the growth-inhibitory activity of OPD were evaluated in human hepatoma cells with different p53 statuses. The cells were treated with various concentrations of OPD for 72 h, and then cell proliferation was determined by the SRB assay. As shown in Figure 5A, wild-type p53 cell lines, such as SK-Hep-1 and HepG2, were more sensitive than the p53-null Hep3B cell line, indicating that p53 plays an important role in the anti-proliferative activity of OPD in human hepatoma cells. To further confirm the involvement of p53 in the antiproliferative activity of OPD, p53 siRNA was transfected into wild-type p53 SK-Hep-1 cells, and the effect of p53 siRNA on the cell proliferation was determined in SK-Hep-1 cells. When the p53 siRNA transfected-SK-Hep-1 cells were treated with OPD (50 μM) for 48 and 72 h, the antiproliferative activity of OPD was decreased compared to that of the control cells (no transfection or scrambled siRNA transfection), suggesting that the anti-proliferative activity of OPD is partly associated with wild-type p53 expression in hepatoma cells (Figure 5B). In addition, the OPD treatment exhibited upregulation of p53 and MDM2 in the control cells. Although p53 expression was not shown in p53 siRNA-treated SK-Hep-1 cells, OPD slightly up-regulated the expression of MDM2 in p53 siRNA-treated SK-Hep-1 cells (Figure 5C).

(A)

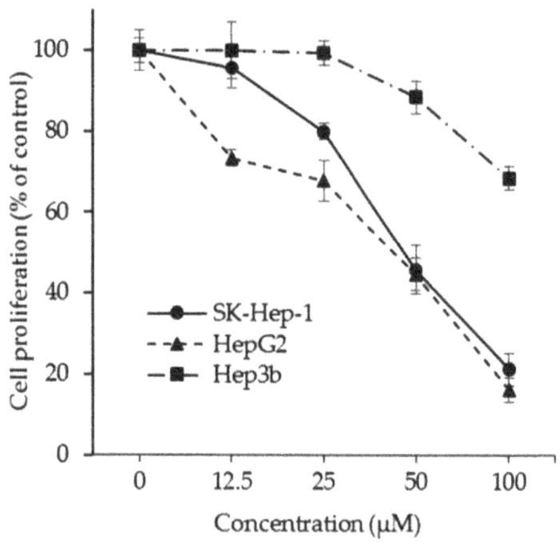

Cell line	IC50 (μM)	p53 status
SK-Hep-1	32.4	wild
HepG2	43.8	wild
Hep3B	>100	null

(B)

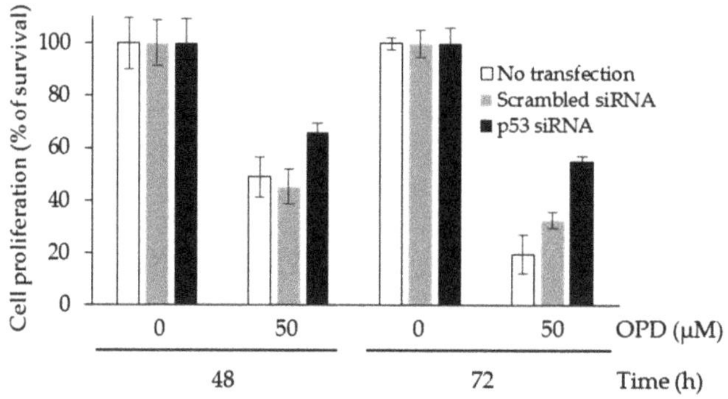

(C)

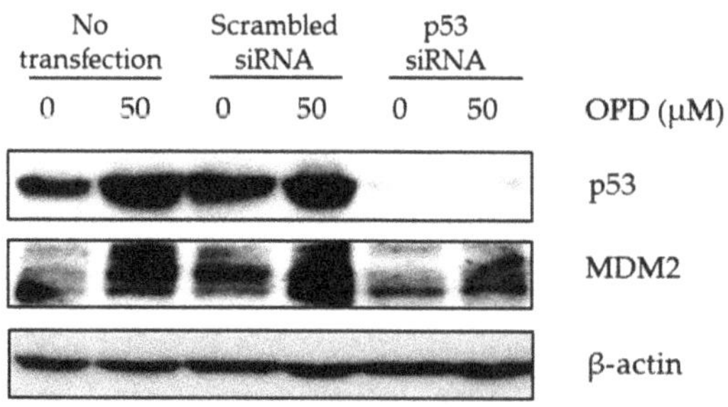

Figure 5. Effects of p53 expression on the cell proliferation of hepatoma cells by OPD. (**A**) SK-Hep-1, HepG2, and Hep3B cells were cultured in a 96-well plate and treated with the indicated concentrations of OPD for 72 h. The cell proliferative effect was determined using the SRB assay. Data are presented as the means ± S.E. (n = 3). (**B**) SK-Hep-1 cells were transfected with 5 nM p53 siRNA or scrambled siRNA for 24 h, and then OPD treatment (50 μM) was given for 48 or 72 h for the measurement of cell proliferation. Data are presented as the means ± S.E. (n = 3). (**C**) The effects of p53 siRNA on the expression level of p53 and MDM2 were analyzed by western blot in control cells and p53 siRNA-transfected SK-Hep-1 cells.

2.5. *Effects of OPD in Combination with Gemcitabine on the Cell Proliferation of SK-Hep-1 Cells*

To further investigate the effect of the combination of OPD with an anticancer agent on the antiproliferative activity of hepatoma cells, we selected gemcitabine, a pyrimidine-based DNA synthesis inhibitor, as a candidate compound based on the use of patients with liver cancer in the clinic. As shown in Figure 6A, cotreatment with OPD and gemcitabine exhibited a synergistic effect (CI < 1.0) on the antiproliferative activity of SK-Hep-1 cells. The combination of the higher concentrations of OPD and gemcitabine showed a relatively stronger synergistic activity. In accordance, when OPD (20 μM) was treated with various concentrations of gemcitabine (0.1–0.4 μM), the combination with the higher concentration of gemcitabine (0.4 μM) was shown to have a stronger synergistic activity (Figure 6).

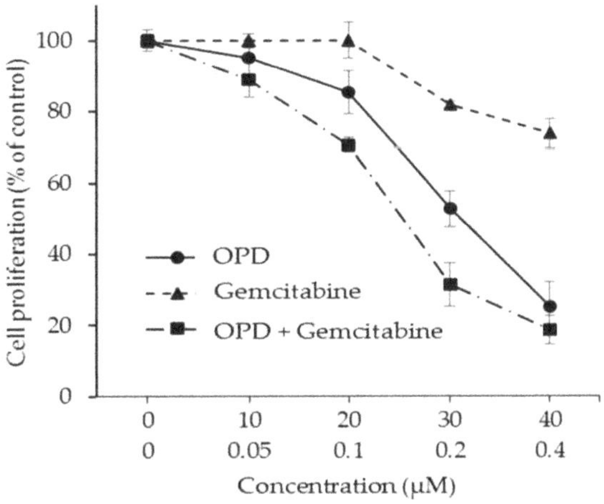

Oxypeucedanin (μM)	Gemcitabine (μM)	Combination index (CI)	Description
20	0.1	1.08	Additive
30	0.2	0.78	Moderate synergism
40	0.4	0.82	Moderate synergism

Figure 6. Combination effect of OPD with gemcitabine on the cell proliferation of SK-Hep-1 cells. (**A**) The cells were treated with the indicated concentrations of OPD and gemcitabine for 72 h, and then cell proliferation was measured by the SRB assay. (**B**) The cells were treated with OPD (20 μM) and various concentrations of gemcitabine (0.1–0.4 μM) for 72 h, and then cell proliferation was measured by the SRB assay. Data are presented as the means ± S.E. ($n = 3$). Based on the cell proliferation data.

Natural products have been used for traditional medicines and also play an important role in drug discovery and development programs. In particular, anticancer drugs are mainly developed based on natural product-originated small molecules. In our continuous efforts to procure small molecules from natural sources in the discovery of antitumor agents, oxypeucedanin (OPD), a furanocoumarin isolated from the root of *Angelica dahurica*, was considered a potential candidate. Previous biological activities of OPD include the effective intervention of sunitinib-induced nephrotoxicity, the hepatoprotective activity of tacrine-induced cytotoxicity in liver cells, and the cytotoxicity against cancer cells such as gastric cancer, prostate cancer, and melanoma cells [27,28]. Although the antiproliferative activities of OPD have been reported in cancer cells, the precise molecular mechanism of OPD in the anticancer activity of human liver cancers remains to be elucidated. This study demonstrates that OPD regulates the induction of G_2/M phase cell cycle arrest and p53-dependent MDM2/p21 signaling pathways in human hepatoma SK-Hep-1 cells.

It is known that the cell cycle is a finely controlled sequence of events in the growth and proliferation of eukaryotic cells. Cell cycle progression occurs in an ordered manner that is monitored by cell cycle checkpoints. Among the checkpoints, the DNA damage-induced G_2/M checkpoint guarantees the fidelity of genomic stability. However, cancer cells have abnormally activated in cell division as a result of diverse factors, including uncontrolled checkpoint protein expression. These defects in the checkpoints lead to genomic instability, cell death, or carcinogenesis. Therefore, the regulation of the G_2/M checkpoint is often applied as a potential therapeutic target to evaluate the efficacy of natural product-derived antitumor agents in cancer cells. In the present study, we found that OPD effectively inhibited the growth of SK-Hep-1 human hepatoma cells. Cell cycle distribution analysis also revealed that the antiproliferative activity of OPD is in part associated with the induction of G_2/M cell cycle arrest in cells. This result was consistent with the previous report of G_2/M phase arrest of OPD in prostate cancer cells [27]. However, a previous study of the antiproliferative activity of OPD on the prostate cancer cells did not investigate in detail the regulatory biomarkers involved in G_2/M phase cell cycle arrest in cancer cells. The present study revealed that the induction of G_2/M phase cell cycle arrest by OPD was correlated with the regulation of Chk1-mediated G_2/M checkpoint proteins, including cdc25c/cdc2 and cdc2/cyclin B1 complex pathways, in hepatoma cells. Chk1 is considered to play an important role in the G_2/M checkpoint via the ATM-RAD3-related (ATR) pathway. Chk1 also regulates the activity of its shared downstream substrate, cell division cycle 25c (cdc25c). OPD effectively modulates the Chk1-cdc25c activation pathway axis, leading to the induction of G_2/M cell cycle arrest in SK-Hep-1 cells. We also found that OPD effectively suppressed the activity of cyclin B1 and its partner cell division cycle 2 (cdc2) expression, which in turn evokes the prevention of entry into the mitosis (M) phase cell cycle transition in hepatoma cells.

Tumor suppressor p53 is mutated, deleted, or rearranged in more than half of all human tumors, and thus, p53 is considered an important target in anticancer drug development [29,30]. p53 is also considered an important factor in the control of the cell cycle at the G_1/S and/or G_2/M transition through diverse mechanisms [31]. In this study, we found that OPD significantly up-regulated the expression of p53 by the accumulation of p53 and increased its stability in SK-Hep-1 cells. The upregulation of p53 levels by OPD led to the activation of downstream target expression such as MDM2, p21 and GADD45α in cells. The association of p53 in G_2/M phase cell cycle signaling was further confirmed by the significant suppression of p53, p21 and MDM2 expression by treatment with caffeine, an ATR/Chk1 inhibitor, in SK-Hep-1 cells. However, OPD did not fully recover the levels of p53 and its downstream target protein expression in the presence of caffeine, indicating that OPD may cause the activation of p53 independently of the ATR/Chk1 pathway. The involvement of p53 in the anti-proliferative activity of OPD in SK-Hep-1 cells was also confirmed using cell types with different p53 statuses and deletion methods. OPD was found to be more effective in p53-wild-type expression cells, and p53 siRNA-transfected cells were less sensitive to the OPD in the antiproliferative activity on liver cancer cells.

The function of p53 is mainly governed by the stability and nuclear localization of p53 in cells. We found that OPD effectively inhibits the degradation of p53 and thus sustains the stability of p53 in cancer cells. In addition, OPD was found to induce the nuclear localization of p53, which may activate the transcriptional activity of its downstream target genes associated with cell cycle regulation in cancer cells.

Gemcitabine (2′,2′-difluorodeoxycytidine), a pyrimidine-based antimetabolite, is currently used to the treatment of pancreatic cancer as well as other cancers [32,33]. Gemcitabine inhibits DNA replication by activating the S-phase checkpoint. A study also showed that gemcitabine activates the ATR/Chk1 pathway [34]. In the present study, we found that OPD in combination with gemcitabine exhibits synergistic anti-proliferative activity in SK-Hep-1 cells. Therefore, OPD might be a promising lead compound in combination with cancer chemotherapeutic agents in advanced liver cancer treatment. In addition, in terms of clinical relevance of furanocoumarins, the bioavailability of oxypeucedanin in plasma samples may be important parameters. In the previous study, Chen et al. [35] reported that the pharmacokinetic parameters of OPD were the Tmax (12 h), T1/2 (2.4 h), and oral bioavailability (F, 10.1%) in rat models by oral administration of OPD. These data suggest that the oral bioavailability of

OPD is a relatively low and thus needed to be further study for improvement of the bioavailability either structural modifications or appropriate formulation of administration of OPD.

3. Materials and Methods

3.1. Chemicals

Dulbecco's modified Eagle's medium (DMEM) and fetal bovine serum (FBS) were purchased from HyClone Laboratories (Logan, UT, USA). Antibiotics-antimycotics solution, Lipofectamine®RNAiMAX, negative control siRNA, and Opti-MEM®Reduced Serum Medium were purchased from Invitrogen (Grand Island, NY, USA). p53-specific siRNA was purchased from Bioneer (Daejeon, Korea). The nuclear extract kit was purchased from Active Motif (Carlsbad, CA, USA). Bovine serum albumin (BSA), dimethyl sulfoxide (DMSO), trichloroacetic acid (TCA), sulforhodamine B (SRB), propidium iodide (PI), ribonuclease A (RNase A), and other agents were purchased from Sigma-Aldrich (St. Louis, MO, CA). Antibodies against p-chk1 (Ser345) (#2348), chk1 (#2360), p-cdc25c (Ser198) (#9529), cdc25c (#4688), p-cdc2 (Tyr15) (#9111), p-cdc2 (Thr161) (#9114), p-p53 (Ser15) (#9284), p21 (#3733), and α/β tubulin (#2148) were purchased from Cell Signaling (Danvers, MA, USA). Antibodies against cyclin B1 (#752), cdc-2 (#54), β-actin, p53 (#126), MDM2 (#965), GADD45α (#797), lamin B1 (#20682) were obtained from Santa Cruz Biotechnology (Dallas, TX, USA)

OPD (Figure 1) and its analogs, isolated from the root of *Angelica dahurica*, were provided by Dr. Jin-Woong Kim (College of Pharmacy, Seoul National University, Seoul, Korea). *Angelica dahurica* (9 kg, dry weight) was purchased from Kyungdong Market Herbal Medicine in Seoul, and ultrasonically extracted three times for 120 min with 100% MeOH. The extract was filtered and concentrated under reduced pressure to obtain MeOH extract (910 g), which was suspended in distilled water to obtain a $CHCl_3$ fraction (229 g). OPD and its analogs were obtained by various column chromatography. Each component was analyzed by ^{1}H-NMR, ^{13}C-NMR, and FABMS, and then identified compared with the literature values of corresponding compounds. OPD and its analogs, dissolved in 100% DMSO.

3.2. Cell Culture

SK-Hep-1, HepG2, and Hep3B cells were purchased from the American Type Culture Collection (Manassas, VA, USA). Cells were cultured in DMEM supplemented with 10% heat-inactivated fetal bovine serum (FBS) and antibiotics-antimycotics (PSF; 100 units/mL penicillin G sodium, 100 μg/mL streptomycin, and 250 ng/mL amphotericin B). Cells were incubated in a humidified atmosphere containing 5% CO_2 at 37 °C.

3.3. Cell Proliferation Assay

Cell proliferation was measured by the sulforhodamine B (SRB) assay [36]. Cells were seeded in 96-well plates (3×10^4 cells/mL), incubated for 24 h, and either fixed (for zero day controls) or treated with various concentrations of test compounds (total volume of 200 μL/well) for 24, 48, and 72 h. After treatment, the cells were fixed with 50% TCA solution and dried at room temperature. Fixed cells were stained in 0.4% SRB in 1% acetic acid, and unbound dye was washed with 1% acetic acid. Stained cells were dried and dissolved in 10 mM Tris (pH 10.0). The absorbance was measured at 515 nm, and cell proliferation was determined as follows: cell proliferation (%) = (average absorbance compound – average absorbance zero day) / (average absorbance control – average absorbance zero day) × 100. IC_{50} values were calculated by non-linear regression analysis using the TableCurve 2D v5.01 software (Systat Software Inc., San Jose, CA, USA).

3.4. Cell Cycle Analysis

SK-Hep-1 cells were plated at a density of 1×10^6 cells per 100-mm culture dish and incubated for 24 h. Fresh media containing various concentrations of test sample were added to the culture dishes. Following a 24 h incubation, the cells were harvested (trypsinization and centrifugation) and fixed with 70% ethanol overnight at 4 °C. Fixed cells were washed with PBS and incubated with a staining solution containing RNase A (50 μg/mL) and propidium iodide (50 μg/mL) in PBS for 30 min at room temperature. The cellular DNA content was analyzed with a FACSCalibur flow cytometer (BD Biosciences, San Jose, CA, USA). At least 20,000 cells were used for each analysis, and the distribution of cells in each phase of the cell cycle was displayed as histograms.

3.5. *Western Blot Analysis*

SK-Hep-1 human hepatoma cells were exposed to various concentrations of OPD for the indicated times. After incubation, the cells were lysed, and the protein concentrations were determined by the bicinchoninic acid method [37]. Each protein was subjected to 6–15% SDS-PAGE. Proteins were transferred onto PVDF membranes (Millipore, Bedford, MA, USA) by electroblotting, and membranes were blocked for 1 h with blocking buffer [5% bovine serum albumin (BSA) in tris-buffered saline-0.1% Tween 20 (TBST)] at room temperature [38]. Membranes were then incubated with indicated antibodies (mouse anti-β-actin, diluted 1:10,000; other antibodies, diluted 1:500–1:1000 in 5% BSA/TBST) overnight at 4 °C and washed three times for 10 min with TBST. After washing, membranes were incubated with corresponding secondary antibodies diluted 1:2000 in TBST for 2 h at room temperature, washed three times for 10 min with TBST, and visualized with an enhanced chemiluminescence (ECL) detection kit (LabFrontier, Suwon, Korea) using an LAS-4000 Imager (Fuji Film Corp., Tokyo, Japan).

3.6. *RNA Interference*

RNA interference of p53 was performed using siRNA duplexes purchased from Bioneer (Daejeon, Korea). The coding strand for p53 siRNA was as follows: sense CACUACAACUACA UGUGUA and antisense UACACAUGUAGUUGUAGUG. For transfection, reverse transfection was conducted using Lipofectamine RNAiMAX (Invitrogen) according to the manufacturer's recommendations. Compound treatments occurred 24 h after transfection. Cells were harvested after 24 h and examined by western blotting.

3.7. *Combination Assay*

Determination of the effect of combination therapy was performed using the SRB assay. On day 1, 3000 cells/well in a volume of 100 μL were plated in 96-well plates. On day 2, gemcitabine (100, 200, or 400 nM) and OPD (20, 30, or 40 μM) were each added in a volume of 50 μL, in all combinations. After 72 h, the cells were fixed with 50% TCA solution for 30 min at 4 °C, rinsed 5 times with water, and air-dried. Fixed cells were colored with 80 μL of 0.4% sulforhodamine B in 0.1% acetic acid) rinsed with 0.1% acetic acid, and air dried. Sulforhodamine was redissolved in 200 μL/well of 10 mM Tris, pH 10, and the absorbance was measured at 515 nm. After calculating the percent of inhibition by OPD and gemcitabine, the combination index (CI) was estimated to evaluate the synergistic effect of OPD and gemcitabine:

$$\mathrm{CI} = \frac{(D)_1}{(D_m)_1[f_a/(1-f_a)]^{\frac{1}{m_1}}} + \frac{(D)_2}{(D_m)_2[f_a/(1-f_a)]^{\frac{1}{m_2}}}$$

where D = dose; Dm = median-effect dose; m = kinetic order; fa = fraction affected.

The combination index (CI) is a quantitative measure based on the mass-action law of the degree of drug interaction in terms of synergism and antagonism (Table 3) for a given endpoint of the effect measurement.

Table 3. Description and symbols of synergism or antagonism in drug combination studies analyzed with the combination index method.

Range of Combination Index	Description	Symbols
<0.1	Very strong synergism	+++++
0.1–0.3	Strong synergism	++++
0.3–0.7	Synergism	+++
0.7–0.85	Moderative synergism	++
0.85–0.90	Slight synergism	+
0.90–1.10	Nearly addictive	±
1.10–1.20	Slight antagonism	−
1.20–1.45	Moderate antagonism	−−
1.45–3.3	Antagonism	−−−
3.3–10	Strong antagonism	−−−−
>10	Very strong antagonism	−−−−−

3.8. *Statistical Analysis*

All experiments were repeated at least three times. Data are presented as the means ± standard error (SE) for the indicated number of independently performed experiments and analyzed using Student's *t*-test. Values of $p < 0.05$ were considered statistically significant.

4. Conclusions

In summary, the present study demonstrates the antiproliferative activities of OPD on SK-Hep-1 human hepatoma cells. The inhibition of proliferation of cancer cells was in part associated with cell cycle arrest at the G_2/M phase and the tumor suppressor p53-mediated signaling pahway (Figure 7). These findings suggest that OPD is a promising new chemotherapeutic candidate for the management of human hepatoma cell treatment.

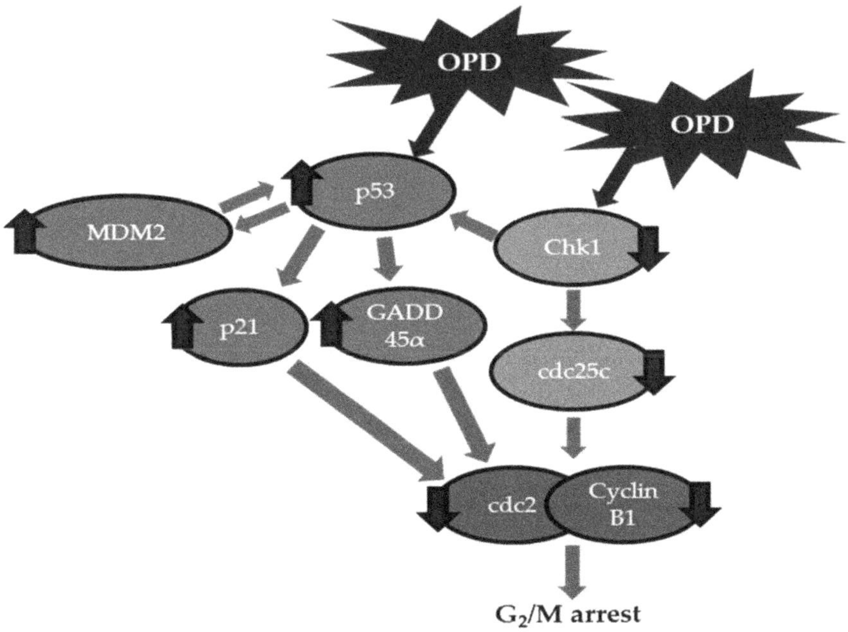

Figure 7. Schematic representation of the mechanisms of action of OPD against SK-Hep-1 human hepatoma cells.

Author Contributions: Conceptualization, S.K.L.; Methodology, S.H.P. and J.-Y.H.; Validation, S.H.P.; Formal Analysis, S.H.P.; Investigation, S.H.P.; Resources, S.K.L.; Data Curation, S.H.P.; Writing-Original Draft Preparation, S.H.P.; Writing-Review & Editing, J.-Y.H., H.J.P. and S.K.L.; Visualization, S.H.P.; Supervision, S.K.L.; Project Administration, S.K.L. All authors have read and agreed to the published version of the manuscript.

References

1. Jemal, A.; Bray, F.; Center, M.M.; Ferlay, J.; Ward, E.; Forman, D. Global cancer statistics. *Ca. Cancer. J. Clin.* **2011**, *61*, 69–90. [CrossRef]
2. Llovet, J.M.; Burroughs, A.; Bruix, J. Hepatocellular carcinoma. *Lancet* **2003**, *362*, 1907–1917. [CrossRef]
3. Bruix, J.; Sherman, M. Management of hepatocellular carcinoma. *Hepatology* **2005**, *42*, 1208–1236. [CrossRef] [PubMed]
4. Bruix, J.; Sherman, M.; Llovet, J.M.; Beaugrand, M.; Lencioni, R.; Burroughs, A.K.; Christensen, E.; Pagliaro, L.; Colombo, M.; Rodes, J. Clinical management of hepatocellular carcinoma. Conclusions of the barcelona-2000 easl conference. European association for the study of the liver. *J. Hepatol.* **2001**, *35*, 421–430. [CrossRef]
5. Llovet, J.M.; Bruix, J. Systematic review of randomized trials for unresectable hepatocellular carcinoma: Chemoembolization improves survival. *Hepatology* **2003**, *37*, 429–442. [CrossRef]
6. Bai, Y.; Li, D.; Zhou, T.; Qin, N.; Li, Z.; Yu, Z.; Hua, H. Coumarins from the roots of angelica dahurica with antioxidant and antiproliferative activities. *J. Funct. Foods* **2016**, *20*, 453–462. [CrossRef]
7. Wall, M.E.; Wani, M.C.; Manikumar, G.; Hughes, T.J.; Taylor, H.; McGivney, R.; Warner, J. Plant antimutagenic agents, 3. Coumarins. *J. Nat. Prod.* **1988**, *51*, 1148–1152. [CrossRef]
8. Cai, Y.; Baer-Dubowska, W.; Ashwood-Smith, M.; DiGiovanni, J. Inhibitory effects of naturally occurring coumarins on the metabolic activation of benzo[a]pyrene and 7,12-dimethylbenz[a]anthracene in cultured mouse keratinocytes. *Carcinogenesis* **1997**, *18*, 215–222. [CrossRef]
9. Oh, H.; Lee, H.S.; Kim, T.; Chai, K.Y.; Chung, H.T.; Kwon, T.O.; Jun, J.Y.; Jeong, O.S.; Kim, Y.C.; Yun, Y.G. Furocoumarins from angelica dahurica with hepatoprotective activity on tacrine-induced cytotoxicity in hep g2 cells. *Planta Med.* **2002**, *68*, 463–464. [CrossRef]
10. Branzei, D.; Foiani, M. Regulation of DNA repair throughout the cell cycle. *Nat. Rev. Mol. Cell Biol.* **2008**, *9*, 297–308. [CrossRef]
11. Goodarzi, A.A.; Block, W.D.; Lees-Miller, S.P. The role of atm and atr in DNA damage-induced cell cycle control. *Prog. Cell Cycle Res.* **2003**, *5*, 393–411. [PubMed]
12. Zhivotovsky, B.; Kroemer, G. Apoptosis and genomic instability. *Nat. Rev. Mol. Cell Biol.* **2004**, *5*, 752–762. [CrossRef] [PubMed]
13. Hartwell, L.H.; Kastan, M.B. Cell cycle control and cancer. *Science* **1994**, *266*, 1821–1828. [CrossRef] [PubMed]
14. Molinari, M. Cell cycle checkpoints and their inactivation in human cancer. *Cell Prolif.* **2000**, *33*, 261–274. [CrossRef]
15. Levine, A.J. P53, the cellular gatekeeper for growth and division. *Cell* **1997**, *88*, 323–331. [CrossRef]
16. Dai, Y.; Grant, S. New insights into checkpoint kinase 1 in the DNA damage response signaling network. *Clin. Cancer Res.* **2010**, *16*, 376–383. [CrossRef]
17. Jessus, C.; Ozon, R. Function and regulation of cdc25 protein phosphate through mitosis and meiosis. *Prog. Cell Cycle Res.* **1995**, *1*, 215–228.
18. Blasina, A.; de Weyer, I.V.; Laus, M.C.; Luyten, W.H.; Parker, A.E.; McGowan, C.H. A human homologue of the checkpoint kinase cds1 directly inhibits cdc25 phosphatase. *Curr. Biol.* **1999**, *9*, 1–10. [CrossRef]
19. Furnari, B.; Blasina, A.; Boddy, M.N.; McGowan, C.H.; Russell, P. Cdc25 inhibited in vivo and in vitro by checkpoint kinases cds1 and chk1. *Mol. Biol. Cell* **1999**, *10*, 833–845. [CrossRef]
20. Porter, L.A.; Donoghue, D.J. Cyclin b1 and cdk1: Nuclear localization and upstream regulators. *Prog. Cell Cycle Res.* **2003**, *5*, 335–347.
21. Chehab, N.H.; Malikzay, A.; Stavridi, E.S.; Halazonetis, T.D. Phosphorylation of ser-20 mediates stabilization of human p53 in response to DNA damage. *Proc. Natl. Acad. Sci. USA* **1999**, *96*, 13777–13782. [CrossRef] [PubMed]
22. Unger, T.; Juven-Gershon, T.; Moallem, E.; Berger, M.; Vogt Sionov, R.; Lozano, G.; Oren, M.; Haupt, Y. Critical role for ser20 of human p53 in the negative regulation of p53 by mdm2. *Embo J.* **1999**, *18*, 1805–1814. [CrossRef] [PubMed]
23. Yuan, J.; Luo, K.; Zhang, L.; Cheville, J.C.; Lou, Z. Usp10 regulates p53 localization and stability by deubiquitinating p53. *Cell* **2010**, *140*, 384–396. [CrossRef] [PubMed]
24. Hall-Jackson, C.A.; Cross, D.A.; Morrice, N.; Smythe, C. Atr is a caffeine-sensitive, DNA-activated protein kinase with a substrate specificity distinct from DNA-pk. *Oncogene* **1999**, *18*, 6707–6713. [CrossRef]

25. Nghiem, P.; Park, P.K.; Kim, Y.; Vaziri, C.; Schreiber, S.L. Atr inhibition selectively sensitizes g1 checkpoint-deficient cells to lethal premature chromatin condensation. *Proc. Natl. Acad. Sci. USA* **2001**, *98*, 9092–9097. [CrossRef]
26. Jin, L.; Li, C.; Xu, Y.; Wang, L.; Liu, J.; Wang, D.; Hong, C.; Jiang, Z.; Ma, Y.; Chen, Q.; et al. Epigallocatechin gallate promotes p53 accumulation and activity via the inhibition of mdm2-mediated p53 ubiquitination in human lung cancer cells. *Oncol. Rep.* **2013**, *29*, 1983–1990. [CrossRef]
27. Kang, T.J.; Lee, S.Y.; Singh, R.P.; Agarwal, R.; Yim, D.S. Anti-tumor activity of oxypeucedanin from ostericum koreanum against human prostate carcinoma du145 cells. *Acta Oncol.* **2009**, *48*, 895–900. [CrossRef]
28. Kimura, Y.; Sumiyoshi, M.; Sakanaka, M.; Taniguchi, M.; Baba, K. In vitro and in vivo antiproliferative effect of a combination of ultraviolet-a and alkoxy furocoumarins isolated from umbelliferae medicinal plants, in melanoma cells. *Photochem. Photobiol.* **2013**, *89*, 1216–1225. [CrossRef]
29. Greenblatt, M.S.; Bennett, W.P.; Hollstein, M.; Harris, C.C. Mutations in the p53 tumor suppressor gene: Clues to cancer etiology and molecular pathogenesis. *Cancer Res.* **1994**, *54*, 4855–4878.
30. Hollstein, M.; Sidransky, D.; Vogelstein, B.; Harris, C.C. P53 mutations in human cancers. *Science* **1991**, *253*, 49–53. [CrossRef]
31. Dai, C.; Gu, W. P53 post-translational modification: Deregulated in tumorigenesis. *Trends Mol. Med.* **2010**, *16*, 528–536. [CrossRef] [PubMed]
32. Carmichael, J. The role of gemcitabine in the treatment of other tumours. *Br. J. Cancer* **1998**, *78* (Suppl. 3), 21–25. [CrossRef]
33. Nabhan, C.; Krett, N.; Gandhi, V.; Rosen, S. Gemcitabine in hematologic malignancies. *Curr. Opin. Oncol.* **2001**, *13*, 514–521. [CrossRef] [PubMed]
34. Arlander, S.J.; Eapen, A.K.; Vroman, B.T.; McDonald, R.J.; Toft, D.O.; Karnitz, L.M. Hsp90 inhibition depletes chk1 and sensitizes tumor cells to replication stress. *J. Biol. Chem.* **2003**, *278*, 52572–52577. [CrossRef] [PubMed]
35. Chen, L.; Jian, Y.; Wei, N.; Yuan, M.; Zhuang, X.; Li, H. Separation and simultaneous quantification of nine furanocoumarins from radix angelicae dahuricae using liquid chromatography with tandem mass spectrometry for bioavailability determination in rats. *J. Sep. Sci.* **2015**, *38*, 4216–4224. [CrossRef] [PubMed]
36. Vichai, V.; Kirtikara, K. Sulforhodamine b colorimetric assay for cytotoxicity screening. *Nat. Protoc.* **2006**, *1*, 1112–1116. [CrossRef] [PubMed]
37. Smith, P.K.; Krohn, R.I.; Hermanson, G.; Mallia, A.; Gartner, F.; Provenzano, M.; Fujimoto, E.; Goeke, N.; Olson, B.; Klenk, D. Measurement of protein using bicinchoninic acid. *Anal. Biochem.* **1985**, *150*, 76–85. [CrossRef]
38. Byun, W.S.; Kim, W.K.; Han, H.J.; Chung, H.-J.; Jang, K.; Kim, H.S.; Kim, S.; Kim, D.; Bae, E.S.; Park, S. Targeting histone methyltransferase dot1l by a novel psammaplin a analog inhibits growth and metastasis of triple-negative breast cancer. *Mol. Ther. -Oncolytics* **2019**, *15*, 140–152. [CrossRef]

Permissions

All chapters in this book were first published by MDPI; hereby published with permission under the Creative Commons Attribution License or equivalent. Every chapter published in this book has been scrutinized by our experts. Their significance has been extensively debated. The topics covered herein carry significant findings which will fuel the growth of the discipline. They may even be implemented as practical applications or may be referred to as a beginning point for another development.

The contributors of this book come from diverse backgrounds, making this book a truly international effort. This book will bring forth new frontiers with its revolutionizing research information and detailed analysis of the nascent developments around the world.

We would like to thank all the contributing authors for lending their expertise to make the book truly unique. They have played a crucial role in the development of this book. Without their invaluable contributions this book wouldn't have been possible. They have made vital efforts to compile up to date information on the varied aspects of this subject to make this book a valuable addition to the collection of many professionals and students.

This book was conceptualized with the vision of imparting up-to-date information and advanced data in this field. To ensure the same, a matchless editorial board was set up. Every individual on the board went through rigorous rounds of assessment to prove their worth. After which they invested a large part of their time researching and compiling the most relevant data for our readers.

The editorial board has been involved in producing this book since its inception. They have spent rigorous hours researching and exploring the diverse topics which have resulted in the successful publishing of this book. They have passed on their knowledge of decades through this book. To expedite this challenging task, the publisher supported the team at every step. A small team of assistant editors was also appointed to further simplify the editing procedure and attain best results for the readers.

Apart from the editorial board, the designing team has also invested a significant amount of their time in understanding the subject and creating the most relevant covers. They scrutinized every image to scout for the most suitable representation of the subject and create an appropriate cover for the book.

The publishing team has been an ardent support to the editorial, designing and production team. Their endless efforts to recruit the best for this project, has resulted in the accomplishment of this book. They are a veteran in the field of academics and their pool of knowledge is as vast as their experience in printing. Their expertise and guidance has proved useful at every step. Their uncompromising quality standards have made this book an exceptional effort. Their encouragement from time to time has been an inspiration for everyone.

The publisher and the editorial board hope that this book will prove to be a valuable piece of knowledge for researchers, students, practitioners and scholars across the globe.

List of Contributors

Victoria Abzianidze, Sofya Zakharenkova and Victor Kuznetsov
Laboratory of Chemical Modeling, Research Institute of Hygiene, Occupational Pathology and Human Ecology, Federal Medical Biological Agency, Kuz'molovsky, 188663 Saint Petersburg, Russia

Petr Beltyukov
Laboratory of Molecular Toxicology and Experimental Therapy, Research Institute of Hygiene,Occupational Pathology and Human Ecology, Federal Medical Biological Agency, Kuz'molovsky, 188663 Saint Petersburg, Russia

Natalia Moiseeva
N.N. Blokchin National Medical Research Center of Oncology, 115478 Moscow, Russia

Jennifer Mejia and Alvin Holder
Department of Chemistry and Biochemistry, Old Dominion University, 4541 Hampton Boulevard, Norfolk, VA 23529, USA

Yuri Trishin
Saint Petersburg State University of industrial technologies and design, Ivana Chernyh str., 4,198095 Saint Petersburg, Russia

Alexander Berestetskiy
All-Russian Institute of Plant Protection, Russian Academy of Agricultural Sciences, Pushkin, 196608 Saint Petersburg, Russia

Tetsuo Tsukamoto
Department of Immunology, Kindai University Faculty of Medicine, Osaka 5898511, Japan

Karlo Wittine, Lara Saftić, Željka Peršurić and Sandra Kraljević Pavelić
University of Rijeka, Department of Biotechnology, Centre for high-throughput technologies, Radmile Matejčić 2, 51000 Rijeka, Croatia

Tomhiro Mastuo, Yasuyoshi Miyata, Tsutomu Yuno, Yuta Mukae, Asato Otsubo, Kensuke Mitsunari, Kojiro Ohba and Hideki Sakai
Department of Urology, Nagasaki University Graduate School of Biomedical Sciences, Nagasaki 852-8501, Japan

Krishan Parashar, Siddhartha Sood, Ali Mehaidli, Colin Curran, Caleb Vegh, Christopher Nguyen, Christopher Pignanelli and Siyaram Pandey
Department of Chemistry and Biochemistry, University of Windsor, 401 Sunset Avenue, Windsor, ON N9B 3P4, Canada

Jianzhang Wu, Guang Liang and Yi Wang
Chemical Biology Research Center, School of Pharmaceutical Sciences, Whenzhou Medical University, University Town, Chashan, Wenzhou 325035, China

Kevin M. Tyo
Department of Pharmacology and Toxicology, School of Medicine, University of Louisville, Louisville, KY 40202, USA
Center for Predictive Medicine, Louisville, KY 40202, USA

Farnaz Minooei and Joel R. Fried
Department of Chemical Engineering, University of Louisville, Louisville, KY 40292, USA

Keegan C. Curry
Department of Biology, University of Louisville, Louisville, KY 40292, USA

Sarah M. Ne Camp and Danielle L. Graves
Department of Bioengineering, Speed School of Engineering, University of Louisville, Louisville, KY 40292, USA

Jill M. Steinbach-Rankins
Department of Pharmacology and Toxicology, School of Medicine, University of Louisville, Louisville, KY 40202, USA
Center for Predictive Medicine, Louisville, KY 40202, USA
Department of Bioengineering, Speed School of Engineering, University of Louisville, Louisville, KY 40292, USA
Department of Microbiology and Immunology, School of Medicine, University of Louisville, Louisville, KY 40292, USA

Hee Jeong Shin, Jang Mi Han and Ye Seul Choi
Department of Life Science and Biochemical Engineering, Sun Moon University, Asan 31460, Korea

Hye Jin Jung
Department of Life Science and Biochemical Engineering, Sun Moon University, Asan 31460, Korea
Genome-based Bio IT Convergence Institute, Asan 31460, Korea
Department of Pharmaceutical Engineering and Biotechnology, Sun Moon University, Asan 31460, Korea

Leah M. Johnson, Sai Archana Krovi, Linying Li and Natalie Girouard
Engineered Systems, RTI International, 3040 E. Cornwallis Road, Research Triangle Park, NC 27709, USA

Zach R. Demkovich and Ariane van der Straten
Women's Global Health Imperative, RTI International, 351 California Street, Suite 500, San Francisco, CA 94104, USA

Daniel Myers and Ben Creelman
PATH, 2201 Westlake Ave, Suite 200, Seattle, WA 98121, USA

Fernando Notario-Pérez, Raúl Cazorla-Luna, Araceli Martín-Illana, Roberto Ruiz-Caro and María-Dolores Veiga
Departamento de Farmacia Galénica y Tecnología Alimentaria, Facultad de Farmacia, Universidad Complutense de Madrid, 28040 Madrid, Spain

Juan Peña
Departamento de Química en Ciencias Farmacéuticas, Facultad de Farmacia, Universidad Complutense de Madrid, 28040 Madrid, Spain

So Ra Kim, Eun Young Lee and Hae Ryoun Park
Department of Oral Pathology, and BK21 PLUS Project, School of Dentistry, Pusan National University, Yangsan 50612, Korea
Periodontal Disease Signaling Network Research Center (MRC), School of Dentistry, Pusan National University, Yangsan 50612, Korea

Da Jeong Kim
Department of Oral Pathology, and BK21 PLUS Project, School of Dentistry, Pusan National University, Yangsan 50612, Korea

Hye Jung Kim
Periodontal Disease Signaling Network Research Center (MRC), School of Dentistry, Pusan National University, Yangsan 50612, Korea

Elisabetta Mazzotta, Gaetano Ragno, Antonio Garofalo and Rita Muzzalupo
Department of Pharmacy, Health and Nutritional Sciences, University of Calabria, Via P. Bucci, 87036 Rende (CS), Italy

So Hyun Park, Ji-Young Hong, Hyen Joo Park and Sang Kook Lee
College of Pharmacy, Natural Products Research Institute, Seoul National University, Seoul 08826, Korea

Index

www.ingramcontent.com/pod-product-compliance
Lightning Source LLC
LaVergne TN
LVHW082129200926
848484LV00008B/2029
* 9 7 9 8 8 8 7 4 0 0 0 5 1 *